RACE IN A BOTTLE

JONATHAN KAHN

RACE IN A BOTTLE

The Story of BiDil and Racialized Medicine
in a Post-Genomic Age

Columbia University Press / New York

Columbia University Press
Publishers Since 1893
New York   Chichester, West Sussex
cup.columbia.edu
Copyright © 2013 Columbia University Press
All rights reserved

Library of Congress Cataloging-in-Publication Data
Kahn, Jonathan.
  Race in a bottle : the story of BiDil and racialized medicine in a
post-genomic age / Jonathan Kahn.
        pages cm
  Includes bibliographical references and index.
  ISBN 978-0-231-16298-2 (cloth : alk. paper)—ISBN 978-0-231-53127-6
(ebook)
    1. Hydralazine—Development—History.   2. Health and race.
3. African Americans—Medical care.   4. Pharmacogenetics—Social
aspects.   5. Pharmaceutical industry—Political aspects—United
States.   I. Title.

  RM666.H7K34   2013
  616.1'2906108996073—dc23

                                                    2012023167

Columbia University Press books are printed on permanent and durable
acid-free paper.

This book is printed on paper with recycled content.
Printed in the United States of America
c 10 9 8 7 6 5 4 3 2 1

Cover design by David Drummond

References to Internet Web sites (URLs) were accurate at the time of writing.
Neither the author nor Columbia University Press is responsible for URLs
that may have expired or changed since the manuscript was prepared.

CONTENTS

Acknowledgments VII

INTRODUCTION:
Race and Medicine: Framing [Is] the Problem
1

1. ORGANIZING RACE:
Paths Toward the Re-Biologization of Race in Modern Biomedical
Research, Practice, and Product Development
25

2. THE BIRTH OF BIDIL:
How a Drug Becomes "Ethnic"
48

3. STATISTICAL MISCHIEF AND RACIAL FRAMES FOR
DRUG DEVELOPMENT AND MARKETING
71

4. CAPITALIZING [ON] RACE IN DRUG DEVELOPMENT
87

5. RACE-ING PATENTS/PATENTING RACE:
An Emerging Political Geography of Intellectual Property
in Biotechnology
124

6. NOT FADE AWAY:
The Persistence of Race and the Politics of the "Meantime"
in Pharmacogenomics
157

7. FROM DISPARITY TO DIFFERENCE:
The Politics of Racial Medicine
193

CONCLUSIONS AND RECOMMENDATIONS
225

Notes   247

Index   303

ACKNOWLEDGMENTS

I FIRST ENCOUNTERED BiDil in March 2002, while hosting sociologist Troy Duster for a talk on race and science at the University of Minnesota. During the course of his presentation, Troy mentioned that a small pharmaceutical company had recently announced its plans to commence a race-specific clinical trial to develop what promised to become the first Food and Drug Administration–approved, race-specific drug. I was intrigued. Soon thereafter I emailed Troy expressing my interest in pursuing the matter further but also wanting to make sure I was not encroaching on anyone else's work. Troy was welcoming and generous; "the more the merrier" was his attitude. Since that time, I have come to get to know and receive help from a myriad of new colleagues and friends across many disciplines interested in similar questions. More people involved have indeed led to a very merry experience in the best sense. With each passing year, I have found an ever-expanding network of remarkably thoughtful and supportive scholars. Perhaps this is no coincidence, given that Troy has been at the hub of many of these networks, particularly an informal LIST-SERV that has provided a tremendous sense of intellectual community over the past few years.

Among the many who have generously shared their thoughts, their work, and their insights with me are: Keith Aoki, Mario Biagioli, Deborah Bolnick, Rene Bowser, Lundy Braun, Dan Burk, Tim Caulfield,

Mildred Cho, Peter Chow-White, Adele Clarke, Richard Cooper, Susan Craddock, Abdallah Daar, Marcy Darnovsky, Lennard Davis, Carl Elliott, Stephen Epstein, Anne Fausto-Sterling, Kim Fortun, Mike Fortun, Jennifer Fishman, Joan Fujimura, Malia Fullerton, Shubha Ghosh, Laura Gomez, Alan Goodman, Joe Graves, Jennifer Hamilton, Evelynn Hammonds, Richard Hayes, Gail Henderson, Sharona Hoffman, David Jones, Nancy King, Barbara Koenig, Sheldon Krimsky, Cynthia Lee, Susan Lehrman, Richard Lewontin, Susan Lindee, Nancy Lopez, Emily Martin, Jonathan Metzl, Steve Miles, Michael Montoya, Ann Morning, Jackson Mugerwa, Alondra Nelson, Osagi Obasogie, Michael Omi, Rayna Rapp, Jenny Reardon, Susan Reverby, Dorothy Roberts, Michael Root, Charmaine Royal, Joshua Sarnoff, Alexandra Shields, Kathleen Sloan, Kim TallBear, Charis Thompson, Richard Tutton, Keith Wailoo, Patricia Wald, Harriet Washington, Patricia Williams, and David Winikoff.

Additionally, Jay Kaufman has been an indispensable guide through the world of epidemiology and statistics. He has been a touchstone for keeping my discussions of anything quantitative on point and comprehensible. He has also been a consistent and remarkable source of references relevant to the uses of race in biomedicine. George Ellison added greatly to my understanding of the complexities of the BiDil story, particularly in the analysis of the relevant clinical trial data. I also remain indebted to him for the London tickets to *Spamalot* he procured for Jon Marks, Mike Fortun, and me. Sandra Lee and I have encountered each other in so many professional settings and share so many of the same interests that we continue to marvel that we have not yet written anything together. Her work and her friendship have greatly enriched my pursuit of our common interests. I did have the pleasure of coauthoring a couple of articles with Pamela Sankar, who has at several points over the years provided invaluable insight into issues with which I was grappling. Pamela demonstrated a remarkable gift for clarifying and getting to the heart of problems on which I was working but was too close to have the sort of critical perspective she provided. Jon Marks has helped me better understand the historical arc of the intersections between science and race with rigor and with humor. David Jones provided invaluable and thoughtful comments on an early draft of the manuscript. Tom Romero read much of the manuscript and provided extremely helpful feedback. As a friend and colleague at Hamline, he introduced me to the world of LatCrit and helped me frame my work at the intersections of critical race theory and health law. Sheila Jasanoff has been wonderfully generous with her insights and support since we first met in Cambridge over a decade ago. Pilar Ossorio provided invaluable help and support in sorting out issues of patent law, genomics, and bioethics. Duana Fullwiley always had remarkable vignettes to share with me that she illuminated and made rich with thoughtful analysis. Dorothy Roberts has shared deep insights into the intersections of law and politics in the arena of racialized medicine. She is also something of a comrade in arms who was with me (as were some of the others listed above) when we were accused at one meeting of "killing people" with our critiques of BiDil. Finally, I owe special thanks to Troy Duster, both for welcoming me into this world at the start of my journey and for continuously providing support and connections for so many of us working in this area. I cannot begin to convey how thankful I am that my work has brought me into the orbit of such a remarkable group of scholars. What is almost as remarkable to me is how consistently kind, generous, and supportive they have been over the years.

My understanding of issues relating to race, health, genomics, law, and commerce has also been greatly enriched by participating in diverse symposia and workshops over the years whose many members are too numerous to list individually.

Material from previously published material may be found scattered throughout the text. These articles include: "Inventing Race as a Genetic Commodity in Biotechnology Patents" (in *Making and Unmaking Intellectual Property: Creative Production in Legal and Cultural Perspective*, ed. M. Biagioli, Peter Jaszi, and Martha Woodmansee, Chicago: University of Chicago Press, 2011, 305–320); "BiDil and Racialized Medicine" (in *Race and the Genetic Revolution: Science, Myth and Culture*, ed. Sheldon Krimsky and Kathleen Sloan, New York: Columbia University Press, 2011, 129–141); "Mandating Race: How the PTO Is Forcing Race into Biotechnology Patents" (*Nature Biotechnology* 29 [2011]: 401–403); "Surrogate Markers and Surrogate Marketing in Biomedicine: The Regulatory Etiology and

Commercial Progression of 'Ethnic' Drug Development" (in *Biomedicalization: Technoscience, Health and Illness in the U.S.*, ed. A. Clarke, Laura Mamo, Jennifer Ruth Fosket, Jennifer R. Fishman, and Janet K. Shim, Durham, N.C.: Duke University Press, 2010, 263–287); "Beyond BiDil: The Expanding Embrace of Race in Biomedical Research and Product Development" (*Saint Louis University Journal of Health Law & Policy* 3 [2010] 61–92); "Patenting Race in a Genomic Age" (in *Revisiting Race in a Genomic Age*, Piscataway, N.J.: Rutgers University Press, 2008): 129–148; "Exploiting Race in Drug Development: BiDil's Interim Model of Pharmacogenomics" (*Social Studies of Science* 38 [2008]: 737–758); "Race in a Bottle" (*Scientific American*, August 2007, 40–45); "Race-ing Patents/Patenting Race: An Emerging Political Geography of Intellectual Property in Biotechnology" (*Iowa Law Review* 92 [2007]: 353–416); "Harmonizing Race: Competing Regulatory Paradigms of Racial Categorization in International Drug Development" (*Santa Clara Journal of International Law* 5 [2006]: 34–56); "Patenting Race" (*Nature Biotechnology* 24 [2006]: 1349–1351); "Genes, Race, and Population: Avoiding a Collision of Categories" (*American Journal of Public Health* 96 [2006]: 6–11); "From Disparity to Difference: How Race-Specific Medicines May Undermine Policies to Address Inequalities in Health Care" (*Southern California Interdisciplinary Law Review* 15 [2005]: 105); "Misreading Race and Genomics After BiDil" (*Nature Genetics* 37 [2005]: 655–656); "How a Drug Becomes 'Ethnic': Law, Commerce, and the Production of Racial Categories in Medicine" (*Yale Journal of Health Policy, Law & Ethics* 4 [2004]: 1–46); "Getting the Numbers Right: Statistical Mischief and Racial Profiling in Heart Failure Research" (*Perspectives in Biology and Medicine* 46 [2003]: 473–483). Support for some of the research behind these articles was received from National Human Genome Research Institute grants 1R03HG004034 and 1R01HG02818. The writing of this book was supported by National Library of Medicine grant 1G13LM010073.

* * *

I dedicate this book to my wife, Karen-Sue Taussig, and our daughter, Emma. In addition to unstinting love and support, Karen-Sue also paved the way for my initial entry into the world of science studies and all things genomic. I would likely never have started down this path but for her. As for Emma, the unbounded joy she provides to my life is wonderfully complemented by her propensity for trying to manage Karen-Sue's and my professional engagements so as to take her to distant parts of the world she would like to see.

RACE IN A BOTTLE

INTRODUCTION

Race and Medicine: Framing [Is] the Problem

This is the patent age of new inventions
For killing bodies and for saving souls.
All propagated with the best intentions.

—LORD BYRON, *DON JUAN*, CANTO I, 132

I N JUNE 2000, at a White House ceremony announcing the completion of the first draft of the human genome, President Clinton declared, "I believe one of the great truths to emerge from this triumphant expedition inside the human genome is that in genetic terms, all human beings, regardless of race, are more than 99.9 percent the same." Following President Clinton, geneticist Craig Venter asserted that this accomplishment illustrated "that the concept of race has no genetic or scientific basis."[1] This was not news to most geneticists and social scientists, but merely confirmed what most had long accepted: "race is not genetic." Yet since the triumphant announcement of 2000, a disproportionate amount of attention has been devoted to the tiny 0.1 percent (since revised to an estimate of 0.5 percent[2]) of the genome where people appear to differ.[3] Despite the grand proclamations of 2000, race has actually been playing an expanding role in genetic research and practice, particularly in the field of drug development.

Less than nine months later, on March 8, 2001, NitroMed, then a privately held biotech firm in Massachusetts, issued a press release triumphantly announcing the receipt of a letter from the Food and Drug Administration (FDA) "describing the regulatory status and ultimate approvability of BiDil®," a heart failure drug meant specifically for African Americans, pending the successful completion of a confirmatory trial.[4]

The trial, known as the African-American Heart Failure Trial (A-HeFT), was successfully completed in 2004. In June of the following year, the FDA approved BiDil as the first drug with a race-specific indication: to treat heart failure in a "black" patient.[5]

This book explores the persistent and expanding use of racial categories in biomedical research and product development in the face of genomic accomplishments that were supposed to render such categories irrelevant. Since the inception of the Human Genome Project, much time and attention has been devoted to insuring that biological knowledge emerging from advances in genetic research is not used inappropriately to make racial categories appear biologically given or "natural." Race is not a coherent genetic concept; rather, it is best understood as a complex and dynamic social construct.[6] Since Richard Lewontin's groundbreaking work on blood group polymorphisms in different groups and races in the 1970s, scientists have understood that race will statistically explain only a small portion of genetic variations. As a 2001 editorial in the journal *Nature Genetics* put it: "Scientists have long been saying that at the genetic level there is more variation between two individuals in the same population than between populations and that there is no biological basis for 'race.'"[7] More recently, an editorial in *Nature Biotechnology* asserted that "race is simply a poor proxy for the environmental and genetic causes of disease or drug response. . . . Pooling people in race silos is akin to zoologists grouping raccoons, tigers and okapis on the basis that they are all stripey."[8]

This is not to deny the reality of human genetic variation. It is, rather, to acknowledge, with geneticists such as Lewontin, that such variation is *clinal*; that is, the tiny portion of the human genome that varies does so in incremental gradations, or clines, generally reflecting geographic or temporal distance between populations. Does a group of average Norwegians have frequencies of certain alleles (different versions of the same gene) that differ from a group of average Nigerians? Yes, probably. But they also probably differ from a group of average Germans, who in turn probably differ from a group of average Italians, and so on. Moreover, there is also relatively greater genetic variation within each of these population groups than between them on average. Genetic variation is real but continuous. In short, people differ, but there is no genetic basis for marking off where one race ends and another begins.

The story told here unfolds around three basic questions: How does race enter biomedical research and practice? What happens to race once it is there? What are the broader social and political implications of racialized biomedicine beyond the immediate contexts in which it is directly in play? In pursuing these three questions, I am particularly attentive to how current biomedical understandings and practices interact with legal and commercial considerations to produce distinctive racial frames for research and product development. The initial framing of a biological condition, such as heart failure, as racial, can shape (and be shaped by) clinical trial design, interpretation of results, legal approaches to patent protection, and commercial strategies for marketing.

Framing has political implications as well. As Paul Farmer and his colleagues have cautioned, an "exclusive focus on molecular-level phenomena has contributed to the increasing 'desocialization' of scientific inquiry: a tendency to ask only biological questions about what are in fact *biosocial* phenomena."[9] As a highly individualistic culture, we tend to cast "natural" differences as an individual problem and an individual responsibility. Making race "natural" has the potential to make racial disparities—not only in health, but also in a whole array of goods from housing and employment to education—"natural," that is, an individual problem and a personal responsibility, and therefore of no concern to the political community at large. In our market-oriented culture, naturalizing race also threatens to privatize race, making it simply another aspect of market relations for which public institutions bear no responsibility. In short, how a problem becomes framed as racial is itself a problem to be explored.

MEETING BIDIL

I use the story of BiDil as a primary entry point for exploring how a larger scheme of institutional, legal, and commercial imperatives is shaping the use of race in biomedicine. One primary concern is that the confluence of these diverse factors is driving the re-emergence of race as a biological construct. This is certainly problematic, given our nation's long history of racial injustice and oppression, but it also has implications both for the responsible conduct of scientific research and for the allocation of scarce resources to deal with the very real problem of persistent health disparities in this country.

BiDil is a combination of two generic drugs used to dilate blood vessels—hence "Bi" (two) and "Dil" (dilators). Its developers combined them into a single pill to treat heart failure. Its origins reach back to the 1980s, and it was not originally racially marked but was intended as a therapy for all. Its turn toward becoming a racial medicine was critically mediated by two patents. The first simply covered the use of the BiDil combination to treat heart failure. It was issued in 1987 and was slated to expire in 2007. The second was almost identical to the first, but covered use in a "black" patient. It was not issued until 2000 and will not expire until 2020.

I first encountered BiDil in March 2002, while hosting sociologist Troy Duster for a talk on race and science at the University of Minnesota. At the time, I was working on a National Institutes of Health (NIH) grant to study the implications of using census categories of race to organize and classify information emerging from the Human Genome Project and related genomic endeavors. During the course of his presentation, Duster mentioned that a small pharmaceutical company had recently announced its plans to commence a race-specific clinical trial to develop what promised to become the first FDA-approved race-specific drug. I was intrigued. I began by asking a question that would become the title of one of my first articles on BiDil: How did this drug become "ethnic"? I mentally placed the word "ethnic" in quotation marks, because it was my sense that the drug's proponents were sometimes trying to elide the difference between social and biological constructions of race by using the less politically charged term "ethnic." My initial work on BiDil opened up into a broader exploration of the complex and varied interplay among science, commerce, and law in the field of racialized biomedicine.

Along the way, a curious thing happened—at least for the historian in me who had previously worked alone in archives to write his first book. I became something of a participant in the unfolding story of BiDil. By 2005, I had published a couple of articles about its development and at the urging of colleagues and family (my wife is an anthropologist of science and hence far more comfortable with the idea of "participant observation" than I), I went to Bethesda, Maryland, to offer my five minutes of testimony before the FDA advisory committee reviewing BiDil for approval. I was among a dozen or so people offering such comments and like many of them, I urged that the committee approve BiDil but without the race-specific indication—that is, as a drug for everyone. It was an interesting proceeding and I suppose the lawyer in me felt relatively comfortable being there. Unsurprisingly, the majority of the committee did not agree with me and granted NitroMed's request for approval with a race-specific indication. Undeterred, I continued to explore the unfolding story of BiDil and to connect it to the larger phenomenon of the expanding use of racial categories in biomedical research and practice. In subsequent years, I sat on conference panels more than once with BiDil's patent holder, cardiologist Jay Cohn, and engaged in published colloquies with representatives of NitroMed and FDA officials regarding the relative merits or problems with race-specific medicines. At one conference, I even had an aggravated NitroMed executive come up to me and say, "When we go to the insurance companies to get preferred coverage for BiDil, they have your articles on their desks!"[10] The story I tell therefore has descriptive, analytic, and normative components to it.

RACE, GENES, AND DRUG DEVELOPMENT

"Race" is a tricky word. My intent is not to provide a fixed normative definition for what I consider to be an inherently flexible and unstable concept, but rather to explore how diverse actors use race in different contexts and to consider how and why race enters practices of biomedicine in different times and places.[11] I generally agree with the sociologists Michael Omi and Howard Winant and their approach to race as "an unstable and 'decentered' complex of social meanings constantly being transformed by *how concept used?*

political struggle."[12] Nonetheless, I also contend that race can have bio-logical consequences, as when it becomes manifest in actual bodies through the historical impact of racialized and/or racist social practices. As epide-miologist Nancy Krieger puts it, race-based health differences can be con-ceptualized as "biologic expressions of race relations."[13] Race then is not "merely" social, as if that means it were somehow not real. Race is real, it matters, but it is not genetic.

As the first race-specific drug ever approved by the FDA, BiDil was touted as a significant step toward the promised era of personalized phar-macogenomic therapies. Upon its approval, the journal *Science* effused, "by backing BiDil, the FDA panel gave another push to pharmacogenomics, an approach that promises to revolutionize both drug discovery and pa-tient care."[14] The new field of pharmacogenomics involves attempts to tai-lor drugs to an individual's genetic profile. It represents one of the most powerfully envisioned applications of the new genetics since the inception of the Human Genome Project. One scientific commentary defines phar-macogenomics as "the study of genetic variability in the way people respond to medicines, traced to the expression of genes related to disease suscepti-bility and drug response at the cellular, tissue, individual and population levels."[15] The great hope of pharmacogenomics is that knowing a person's genetic make-up will allow doctors to optimize drug selection and dosage. While the multi-billion-dollar Human Genome Project has been slow to deliver on so-called genetic therapies, it has produced information that undergirds current attempts by a wide array of biomedical researchers and pharmaceutical corporations to develop pharmacogenomically tailored medicines.[16] Around the time of BiDil's approval in 2005, one leading researcher at Roche Pharmaceuticals opined that "we're at the beginning right now, and [pharmacogenomics is] going to absolutely be integrated into the entire drug discovery and development process in the future. Ten years from now, it will just be part of the woodwork."[17]

Since NitroMed's initial announcement, BiDil has emerged as a central player in ongoing debates over whether and how to use race and ethnicity as categories in biomedical research. It has also played a significant role at the forefront of broader political and legal discussions of the legitimacy of

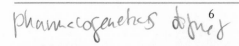

identifying and acting upon perceived biological or genetic differences among the races. This is hardly surprising, given NitroMed's own emphasis on "ethnic differences in the underlying pathophysiology of heart failure."[18] More surprising, however, is the lack of attention paid to just how BiDil became ethnic. Claims couched in scientific rhetoric and supported by the imprimatur of peer-reviewed journals are frequently afforded deference, and BiDil is no exception. Both the general news media and a number of science and medical journals covered BiDil extensively without any substantial effort to investigate the claims made in press releases and medical reports.[19] The story they tell is of the path-breaking development of a new therapy for heart failure to help an underserved racial population.

However, when one investigates the origins and development of BiDil, a different and far more complex story emerges. At the most basic level, it turns out that BiDil became an ethnic drug through the interventions of law and commerce as much as through medical understanding of biological differences that correlate with racial groups. This part of the story has been masked both by well-meaning concerns about perceived health disparities and by an imprudent reliance on erroneous or incomplete statistical data. One of the foremost ironies of BiDil is that it was approved based primarily on the data produced by a race-specific clinical trial that enrolled only African Americans. With no comparison population enrolled, there is no basis to make any claims that the drug worked differently or better in blacks than in anyone else. By obtaining approval of BiDil as a drug solely to treat African Americans, NitroMed opened up a Pandora's Box of racial politics without fully appreciating the implications of what it was doing.

GENETICS IS COMPLEX, SO IS RACE

In my years of writing about and discussing issues of race and medicine, I have found the lack of attention to the complexities of race to be one of the most persistent and widespread problems underlying confusion about the appropriate use of racial categories in medical research and clinical practice.

I believe that underlying such confusion is an even deeper set of assumptions about the nature of race and more broadly of social science in relation to the natural sciences. These assumptions are grounded in the acceptance of race as a social category that is aligned with a near-simultaneous marginalization of race as "merely" social and hence not deserving of the same sort of care of consideration devoted to "real" natural phenomena, such as genetics. Biomedical experts have spent years developing expertise, special knowledge, and skills that set them apart. They can speak a language to which most people do not have access. Race, in contrast, is a language open to all. We all live and talk about race in various ways in our daily lives. Race therefore appears obvious, intuitive, and in need of no special knowledge to discuss or analyze. In some contexts this may be true, but biomedicine is not one of them. When I speak to doctors or geneticists about issues of race and medicine, my take-home message for them often is: "Yes, genetics [or cardiology, oncology, etc.] is complex and requires specialized skills and knowledge. But race too is complex. Using race in biomedical contexts requires great care and expertise, just like genetics." My aim is not to bash science but to make it better by putting it in context. Biomedicine is not just a technical enterprise. It is embedded in complex social, political, economic, and legal webs of meaning and power, each shaping and constructing the other. Only by building connections across these domains and the disciplines that study them can we arrive at more productive and responsible uses of race in biomedicine.

SOME BASICS ON GENETICS AND HUMAN VARIATION

To appreciate the significance of the use of race in biomedical contexts, it is helpful to have an understanding of some basic concepts of genetics. The human genome is comprised of all the deoxyribonucleic acid (DNA) a person possesses.[20] DNA is composed of ordered combinations of four nucleotide bases: adenine, guanine, thymine, and cytosine—generally abbreviated as A, G, T, and C.[21] The human genome contains an estimated three billion nucleotide bases.[22] A single nucleotide polymorphism, or SNP, is a DNA sequence variation that occurs when a single nucleotide (A, T, C, or G) in the genome sequence is altered.[23] Genes are arrays of nucleotides that code for the production of proteins.[24] An allele is an alternative form of any particular gene.[25] Although humans are 99.5% genetically the same, that 0.5% variation amounts to about fifteen million variations.[26] With so many variations, it is often possible to find certain variations occurring in different frequencies between different groups of individuals. As Troy Duster has noted:

> It is possible to make arbitrary groupings of populations (geographic, linguistic, self-identified by faith, identified by others by physiognomy, etc.) and still find statistically significant allelic variations between those groupings. For example, we could examine all the people in Chicago, and all those in Los Angeles, and find statistically significant differences in allele frequency at some loci. Of course, at many loci, even most loci, we would not find statistically significant differences.[27]

Given that it is theoretically possible for researchers to find differences in allele frequencies between Chicagoans and Los Angelenos, it is hardly surprising that they may find differences between groups somehow marked as "black," "white," or "Asian." The difficulty comes when people try to assign particular meanings to such variation.

In recent years, the terms "race" and "ethnicity" have come to be used interchangeably in many discussions of race and biomedicine. I tend to favor the use of the term "race" over "ethnicity" because of my perception that "ethnicity" is increasingly being used to elide the resonance and significance of the concept of race as it relates to historical practices of racism. It is worth noting that even those who try to develop more refined definitions of the two often end up defining one in terms of the other. Thus, for example, the journal *Nature Genetics*, in a very well-meaning editorial requiring authors to explain how and why they use racial categories in science, provides as one of several definitions of race: "A distinct *ethnic* group characterized by traits that are transmitted through their offspring"; while providing as one of several definitions of ethnicity: "A social group or category of the population that, in a larger society, is set apart and bound together by common ties of *race* [italics added], language, nationality or culture."[28] Writing about similar difficulties in using the terms "race" and "ethnicity," sociologist Steven Epstein notes that "It follows from these definitions that a race may or may not also be an ethnic group, and vice versa. In neither case, however, are we speaking of differences that are predetermined by human biology. Rather, ethnic and racial groups emerge out of a process of collective attribution."[29]

The terms "black" and "African American" exemplify some of the difficulties in sorting out usages of racial and ethnic categories. The U.S. Census lumps them together as "Black or African American." In practice, self-identifying as "black" or "African American" in the United States has often meant the same thing. But as the number of new immigrants from the Caribbean, South America, and Africa rises, the conflation of these terms can be problematic. In the course of this book, I sometimes alternate between these terms as well. This reflects, in part, the difficulty in settling on one fixed term. It also reflects the variable ways in which the diverse actors encountered in these stories employ the terms. Thus, for example, the abstract to the race-specific patent on BiDil refers to an "African American" patient; but the FDA-approved label for the drug refers to "black" patients.

WHAT IS RACIALIZED MEDICINE?

The use of race in medical practice is not necessarily the same thing as racialized medicine. For example, it may be entirely appropriate, even necessary, to use race when tracking and addressing broad issues, such as health disparities in American society. Understanding race as a social construct is entirely consistent with recognizing and addressing race-based inequalities in access to or quality of medical care in our society. Such inequalities reflect the biological implications of the social and historical phenomenon of racial discrimination.

In contrast, *racialized* medicine is premised on an implicit, and sometimes explicit, understanding of race as a genetic fact. Such an understanding is both scientifically flawed and politically dangerous. History teaches us that constructing races as genetically bounded and discrete categories is only one short step from constructing races as inferior and superior. Racism feeds on biologically reductive constructions of racial difference. In this book, I argue that it is imperative to recognize the significance and complexity of race to understand and address the real and persistent health disparities that plague our country. But, as numerous studies have indicated, these disparities are the result of social, economic, and political histories of injustice, not genetics.[30] They demand social, economic, and political responses. If we mistakenly reduce health disparities among socially defined racial groups to a function of genetic difference to be addressed through race-specific medicine, we risk diverting valuable resources from developing policies and practices to confront the true causes of health disparities.

Unlike *racialized* medicine, which treats race as genetic, the *use* of race in medical practice has many legitimate and important places. Collecting broad-based epidemiological data is perhaps foremost among these. Only by using social categories of race is it possible to identify and track racial disparities in health, health-care access, and outcomes. Such information is needed to address ongoing issues of racial injustice in society. It may also be appropriate for individual health practitioners to take race into account under certain circumstances when trying to assess the needs of their patients. To the extent that health practitioners understand race as a social phenomenon that has biological consequences, it may be legitimate and important to consider its implications when formulating appropriate medical interventions.

Social understandings of race vary over time and across space. In the past, the U.S. Census has included racial categories ranging from Mulatto to Hindu. In the Jim Crow South, children of Armenian or Greek immigrants were sometimes mandated to go to schools designated for black children. Today, someone of light brown complexion who is socially identified as "black" in the United States (for example, someone with a white mother

Haiti 9x.

from Kansas and a black father from Kenya) might be identified as "white" in Jamaica or Brazil. Legal scholar Patricia Williams provides a revealing anecdote of this phenomenon in action, relating an exchange between a Haitian statesman and an American official in the 1930s:

> "What percent of Haiti's population is white?" asked the American. "Ninety-five percent," came the answer. The American official was flustered and, assuming that the Haitian was mistaken, exclaimed, "I don't understand—how on earth do you come up with such a figure?"
>
> "Well, how do you measure blackness in the United States?"
>
> "Anyone with a black ancestor."
>
> "Well, that's exactly how we measure whiteness," retorted the Haitian."[31]

Since the 1960s, the concept of "self-identification" has become the norm in assigning racial identities to individuals in the United States. As a social practice for collecting census data relating to social and economic phenomena, such as employment or education, this makes sense; but as a medical or scientific practice, if connected to ideas of biological difference, it becomes far more problematic.

Often, when discussing the relationships among race, health, and genetics, I am met with questions about sickle cell anemia. Historically, sickle cell is perhaps the most powerfully racialized genetic condition in the United States, where it is invariably cast as a "black" disease. It actually provides an excellent example of the complexities of uncritically associating race, genes, and disease. Sickle cell anemia is a condition that impairs a person's red blood cells from carrying oxygen. It can cause mild or severe pain in organs, joints, or muscles, and in extreme cases even death. A "carrier" of the sickle cell "trait" has one copy of the sickle cell gene (in the language of biology, the carrier is "heterozygous"); individuals with the actual disease have two copies of the gene, one from each parent (known as "homozygous"). People with the trait (i.e., one gene) but not the actual disease generally do not manifest any ill health effects. Indeed, it is understood that having one gene may enhance a carrier's resistance to malaria.

In the United States, approximately one in twelve blacks carries the sickle cell trait. The prevalence of the sickle cell trait is higher in populations identified as African American than in populations identified as Caucasian American, but the trait most emphatically is not exclusive to blacks or Africans. Rather, it is currently understood by the medical and scientific community as an artifact of populations descended from regions of the world with a high incidence of malaria, such as West Africa. For example, the trait is also found at relatively high frequencies among many Mediterranean populations, including especially Greeks and Sicilians, as well as certain Arab and Asian Indian populations, whereas it is rare in South African blacks.[32] If the trans-Atlantic slave traders had raided the shores of Greece instead of West Africa, we in the United States might today be (mistakenly) characterizing sickle cell anemia as a "Greek" disease. Similarly, if southern Africa rather than West Central Africa had been the major focus of the slave trade, today's African American descendants of those original enslaved Africans would likely have no higher prevalence of sickle cell anemia than most Americans descended from Europeans.

When using race in medical practice, what matters is our shifting understanding of the correlations between such evolving social identities and the economic, political, and environmental conditions to which they may be related. For example, what are we to make of the fact that African Americans suffer from disproportionately high rates of hypertension, but Africans in Nigeria have among the world's lowest rates of hypertension, far lower than the overwhelmingly white population of Germany? The analysis making these findings reviewed studies of hypertension from around the world with a total of 85,000 subjects. Its conclusion: "these data demonstrate that the consistent emphasis given to the genetic elements of the racial contrasts may be a distraction from the more relevant issue of defining and intervening in the preventable causes of hypertension, which are likely to have a similar impact regardless of ethnic and racial background. Once the problem of ethnic/racial contrasts is characterized more closely as a special instance of environmental influences at the population level, it could become more tractable in both the realms of research and practice."[33] Genetics certainly plays a role in hypertension. But as this study shows, any role it plays in explaining racial differences in hypertension must surely be vanishingly small. Moreover, in a direct study of the value of using race as a surrogate for genetics in a clinical context, a recent paper in the online journal *PLoS One* found that evidence "suggest[s] that in the genomic era conventional racial/ethnic labels are of little value."[34]

There may be occasions when race can be productively used in genetic research, but in such cases it is very important to differentiate between using a racial group to characterize a gene versus using a gene to character-ize a racial group. Thus, for example, a researcher trying to understand the genetics of diabetes may choose to study the Pima Indians in the southwest-ern United States, because that group has a very high incidence of diabetes. This is an example of using a socially identified racial or ethnic group in order to try to characterize a gene (here for diabetes). It is quite another thing, however, for a researcher who finds such a gene to use it to character-ize the identity of Pima Indians as a group with "the gene for diabetes." This approach *racializes* the genetic basis for diabetes as inherent to Pima Indians. Using racial or ethnic groups to find genes associated with diabetes does not necessarily stigmatize such groups or reduce them to bounded genetic entities; characterizing racial or ethnic groups in terms of genes does.[35]

Medical practitioners need not, indeed often should not, ignore race. The issue is not primarily one of *whether* to use racial categories in medical prac-tice but *how*. Carefully taking account of race to help understand broader social or environmental factors that may be influencing health disparities can be warranted in certain situations. But it is always important to under-stand that race itself is not an inherent causal factor in such conditions and that race is itself a socially constructed term, not a biological reality.

FIVE THEMES

Below I elaborate five themes that inform much of this book. Each runs throughout the story, with different ones setting the dominant tone in different places in the text. At times, multiple themes may be playing off one another, while others may fade into the background. I list the themes in a sequence that roughly matches their foremost emergence through the arc of the book, mirroring my concern to explore how race enters biomedicine, what happens to it once it is there, and what the broader implications of this phenomenon are.

INSTITUTIONAL MANDATES

My first theme involves institutional mandates that promote the introduction of race into biomedical research and practice. Foremost among these is a mandate of classification, promulgated by the U.S. Office of Management and Budget (OMB), which sets forth the racial and ethnic categories used by the federal government in collecting and organizing demographic data. These categories are most familiar to us through the census form, but they also direct researchers in the collection and organization of clinical data and drug-approval applications. The federal government also shapes the conceptualization and use of biomedical knowledge and racial categories by the way in which it organizes and classifies vast amounts of genetic information stored in massive biobanks used by researchers worldwide. Additionally, the U.S. Patent and Trademark Office (PTO) plays a distinctive and subtly powerful role as a site where mandates from particular federal officials may be influencing the introduction of race into biomedicine. What often results is a collision of categories—social categories of race constructed for the census with biological categories of population intended for biomedical research—that may unintentionally promote the conflation of race and biology in highly problematic and sometimes misleading ways.

CARE OF THE DATA AND THE INERTIAL FORCE OF RACE

This brings me to my second theme, which I call "care of the data" (a term I borrow from historian Mike Fortun). From clinical bench to bedside, the most consistent attribute of those using race is a perplexing inattention to the complexities of the category. It is perhaps the very givenness of our social understandings of race that enables such a casual approach to race in these diverse forums. I have generally found a great contrast between the care and attention biomedical professionals devote to the technical aspects of their work and their casual, almost unthinking use of racial categories in collecting and organizing their data. Thus, for example, articles published in biomedical journals may discuss at length genetic sequencing platforms or assays and may describe statistical methods in exhausting detail, but when it come to race, definitions are often absent or at best consigned to a perfunctory statement that race was "self-identified."

"Self-identification" may serve for collecting census data, but it is often inappropriate or misleading in a biomedical context. It has become a fig leaf that covers a broad array of implicitly biologized conceptions of race. Too frequently, an implicit assumption to the effect that "genetics is complex, race is obvious" informs genetic research and practice. Throughout the book, I argue that we need to inject the same sort of care that scientists show for genetic data into their production, interpretation, and circulation of racial data.

This will not be easy. I also argue that there is a tremendous inertial force to racial categories in biomedicine. Race is a powerful, deeply embedded, and pervasive part of American history, culture, and politics. Once introduced into a conceptual system, it is very hard to dislodge it or even to alter or refine its use. Here, the intersections with the themes of federal mandates and commercial imperatives is especially salient, as the latter have created powerful incentives that direct biomedical professionals to introduce race into their work at many levels.

THE BALANCE OF COMMERCE AND SCIENCE

My third theme focuses on the balance between science and commerce. In the United States, the two have always gone hand in hand. Some people have responded to my criticisms about commercial considerations driving the use of race in biomedicine by saying, "We have a capitalist system. Of course drug companies want to make money; that's how it works, and that's how we get valuable drugs to market." Fair enough. But to understand the use of race in drug development, the issue is not whether we do (or should) have a capitalist system; it is how commercial considerations affect the choices being made in framing research protocols, conducting clinical trials, interpreting scientific results, seeking regulatory approvals, and developing marketing campaigns. Stating the obvious fact that drug companies are profit-seeking entities does not address these concerns. Accepting that biomedicine is bound up with commerce, we still must examine with specificity the nature of the relationship and consider whether it is properly balanced. When commercial considerations move beyond selecting potentially profitable drugs for development into the realm of actually shaping trial design and framing the interpretation of results, then one may legitimately argue that the balance between commerce and science is out of whack and demands scrutiny both by the clinicians participating in the trials and by the regulatory agencies reviewing their results.

I argue that there is a big difference between choosing to develop one drug over another because it has greater commercial prospects versus choosing to ignore or distort data because it threatens a drug's commercial prospects. As I explored the diverse uses of race in biomedicine, I found that race increasingly is being exploited in problematic ways for commercial purposes. In this relationship, commerce, not science, has been framing the scientific questions being asked and the interpretation of results. This is a relationship out of balance.

THE PERSISTENCE OF RACE AND THE POLITICS OF THE MEANTIME

My fourth theme is the persistence of race in the face of genomic discovery and a related phenomenon, which I call the "politics of the meantime." From BiDil onward, researchers, clinicians, government officials, and corporate executives have all consistently referred to race as a "surrogate," a "stepping-stone," or a "placeholder" for as yet unknown genetic variation. Many even concede that race is a "crude surrogate." They argue, however, that it is the best thing we have to get us through the present period of limited genetic knowledge and to keep us going down the road to an era of truly individualized personal genomic medicine. The politics of the mean-time involves the choices regarding allocation of resources and framing of health-related priorities that such claims enable. In particular, casting race as a stepping-stone enables the casual use of racial categories in biomedical research, practice, and product development by casting such use as merely instrumental and temporary at worst, and at best a means to bring us to a genomic promised land. Even as genomic milestones are being reached and surpassed, the use of race is persisting. I argue that genomic progress alone will never lead race to fade away. The combined incentives of institu-tional mandates and commercial advantage continue to support the use of race. The inertial power of racial categories also carries forward their use, even after the initial rationale for their introduction has passed.

THE POLITICS OF RACE, GENETICS, AND DISPARITIES

Finally, beyond particular cases or practices, the intersections of race, law, and commerce in the domain of biomedicine have broader political impli-cations for how we, as a society, conceive and approach health disparities and racial injustice. Racial disparities in health are real and significant. Their causes are complex and varied. Do genes play a role? Yes, certainly; genes play a role in just about everything having to do with health. If we are interested in genetics, the question is (or should be): "What role do genes play in disparities relative to other forces, such as social conditions, environment, economic status, political power, etc.?" Posed in that man-ner, it is clear that while genetics may play a very significant role in many diseases, it plays a diminishingly small role in actual health *disparities*. Yet, one corollary of race-specific medicine has been a concerted drive to locate the causes of disparities at the molecular level in the purportedly defective genes of racialized individuals. The implications of this focus are many. Most immediately, it diverts attention and resources away from the broader social and political causes of disparities that are deeply embedded in our nation's troubled history of racial injustice. It promises a neat technological fix for what are inescapably difficult (and messy) problems of racism, political power, and socioeconomic status.

APPROACHING RACE AND MEDICINE

As I approach the intersections of race, science, law, and commerce, I begin in Chapter 1 by considering how and where race enters modern biomedicine, paying particular attention to the role of federal regulatory frameworks and mandates in incentivizing the introduction of racial categories in research and practice. Foremost among these are initiatives such as the National Institutes of Health Revitalization Act of 1993, which affirmatively mandates the use of the census racial categories in producing and organizing clinical data, and others such as the Food and Drug Modernization Act (FDMA) of 1997, which strongly encourages it. This chapter also considers the implications of how federally sponsored biobanks, which compile genetic data from around the world, frequently organize their vast data sets using population groupings that often become collapsed into racial categories reflecting the OMB mandate. This sets the stage for exploring what happens to race after it enters biomedical research and practice by looking for where it travels, how and by whom it is taken up, and what diverse purposes it serves—both intentional and unintentional.

I then turn to telling the story of BiDil in depth. Chapter 2 explores the origins of BiDil as a drug for everyone and considers how it became racialized primarily in response to an FDA ruling that placed in jeopardy the value of its owner's original nonracial patent. I argue that obtaining a second, race-specific patent was driven primarily by concerns to extend the commercial life of the product. I begin by elaborating the case for BiDil made by its promoters and then move on to deconstruct that case by looking closely at the origins of the drug in the 1980s as a nonracial drug to treat heart failure in anyone, regardless of race. I analyze the critical moment in

NIH Revitalizu Act of 1993   FDMA § 1997

1999 when BiDil's patent holders transformed it into a racially marked therapy and then explore the distinctive role of law, particularly patents, in driving BiDil's racial turn.

Chapter 3 unfolds around the story of an inaccurate statistic claiming that African Americans suffered mortality from heart failure at a rate twice that of whites. It traces the origins and circulation of this statistic, providing a sustained analysis of the power of race to take on a life of its own once introduced into a conceptual system for making sense of health disparities. It then examines how BiDil's proponents used this statistic, in conjunction with equally problematic assertions that angiotensin-converting enzyme (ACE) inhibitors (another class of drugs to treat heart failure) do not work well in blacks, to create a racial frame for BiDil that played a central role in driving the drug toward its race-specific approval by the FDA.

A close reading of the FDA hearing that approved the race-specific indication for BiDil is at the center of Chapter 4. I argue here that the racial frame played a critical role in shaping how the committee reviewed the data before it. This chapter examines how the story of BiDil presented a new model for development of targeted therapeutics that exploited race to cast the drug as an advance toward the promised land of individualized pharmacogenomics. Specifically, this chapter considers how BiDil's proponents used race: first, to resurrect the fortunes of an apparently failed drug; second, to gain faster and cheaper FDA approval; and third, to expand its potential market by informally promoting off-label use of the product to the general population. The chapter then moves on to examine the broader marketing of BiDil, both to capital markets and to the public at large, situating BiDil at the forefront of a drive to bring the long-established corporate practice of "ethnic niche marketing" into the world of pharmaceuticals. I argue that NitroMed used the FDA's race-specific approval of a drug to treat a biological condition to create a market based on the racially marked social group of African Americans. The chapter then analyzes the myriad factors contributing to NitroMed's ultimate failure to capitalize on the early promise of its racialized reinvention of BiDil. This necessarily raises the question of whether BiDil was a harbinger of things to come or merely an anomaly. The answer, of course, is a little of both. Its distinctive history is unlikely to be precisely repeated, but the remainder of the chapter makes the case that the BiDil model is being emulated, looking at other efforts to use race to exploit niche markets and differentiate other pharmaceutical products in a crowded marketplace.

Chapter 5 expands upon the implications of BiDil as a harbinger by situating it in the larger context of the rising use of racial categories in biotechnology patents. A central theme here is to explore the interplay among commercial interests, regulatory structures, and scientific practice in generating distinctively racialized conceptions of biomedicine in the field of intellectual property. This chapter provides a basic introduction to some of the core concepts and rationales of patent law and then lays out the results of a study showing the steady rise of racial biotechnology patents over the past decade. It then examines exactly *how* race is being used in these patents, considering how such use is often premised on an unstated white norm underlying a characterization of some sort of racial difference at the genetic level. It argues that while race may be used as a surrogate for statistical correlations and genetics frequencies in the body of the patent, it often becomes solidified into a static and bounded genetic category in the legally operative claims section of the patent. It argues that far from adding anything of substantive scientific value to most patents, the use of race is driven by *legal* purposes of obtaining additional layers of potential patent protection for particular biotechnological inventions. The chapter concludes with an analysis and critique of recent practices within the PTO, whereby federal patent examiners have been actively *requiring* the introduction of racial categories into certain biotechnology patent applications. I then extend my analysis to consider some of the broader implications of racial patents, arguing that the introduction of race into patent law is producing a new political geography of intellectual property in which racial identity itself is becoming a patentable commodity in a manner that is transforming social race into a (legally) genetic fact. Pursuing an analogy to other forms of property, I suggest that the racialized territory of these biotechnology patents is creating a new "segregated genome," with racially identified neighborhoods whose value is being appropriated and exploited in capital markets.

Moving outward from the focus on patent law, Chapter 6 examines the broader forces driving the persistent use of race in biomedical research and practice. It explores "the politics of the meantime" in pharmacogenomics, arguing that debates over the appropriate use of race in biomedicine are being obscured or sidestepped by appeals to use race as an interim surrogate for genetic variation and that the need for race will "fade away" once the promised land of truly individualized pharmacogenomic medicine is attained. I argue that there is a distinctive politics to this claim that allows racialized medicine to persist and flourish in the face of the very same genomic advances that are supposed to render it irrelevant. I examine the story of the blood-thinning drug warfarin as one of the clearest examples of this phenomenon. In this case, race has persisted as a central component of dosing guidelines and diagnostic testing, even as specific genomic markers for warfarin response have been identified and confirmed. Beyond the legal and institutional mandates discussed in previous chapters, I argue that there are also three dynamics more internal to biomedicine that mitigate against race fading away of its own accord: First, genetics will never explain all biological variation in response to drugs or the manifestation of disease. There will always be something we do not know, and that unknown something will always be susceptible to racialization. Second, race has acquired an inertial force that carries it forward as part of the common sense of biomedical research and practice. Third, race continues to have a commercial value in differentiating products in a crowded biomedical marketplace.

Chapter 7 engages issues of framing systematically to situate the rise of racialized medicine yet more broadly in the context of ongoing political debates about the balance between state versus market interventions to address racial health disparities. This chapter argues that the focus on genetic difference effectively privatizes race in a manner that renders it susceptible to commercial exploitation. It also makes use of and contributes to broader, more conservative initiatives to remove race and racial justice from the public sphere as legitimate concerns of the political community. I argue that backlash against affirmative action and efforts to develop race-specific medicines both look to unfettered market mechanisms as the best means to address imbalances in access to goods such as jobs or health. They locate the source of the problem in the individual—either in terms of individual "merit" or in terms of individual genes. They reject or obscure the need for state intervention to solve the problem, focusing instead on individual responsibility to take action in private markets—working harder to get a good job or purchasing the proper pharmaceutical product to treat a disease. This scheme recasts historically rooted and politically sustained disparities in health care into mere "differences" rooted in genetics.

Finally, the conclusion elaborates some preliminary recommendations about how best to approach the use of racial categories in biomedical theory and practice. I intend these recommendations largely as a means for opening a discussion to consider implementing some structural incentives to promote greater care of racial data and thereby provide a modest counterbalance to the myriad forces, particularly commercial and political, mitigating against such care. This could be a modest but significant step toward addressing some of the problems discussed in this book and providing a more productive and equitable approach to the use of race in biomedical research and practice.

THREE CLICHÉS

Throughout this book, I am sensitive to the complex double edge of using race in biomedicine. The sky has not fallen since the approval of BiDil, and many good people are using race in biomedical research and product development with the best of intentions. But they are largely acting without taking sufficient care to understand the potential of such use to reify race as genetic and to reinforce stigmatizing racial stereotypes. Often when speaking about the implications of a race-specific drug such as BiDil,

I have framed my concerns in terms of three (historically informed) cli-chés: race-specific medicine may be a case of 1) the road to hell being paved with good intentions, because of 2) the law of unintended consequences, which is leading to 3) an accident waiting to happen. Alternatively, I sometimes analogize the use of race in medicine to another drug for heart disease: nitroglycerin. Like this volatile compound, race, if used with care and attention, can produce valuable results; but used carelessly, casually, or clumsily, it can explode in your face.

1

ORGANIZING RACE

Paths Toward the Re-Biologization of Race
in Modern Biomedical Research, Practice,
and Product Development

ACE ENTERS BIOMEDICINE through many pathways. Foremost among
these are federal initiatives that shape the production and use of racial categories in biomedical research. Recent debates over the appropriate use of racial and ethnic categories in biomedical contexts have
often concentrated on the practices of individual researchers with the
aim, in part, to help researchers appreciate the nuances and complexities of
the racial categories they use.[1] A focus on individual practices, while necessary, overlooks the myriad structural forces that teach researchers and
clinicians to see and use race in particular and often problematic ways.
Prominent among these forces are a wide array of federal mandates that
dictate the characterization and application of genetically based biomedical interventions, such as pharmaceuticals and diagnostic tests, in relation
to socially defined categories of race. Key federal mandates include: the
NIH Revitalization Act of 1993,[2] which directs the NIH to establish guidelines for including women and minorities in clinical research; the FDMA
of 1997, which in the context of drug development directs that "the Secretary [of Health and Human Services] shall, in consultation with the director of the National Institutes of Health and with representatives of the
drug manufacturing industry, review and develop guidance, as appropriate, on the inclusion of women and minorities in clinical trials;"[3] and two

subsequent FDA guidances for industry. The first, a 1999 guidance entitled "Population Pharmacokinetics,"[4] made recommendations on the use of population pharmacokinetics in the drug-development process to help identify differences in drug safety and efficacy among population subgroups, including race and ethnicity.[5] The second, a 2005 guidance entitled "Collection of Race and Ethnicity Data in Clinical Trials," recommends a standardized approach for collecting and reporting race and ethnicity information in clinical trials that produce data for applications to the FDA for drug approval.[6]

The NIH Revitalization Act had its origins in the mid-1980s, when concerns of the Congressional Caucus for Women's Issues led to a U.S. Government Accountability Office study that ultimately found the NIH was failing to follow its own policies regarding the inclusion of women and minorities in clinical trials. After the report was released in 1990, the Congressional Black Caucus took an interest in the issue, which led to the eventual passage of the NIH Revitalization Act in 1993. The act itself required that women and minorities be included as research subjects in NIH-funded research beginning in 1995. Researchers would, in effect, have to certify that they had enrolled adequately diverse populations, had made sufficient efforts to enroll diverse populations, or could provide a biomedical justification for not enrolling diverse populations (for example, not enrolling women in a study of prostate cancer).[7]

Sociologist Steven Epstein identifies five frames underlying arguments for the drive to racial and gender inclusion in biomedical research. First, "underrepresentation," the basic observation that women and minorities were underrepresented in clinical trial research populations; second, "misguided protectionism," an argument growing out of AIDS activism, that patients had a right to assume the risks of research; third, "false universalism," challenging the idea that the experience of the dominant group in society (white men) should be taken as the universal experience for all groups in society; fourth, "health disparities," demanding a targeted redress that took account of race; and fifth, "biological difference," which built on the idea of false universalism to argue that embodied differences in women and minorities needed to be taken into account in conducting biomedical research.[8]

Epstein was struck by the fact that proponents of the "biological-differences" frame "appeared to be relatively unbothered by the risk . . . that difference might be conceived of in pejorative terms and used to bolster arguments about social inferiority."[9] Nonetheless, he notes that at the time of its passage, Otis Brawley, then director of the National Cancer Institute's Office of Special Populations Research, worried that the NIH Revitalization Act's "emphasis on potential racial difference" possibly "fosters the racism that its creators want to abrogate by establishing government-sponsored research on the basis of the belief that there are significant biological differences among the races."[10] Along with the NIH, the FDA showed an increasing interest in issues of inclusion in the late 1980s and early 1990s.[11] The FDMA and related guidances for industry, however, do not mandate the same sort of subgroup analyses as the NIH Revitalization Act. They simply urge that companies collect data by sex, race, and ethnicity, and be on the lookout for "differences of clinically meaningful size."[12]

PRODUCING AND ORGANIZING SOCIAL DATA ON RACE AND ETHNICITY: OMB DIRECTIVE 15

These federal mandates have had a profound effect upon the use of racial categories in biomedical research, clinical practice, product development, and health policy. Their construction and definition of racial categories is structured by the OMB Revised Directive 15 on "Standards for Maintaining, Collecting, and Presenting Federal Data on Race and Ethnicity." The standards were developed "to provide a common language for uniformity and comparability in the collection and use of data on race and ethnicity by Federal agencies."[13] By conditioning grants and approvals on the collection of data according to the OMB categories, they provide powerful incentives to introduce race into biomedical contexts, regardless of its relevance.[14]

FDA

FDMA 1. NIH (Revitalization Act)

The U.S. government has long collected data based on categories of race and ethnicity. The census is a prime example. Since the first census in 1790, racial categories have changed over time to reflect the social and political concerns of the day. The first census had four categories: Free White Male, Free White Female, Other Free Person, and Slave. During the nineteenth century, additional categories that fell in and out of use included Free Colored Person, Black, Mulatto, Quadroon, Octoroon, Indian, Chinese, and Japanese. The twentieth century saw a new proliferation of categories, including Hindu, Korean, and Negro. Then, in the 1970s, various federal agencies responsible for collecting data relating to race and ethnicity beyond the census, led by the Office of Education and the Department of Health, Education, and Welfare, came to the OMB looking for assistance in developing government-wide standards for data on race and ethnicity.[15]

In 1977, the OMB produced "Statistical Policy Directive No. 15, Race and Ethnic Standards for Federal Statistics and Administrative Reporting." After several revisions and much debate over the following two decades, the OMB standards now provide set categories as a minimum standard for maintaining, collecting, and presenting data on race and ethnicity for all federal reporting purposes. The directive sets forth the following basic racial categories for organizing such data: American Indian or Alaska Native, Asian, Black or African American, Native Hawaiian or Other Pacific Islander, and White. There are two categories for data on ethnicity: "Hispanic or Latino," and "Not Hispanic or Latino."[16] Beyond this minimum standard, agencies and researchers have some latitude as to specifically how they will use the categories. Thus, for example, in the 2000 census, the Census Bureau allowed individuals to self-identify and to select multiple categories of race/ethnicity.[17]

The power of the OMB data standards to affect understandings of identity and group status is profound. As a consequence of major governmental programs and legal initiatives instituted since the 1960s, the OMB standards provide the basis both for census information and also for access to a variety of significant governmental goods and services that are contingent upon falling into a particular racial or ethnic group.[18] Federal users of racial data provided by the census include: the Department of Education, the Department of Justice (DOJ), the Department of Labor, the Equal Employment Opportunity Commission, the Federal Reserve, the Department of Health and Human Services (DHHS), Housing and Urban Development, the Department of Agriculture, and the Veterans Administration.[19] To make claims for resources or to demonstrate discrimination, groups must be counted.[20] It is in this context that federal initiatives have created a new possessive interest in hitherto marginalized and subordinated racial identities. The OMB categories (as a basis for classifications used in the census and other areas) have also shaped individuals' conceptions of their very identity as Americans.[21]

In local contexts, most state and local public health agencies organize their practices around the OMB categories.[22] The same may be said of all federally funded research and practice that touches on health-related issues, an area in which the OMB Directive 15 has become the de facto standard for the collection and organization of racial data.[23]

PRODUCING AND ORGANIZING GENETIC INFORMATION: FEDERALLY SPONSORED GENETIC DATABASES

The challenges of managing racial data become even more complex as biomedical researchers and clinicians use the social categories of race mandated by OMB Directive 15 alongside purported genetic population groupings produced and organized by federally sponsored genomic initiatives. As genetic research has grown over the past three decades, the federal government has sponsored an array of data banks that collect, store, and classify genetic information for use by biomedical researchers. Such data banks include the National Institute of General Medical Sciences (NIGMS)—Coriell Human Genetic Variation Collections, the DNA Polymorphism Discovery Resource (PDR), the database of single-nucleotide polymorphisms (dbSNP database), and the International Haplotype Map Project (IHMP, also known as the "HapMap"). Acting as an umbrella over these collections is a repository maintained by the federal government's National Center for Biotechnology Information (NCBI), known as "GenBank," which contains a web-based annotated collection of all publicly available DNA sequences. GenBank, in turn, is part of the International Nucleotide Sequence Database Collaboration, which also encompasses the DNA DataBank of Japan (DDBJ) and the European Molecular Biology Laboratory (EMBL) database. Each of these databases organizes genetic information into highly problematic population groupings that are adapted and used by researchers as correlates for racial categories. These databases are powerful not only because of their method of internally categorizing genetic information, but also because, as examples of authoritative scientific research, they provide working models of acceptable categorization by which any scientist may organize genetic data.[24]

Maintained by the independent, nonprofit Coriell Institute for Medical Research, the NIGMS "Human Genetic Cell Repository" aims to provide "scientists with the materials for accelerating disease-gene discovery."[25] As organized in its Human Genetic Variation Collection, the NIGMS classification of genetic data includes dozens of "population" groups from all over the world. The multifarious classifications used to organize this data range from "Caucasians" and "African Americans" in North America, to "Basque" and "Greek" in Europe, to "Indo Pakistani" and "Khmer—Cambodia" in Asia.[26]

As a comprehensive database, the NIGMS collection also includes access to data from the PDR, dbSNP, and the IHMP. It classifies genetic samples according to a wide array of categories that freely mix race, ethnicity, religion, geography, and citizenship—implying that each has distinctive and legitimate relations to genetic variation. The PDR is maintained by the National Human Genome Research Institute (NHGRI), in collaboration with the Centers for Disease Control and Prevention (CDC) and the NIGMS. This resource is "designed to reflect the diversity in the human population. . . ."[27] It includes samples designated as "European-American," "African-American," "Mexican-American," "Native American," and "Asian-American."[28]

The NHGRI and the NCBI maintain the publicly accessible dbSNP database.[29] The dbSNP database contains information on more than 2.7

million SNPs that researchers use to explore the structure of human variation and to design genetic association studies. This database had grouped
its genetic data into a perplexing amalgam of diverse categories that employ
racial and ethnic constructs (e.g., U.S. Caucasians, African Americans, and
Hispanics), geographic constructs (e.g., North Africa, East Africa), political nation states (e.g., Russia and satellite republics), mixes of geography
and nation states (e.g., Sub-Saharan Nations bordering the Atlantic North
of the Congo River), and mixes of all three ("All samples north of Tropic
of Cancer. This would include defined samples of U.S. Caucasians, African
Americans and Hispanics."). Thus, as biomedical researchers mine the
dbSNP data, they are accessing and organizing terms that juxtapose or directly classify genetic data in terms of race, ethnicity, nation, and/or geography. When used in studies or trials covered by federal mandates, the
diverse and sometimes contradictory population classifications employed
variously by the NIGMS, PDR, and dbSNP databases cry out to be sim-
plified and reclassified in terms of the basic OMB Directive 15 social categories of race and ethnicity.[30]

A potentially different, but still problematic, model of federally sponsored genetic database production and organization is the IHMP. Led by a
consortium of government-supported researchers in Japan, the United
Kingdom, Canada, China, Nigeria, and the United States, the IHMP was
premised on a recognition that identifying the significance of each individual SNP would be a daunting task, because there is approximately one
SNP for every 1,000 bases of DNA, with an estimate of perhaps 4 million
common SNPs.[31] Recent research has found, however, that SNPs travel
across generations in rather large blocks, often 10,000 to 50,000 nucleotide bases each. These blocks are known as haplotypes. The IHMP aims to
greatly increase the efficiency of genetic research by enabling scientists to
search through bundles of 10,000 to 50,000 bases rather than going through
an entire genome one base at a time to discover specific SNPs.[32]

The first phase of the IHMP cataloged more than one million SNPs
in the genome sequences of 269 people who were classified into four population groups: "(1) 90 individuals . . . from the Yoruba in Ibadan, Nigeria . . . ;
(2) 90 individuals . . . in Utah, USA . . . ; (3) 45 Han Chinese in Beijing,
China . . . ; [and] (4) 44 Japanese in Tokyo, Japan."[33] In contrast to the

population categories in other federally sponsored genetic databases, the Consortium was careful to emphasize that "because none of the samples was collected to be representative of a larger population such as 'Yoruba,' 'Northern and Western European,' 'Han Chinese,' or 'Japanese' (let alone all the populations from 'Africa,' 'Europe,' or 'Asia'), we recommend using a specific local identifier (for example, 'Yoruba in Ibadan, Nigeria') to describe samples initially."[34]

And indeed, the samples subsequently deposited with the NIGMS/ Coriell Human Genetics Variation Collection are so identified.[35] This unusually careful characterization of data resulted, in part, from the Consortium's deliberate attention to what it termed "integrating ethics and science in the International HapMap Project."[36]

Yet, as the data from the HapMap was taken up and circulated both in the popular press and in scientific journals, these careful classifications were repeatedly conflated with the broad, racially marked continental categories of "African," "Asian," and "European." For example, prominent popular reports of the completion of the first phase of the HapMap described the samples variously as "people from Africa, the Far East, and western Europe";[37] "people from Asia, Africa and the United States";[38] and "people from Africa, Asia, and the European population."[39] Among scientific journals, a typical article on linkage disequilibrium in the *American Journal of Human Genetics* refers to the HapMap as sampling "four populations with African, Asian, and European ancestry."[40]

The International Haplotype Map Consortium (IHC) itself bears a measure of responsibility for such easy conflation. The initial justification for selecting geographically dispersed populations was to capture greater genetic variation.[41] But one could argue that since the greatest genetic diversity is to be found among populations within Africa, a more revealing map might have been developed by sampling geographically dispersed populations within Africa. Alternatively, the IHC could have chosen not to mark the samples according to their points of origin. Moreover, in its actual sampling and classification strategy, the IHC sent conflicting messages regarding the local specificity of the populations. Most prominently, in sampling 45 Han Chinese and 44 Japanese, the project design implicitly asks for these two groups to be amalgamated into a larger "Asian" category to parallel the 90 samples each from the Ibadan, Nigeria, and Utah, United States, collections. The IHC's otherwise responsible and careful post hoc characterization of the samples thus operated in tension with the message sent by the underlying structure of the project design.[42]

THE ETHICS OF CLASSIFICATION

Each of these genetic databases is a state-sponsored technology of classification. They provide means to organize a vast array of genetic information into more comprehensible and usable forms. Systems of classification, however, are artifacts that embody ethical choices. As Geoffrey Bowker and Leigh Star have noted, "each standard and each category valorizes some point of view and silences another. This is not inherently a bad thing—indeed it is inescapable. But it *is* an ethical choice, and as such it is dangerous—not bad, but dangerous."[43] In the realm of genetics, where such systems address the human body, new biologically based categories can profoundly affect people's identities, aspirations, and dignity. Genetic classification is powerful but it is also dangerous, because it involves biological categories that may be confused and conflated with race. Any resulting reification of social categories of race as biological constructs risks new forms of exclusion and stigma.[44]

In a different but related context, Bowker and Star note how psychiatrists increasingly use the language of the *Diagnostic and Statistical Manual of Mental Disorders* (DSM) "to communicate with each other and their accounting departments, although they frequently do not believe in the categories they are using." For many federally funded researchers and practitioners who use genetic information, the government mandates the collection and organization of biological data according to socially constructed categories of race and ethnicity. As a result, many researchers who might not otherwise believe in any biological basis for race may easily default to using racial categories in biological contexts, especially when directed to do so by federal mandate.[45]

As scientists and health professionals increasingly use federally maintained genetic population categories alongside the federally mandated social categories of race and ethnicity, these two powerful systems of categorization are colliding in practice and becoming confused in everyday discourse, with consequences that are difficult to foresee. The power of social categories to shape scientific and professional practice is leading to the convenient use of racial and ethnic categories in inappropriate and harmful ways.[46] Genetic databases and OMB Directive 15 are seemingly "technical" methods of categorization, but such apparent neutrality is precisely what drives and lends the aura of legitimacy to the casual and often reflexive conflation of race and genetics in a variety of biomedical contexts.

Certain health effects do correlate with social categories of race and ethnicity, and scientists may legitimately use the collection of health data according to these categories, so long as the categories are understood as social and not genetic.[47] In the field of public health research in particular, racial and ethnic data play a central role in developing policies and interventions to combat inequities in the delivery of health care.[48] One of the primary goals of the federal government's "Healthy People 2010" initiative was "to eliminate health disparities among different segments of the population."[49] Thus, an ongoing tension exists between the need to resist the reductive tendency to naturalize race as a genetic category and the practical reality that race, as a social category, may end up influencing levels of stress, access to care, or other factors having biological consequences that need to be addressed.[50]

RACIAL "RECURSION": THE RETURN OF THE REPRESSED

The experience of reracializing the HapMap population categories points up a broader phenomenon, common throughout biomedical research, that I refer to as *racial recursion.* Racial recursion is the tendency of categories employed to avoid racial classifications to loop back to race as they travel over time and across domains. Thus, the carefully crafted, locally specific population categories used by the HapMap project soon came to stand for continental groups, which then came to be understood as the equivalent of racial groups. The most common term used to avoid race has been "ethnicity." Though rarely defined, ethnicity has been emerging as a default term increasingly used to avoid "race," but in effect meaning the same thing. Thus, for example, a rising number of biomedical studies refer to African, European, and/or Asian ethnicity.[51] Race-specific patent applications have also shown a marked rise in the term "ethnic" over "race" in making claims.[52] Developers of genetic ancestry-tracing products have been promoting the term "biogeographical ancestry" in place of racial designators. The term seems to join concepts of ancestral descent and geographic location. When examined more closely, however, it is defined as "the heritable component of race."[53] Results provided to consumers using this technology are invariably given in terms of classic racial categories of African, Asian, and European (and occasionally Native American).[54] The circle of racial recursion is complete: from race, to ethnicity, to biogeographical ancestry, to continental ancestry, and back again to race.

In her charting of three roughly equal phases of U.S. biological kinship categories across the twentieth century, Donna Haraway notes shifts from race to population to genome as "key objects of knowledge." She identifies concomitant shifts in the "status of race as an epistemological object in science and popular culture," moving from race being viewed as real and fundamental to race being understood as an "illusory object constructed by bad science," to a reemergence of race during the genomic era (since 1975) as a central component of "medical discourse on organ transplantation and drug testing."[55] These shifts are themselves a sort of historically informed example of racial recursion. As Anne Fausto-Sterling noted in commenting on Haraway's schema, "the race term always lurks in the wings." Fausto-Sterling goes on to consider how "in the current literature, a variety of words, singly and in combination, both technical and popular, pepper scientific discussions of human variation. Examples include: race, diversity, ethnic, group, population, community, descent, ancestry, geographic origin, minority, gene frequency, haplotype, language communities, stocks, single nucleotide polymorphisms."[56] Each of these terms describes aspects of human variation, but just as biomedical professionals are professing to use race as mere surrogate until better genetic information is obtained, so too are they using these substitute categories, such as ethnicity or biogeographical ancestry, as a sort of surrogate for race, hoping to avoid a direct engagement with the difficult issues race presents.

RESEARCHERS RESPOND

In his study of Werner Kalow, one of the fathers of modern pharmacogenomics, historian David Jones explores "the deep roots of the genetic and racial preoccupations in pharmacology."[57] Tracing Kalow's career from the 1930s to the 1990s, Jones argued that its trajectory "shows how race emerged as a central concern at the origins of the field and has remained an irresistible attraction for pharmacologists."[58] Jones notes in particular an intriguing tension in Kalow's work as he continued to make use of race into the 1970s, even after he became aware of the work of anthropologists, such as Ashley Montague, who offered trenchant critiques of biological conceptions of race.[59] The fascination of race as genetically significant in pharmacology seemed to persist even in the face of mounting evidence to the contrary.

More generally, the use of the terms "race" or "ethnicity" in biomedical journal articles has grown steadily since 1960—the year after the term "pharmacogenetics" was first coined.[60] A review of articles indexed at the federally managed PubMed database of biomedical journals using combinations of the terms "race," "ethnicity," "pharmacogenetics," and "pharmacogenomics" (coined in 1998)[61] indicates a steady rise in attention paid to racial categories in medicine. Far from abating in the face of genomic discovery, the use of racial categories has steadily increased in the genomic era—indeed, far outpacing its use in the period before the advent of the Human Genome Project (see Figure 1.1).[62] The rising use of race is less pronounced but still significant when viewed as a percentage of all articles indexed by PubMed (see Figure 1.2).

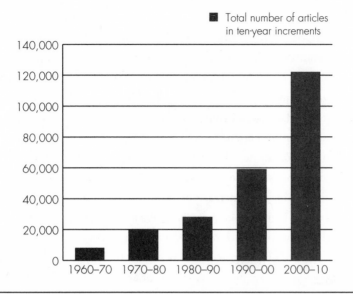

FIGURE 1.1 Journal articles using "race" or "ethnicity."

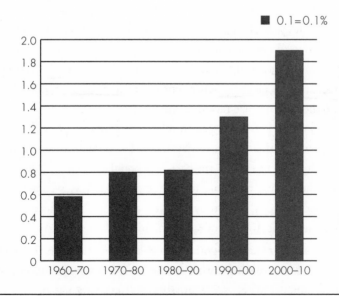

FIGURE 1.2 Articles using "race" or "ethnicity" as percent
of total articles published.

Most striking is the doubling and then more than redoubling of the use of "race" and "ethnicity" in absolute terms over the past two decades. The initial doubling coincides with the implementation of the NIH Revitalization Act inclusion mandate and the FDA's increasing emphasis on gathering racial data for drug submissions. The subsequent redoubling occurs in the decade following the completion of the first draft of the human genome.

When we look at the subset of journal articles dealing specifically with pharmacogenomics, we see an even more well-marked trend in absolute terms, with a nine-fold increase between the 1980s and the 1990s, and a nearly five-fold increase between the 1990s and the 2000s (see Figure 1.3). Again, the trend is less pronounced when viewed as a proportion of all articles published on pharmacogenomics. Nonetheless, part of the dip in the 2000s is accounted for by the explosion of articles on all aspects of pharmacogenomics, as several new journals devoted explicitly to that topic were founded (see Figure 1.4).

How, then, is race being used in these articles? Short of a full content review of thousands of articles, a study by Sankar, Cho, and Mountain provides valuable insight into this question. They examined 330 randomly selected articles published between 2001 and 2004 that reported on genetic research and used one or more words from a defined list of race, ethnicity, or population terms. Just over half of the articles reviewed "used race or ethnicity terms as either a dependent or independent variable. Another quarter either did not use race or ethnicity terms at all or used them only to refer to populations discussed in related research."[63] They found additionally, however, that "the majority of articles did not justify the use of a labeled population or explain the basis of a population label."[64] More troubling was the finding that no article among the 330 reviewed actually defined race or ethnicity. The study thus reveals an almost reflexive and certainly non-self-reflective use of race in biomedical research. As the authors modestly assert, "These findings lend credence to concerns that genetics researchers neither address what they mean by race and ethnicity terms nor explain the relevance of race or ethnicity to their research."[65]

Similar results have been found in other studies of published biomedical research that makes assertions about associations among genetics,

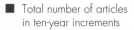

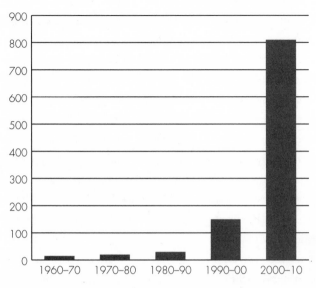

FIGURE 1.3 Journal articles using "pharmacogenetics" and "race" or "ethnicity."

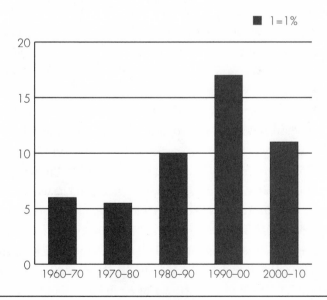

FIGURE 1.4 Articles using "pharmacogenetics" and "race" or "ethnicity" as percent of total articles published using "pharmacogenetics."

health outcomes, and race or ethnicity. When viewed in relation to the charts showing a rise in the use of race in biomedical research, the concordant findings of these multiple studies lead to the seemingly paradoxical conclusion that race is becoming increasingly salient even as it is apparently drained of substance.[66]

The paradox may resolve itself if we consider that it is precisely the lack of adequate definition that facilitates the expanding use of racial categories in biomedical research. In this regard, the common use (or mis-use) of racial categories may be viewed, in part, as analogous to the role a symbol may play in helping to build and sustain community. Anthropologist Anthony Cohen notes that symbols are effective in this capacity "because they are imprecise."[67] The imprecision of most symbols allows diverse members of the community to attach different meanings to them while still sharing the symbols themselves. In a similar manner, biomedical professionals share the basic symbol of "race" while attaching diverse (and usually unarticulated) meanings to it. They are all able to research "race" without considering the tensions inherent in their various deployments of the concept.

The imprecision of the symbol "race" also allows researchers to blur the social and biological meanings they ascribe to it. Ironically, this blurring was, in part, enabled by the work of geneticists, such as Richard Lewontin, who, together with a wide array of social scientists, have worked diligently since World War II to reconfigure race from a biological construct into a social construct.[68] In its 1998 "Statement on Race," the American Anthropological Association asserted that "racial beliefs constitute myths about the diversity in the human species and about the abilities and behavior of people homogenized into 'racial' categories."[69] The social science literature on race as a social construct is enormous, and its terminology has penetrated the life sciences. For example, the glossary of terms at the website for the NHGRI defines race as "an ideology and for this reason, many scientists believe that race should be more accurately described as a social construct and not a biological one."[70] Race as a social construct, however, has itself become something of a symbol. It has been deployed casually and without precision in a manner that has allowed an easy elision of detailed definition or (as indicated by the Sankar, Cho, and Mountain study) any definition at all. As "merely" social, it does not command attention in the life sciences, with their focus on purportedly "natural" and "objective" phenomena. Hence, ironically, as biomedical researchers accept race as a social construct, they may also disavow (consciously or not) responsibility for rigorously interrogating the racial categories they employ.

RACE, TECHNOLOGY, AND "CARE OF THE DATA"

The casual and often perfunctory assignment of social categories of race stands in marked contrast to the meticulous care taken concerning the more technical aspects of biomedical research and analysis.[71] One influential article on the pharmacogenomics of the blood-thinning drug warfarin, published by the International Warfarin Pharmacogenomics Consortium (IWPC) in the *New England Journal of Medicine*, provides an instructive example. In recent years, warfarin emerged as something of a poster child for pharmacogenomics, because several specific genetic variations have been identified as having a significant impact on warfarin metabolism. In February 2009, the IWPC published a study presenting an algorithm using genetic information to help guide doctors in calibrating doses of warfarin.[72] The IWPC, composed of eminent biomedical researchers and institutions from around the world and based in Stanford, California, operates under the auspices of the Pharmacogenomics Knowledge Base (PharmGKB).[73] To develop a genetic dosing algorithm, it analyzed warfarin dose-response information from over twenty-one sites in nine countries. The study was not the first to show the advantage of incorporating genetic information into prescribing patterns, but it was by far the largest and most inclusive to date, with information on more than 5,000 patients.[74]

The study was based on the perceived need to develop a dosing algorithm using both genetic and clinical data gathered from a "diverse and large population."[75] In this context, "diverse" included the concepts of race or ethnicity. From the outset, the study's use of these concepts was problematic.

As stated in the methods section, "Information of race or ethnic group was reported by the patient or determined by the local investigator."[76] This may reflect the simple reality of using data collected from numerous sites across the globe, but both self-reporting and external ascription of race raise significant issues in a biomedical context.

The contrast between the study's perfunctory discussion of race and its detailed elaboration of the technical methods of biomedical analysis is striking. The published report was accompanied by a twenty-one-page appendix of supplementary information that extensively covered such areas as "Variables Included in the Regression Analysis and Warfarin Dosing Algorithms" and "Sensitivity Analysis Testing Performance of Various Dosing Approaches Using Different Cut-Points to Create Low, Intermediate and High Dose Groups." It also included two pages on "Detailed Definitions of Stable Warfarin Definitions for the Collected IWPC Data." Yet the sum total of consideration devoted to definitions of race in the twenty-one-page appendix is limited to "Self-Reported Information and Racial Categories Used as Defined by the U.S. Office of Management and Budget."[77] Notably, even this brief mention of race is inconsistent with the statement in the article itself that race was either "reported by the patient or determined by the local investigator."[78]

In biomedical studies of the interaction of social and biological factors, self-reporting, as a fundamentally subjective social practice, may capture valuable social variables that affect health. Such is the case for many epidemiological studies seeking to track health disparities and understand how social, environmental, historical, economic, or other social factors affect the heath of particular racial groups. In a focused study of genetic polymorphisms, however, self-reporting of race is far more problematic. In the epidemiological example, self-reporting captures social experience, which may be relevant to the study. In the genetic example, self-reporting is meant to stand in for genetic ancestry linked to continental populations. This is not how most people conceive of race when they "self-report." The social experience of racial identity is not necessarily coincident with continental ancestry. For example, a white South African, whose ancestors

Compare: determining race & ...

emigrated to Africa hundreds of years ago, might consider herself to be of African ancestry. Similarly, a direct descendant of Alexandre Dumas, whose mother was an Afro-Caribbean Creole, might self-identify as being of European ancestry. Or, more recently, there is the case of the literary critic Anatole Broyard, himself of New Orleans Creole background, who identified as African American while a child and then reconfigured his identity as white while an adult. Stories of "passing" permeate American history.[79] Moreover, one U.S. study found that one-third of people change their own self-identified race or ethnicity in two consecutive years.[80]

Such examples bring into relief the fact that definitions of race involve not only geography or descent; they also implicate *time.* The question underlying many definitions of race is not simply *where* is a person from, but *when* are they from? The child Broyard was black, the adult was white. The white South African is African, unless we choose to fix her identity at a time predating the emigration of her ancestors from Europe. We are all "African" if we choose to locate our ancestral origins back far enough in time. The operative concept here is "choice." We do not have a single "true" ancestral identity that can be connected to a race. How we characterize it depends in large part on the choices we make regarding which time frame is most relevant to suit our particular purposes.

Complicating matters still further, another study found people often have very incomplete knowledge of their biological ancestry. Of a sample of 224 subjects interviewed for a study on attitudes toward race-based pharmacogenomics (the tailoring of drugs to genetic profiles), nearly 40 percent did not know the race of all four of their biological grandparents.[81] In such situations, self-declared race may fail to capture significant variation in biological ancestry.

A vignette from the story of BiDil highlights this problem. One news account of enrollment for the A-HeFT study related the story of Elyse Frazier, a fifty-six-year-old woman with heart failure who was asked to enroll in the trial. The research coordinator asked Frazier if she considered herself African American (a requirement for inclusion in the trial). Frazier was puzzled because, although she considered herself black in matters of politics, she had not considered the question before in a medical context. By her reckoning, her mother was half black, half Cherokee Indian; her father half black and half Blackfoot Indian. To the research coordinator's question, Frazier ultimately answered "yes" and was included in the trial. The news article concluded with Frazier wondering about whether future generations would be eligible for BiDil: "Based on her calculations, one of her grandsons, she points out, is 3/8 black, 1/16 Cherokee, 1/16 Blackfoot, 1/4 white and 1/4 Mexican."[82]

Such problems are only compounded in situations in which race is externally ascribed by a local investigator. Robert Hahn, for example, conducted a series of studies in the field of public health showing how external ascriptions of race are often unreliable and also may change over time.[83] Additionally, a British study showed that external ascriptions of racial identity by law enforcement authorities correspond very poorly with underlying patterns of genetic variation.[84] The article notes that in the British study, "classifications into the five 'ethnic' groups [Caucasian, Afro-Caribbean, Indian subcontinental, Southeast Asian, and Middle Eastern] were assigned by police officers by visual characteristics, based on [perceptions of outward] appearance rather than any knowledge of an individual's ancestry."[85] The actual correspondence of these external ascriptions to the "true" ancestry of the individuals ranged from 30 percent for the Middle Eastern category up to 67 percent for Afro-Caribbean, with Caucasian falling at 56 percent.[86]

Moving back into the arena of biomedicine, Duana Fullwiley's ethnographic study of two laboratories in which researchers were focused on the intersection of pharmacogenomics and race further elaborates the complexities of using social categories of race in a biological context. After months of observing researchers organize DNA samples by race, Fullwiley asked, "How do you define race?" Most of her informants

drew a blank at the question, leading to a pause in the interview that lasted anywhere from 5 to 30 seconds before they then offered responses that were often unsure. . . . Yet for the most part, it was simply due to confusion about what race is. When probed about its relationship to genetics, and to their projects in particular, their usual intellectual rigor was replaced with nervous laughter and, in some cases, embarrassment. As one exclaimed, they simply "did not understand what race is!"[87]

This anecdote well illustrates the relative lack of consideration researchers give to racial ascription in their work.

In a separate article, Fullwiley explored a curious situation in which scientists conducting a "Study of Pharmacogenetics in Ethnically Diverse Groups" (SOPHIE) found significant discrepancies among three genetic data sets typed according to racial identification of the samples.[88] One of the SOPHIE projects involved comparing DNA from donors at the Parkinson's Institute in Sunnyvale, California, to DNA samples from SOPHIE's own data set and samples from the Human Variation Panels maintained by the Coriell Institute for Medical Research on behalf of the NIGMS.[89] The researchers found that the two data sets marked "Caucasian" by different labs had different frequencies of a particular allele related to Parkinson's disease.[90] Fullwiley goes on to provide the response of one of the project directors (a professor in the Department of Biopharmaceutical Sciences at the University of California, San Francisco) to this discrepancy:

I did try and find out the ethnic stratification of the Caucasian DNA that we collected here in SOPHIE as well as in Coriell, but that's not easy to get. They're just "European-Americans." So whether in fact the ones from Coriell came from Ireland or Finland, and ours are all from Italy and Spain, I don't know. . . . One of the main differences between Coriell and SOPHIE is the way that they were collected [self-report vs. family history of identifying as that group for three generations]. I would say we should take a close look at this because people may not want to be using Coriell if it is contaminated.[91]

The Coriell Repository is used worldwide as a basic resource for genetic research. Both it and the Department of Biopharmaceutical Sciences at the University of California, San Francisco, can be presumed to be at the forefront of responsible practices in the analysis of DNA samples. Yet even here, at the pinnacle of biomedical research, there appeared to be significant discrepancies in the allele frequencies for two data sets, both marked "Caucasian." The explanation might be found in the way race was assigned to the samples, or the way they were handled—or it may simply be that correlating genetic variation with broad census-based racial categories such as Caucasian is inherently problematic.

The point here is not to assess (or even necessarily understand) the intricacies of the IWPC study of the technical analysis performed by the SOPHIE project on their DNA samples. Rather, it is to contrast the extreme care and detail devoted to elaborating laboratory or statistical techniques with the casual and perfunctory discussion of how the samples come to be racially marked in the first place. Scientists and medical doctors understandably go into greatest detail with respect to those very techniques and practices in which they are professionally trained and proficient. This detail reflects their reasonable understanding that the analysis of DNA takes great care and expertise. The contrasting lack of care taken in characterizing the racial identity of individuals or genetic samples indicates an implicit assumption that such characterizations are obvious, uncomplicated, and take no special expertise. This contrast may be understood more broadly as reflecting a conceptual separation of the world of the "social" from that of the "natural," wherein the former is understood to contain transparent categories accessible to all, while the latter requires specialized knowledge and expertise for proper analysis and interpretation. In other words, race is seen as easy and obvious; DNA is seen as difficult and complex. There is an utter failure to consider that social objects such as race may demand similar rigor, expertise, and care in handling as do scientific objects such as DNA.

CONCLUSION

Institutional mandates employing the OMB Directive 15 racial categories have had a profound effect upon the production and organization of biomedical knowledge over the past twenty years. Federally maintained databases have further structured the racial characterization of genetic information. Together they constitute a formidable framework that incentivizes and shapes the introduction of race into contemporary biomedicine. The widespread relative lack of care given to racial data is perhaps testimony to the likelihood that much of its recent use is less an organic outgrowth of researchers' intrinsic scientific interests than an adaptive response to external directives.

The dynamic relation between race and biomedicine becomes even more complex when commercial imperatives are introduced into the mix. The story of BiDil emerges from the context of mandated collection of racial data, but as the next several chapters show, race comes to take on new significance and travel to new domains as it becomes invested with capital value in the context of patenting and drug development.

2

THE BIRTH OF BIDIL

How a Drug Becomes "Ethnic"

O N JUNE 23, 2005, the FDA approved BiDil to treat heart failure in African Americans, and *only* African Americans. BiDil was not a new drug but a combination in a single pill of two existing generic drugs that had been used to treat heart failure, regardless of race, for over a decade based on evidence from two clinical trials conducted in the 1980s. BiDil was brought to the FDA by NitroMed, a small Massachusetts biotech company with no other products on the market. NitroMed explicitly requested race-specific FDA approval for its drug based on clinical data produced by its African-American Heart Failure Trial (A-HeFT) on the grounds that the trial population happened to all be self-identified African Americans.

A-HeFT provided strong evidence that BiDil was effective in treating heart failure—a debilitating and ultimately fatal disease afflicting several million Americans. It did not, however, provide evidence that race had anything to do with how BiDil works. This is for the simple reason that A-HeFT enrolled *only* "self-identified" African Americans. With no comparison population, the trial provided no scientific basis for claiming that BiDil works differently or better in African Americans than in anyone else.

Why then did NitroMed seek race-specific approval for its drug? One would have thought a corporation would want the broadest possible market for a drug, yet here was NitroMed deliberately seeking to narrow the scope of its labeling. At the FDA approval hearing much was made of following the "signal" from the two trials conducted in the 1980s that first tested the generic components of BiDil as a treatment for heart failure. As discussions at the hearings progressed, however, it became clear that reviewers were relying primarily on data from the first trial, which placed only forty-nine African Americans on the two BiDil generic components. Given that most valid clinical trials test a drug in thousands of subjects, results from forty-nine African Americans seem a slender reed indeed upon which to weigh the value of a new drug. I argue that the answer may lie less in such tenuous medical evidence than in stouter commercial considerations. It turns out that NitroMed held two key patents for BiDil, both acquired from cardiologist Jay Cohn of the University of Minnesota. The first covers the non-race-specific use of BiDil. When NitroMed acquired the rights to this first patent in 1999, however, the patent was set to expire in 2007—a mere two years after the FDA ultimately approved BiDil. The second patent is race-specific and lasts until 2020. This extra thirteen years of patent protection presented a compelling commercial reason for seeking to cast BiDil as a racial drug—but it was not supported by the medical evidence.

The FDA, however, accepted NitroMed's argument that the drug should be labeled as indicated only for African Americans because the trial population was entirely African American. This sent the troubling and unsubstantiated message that the subject population's race was somehow a relevant biological variable in assessing the safety and efficacy of BiDil. Ominously, it also gives the federal government's imprimatur to the use of race as, in effect, a genetic or biological category. I say "ominously" because, like BiDil, most drugs on the market today were also approved based on data from single-race clinical trials—in white people. We do not call these "white" drugs—nor should we. Rather, the operating assumption for approving these drugs was that the racial category of "white" was coextensive with the category "human being." That is, a drug tested on white people was good enough for everybody. In approving BiDil as a drug only for African Americans, the FDA also implicitly adopted an assumptio that drugs tested in black people are only good for black people. This sends the clearly unintended but nonetheless powerful message that black people are somehow less fully representative of humanity than are white people.

This chapter begins by outlining the case for BiDil as made by its promoters. Their claims were built around assertions of differential rates of heart failure among blacks and whites, observed differences in average levels of nitric oxide in blacks and whites, and hypothesized underlying genetic differences between blacks and whites that may account for such interracial variation. These are the claims that framed NitroMed's approach to the FDA for approval of the race-based trial. The chapter then moves on to deconstruct the case for BiDil by going back to the drug's origins and development in the 1980s as a nonracial drug. It concludes with an analysis of the critical moment in 1999 when BiDil made its turn toward "ethnicity."

THE CASE FOR BIDIL

Congestive heart failure is a debilitating chronic disease that affects an estimated five million Americans, with approximately 400,000 to 700,000 new cases each year. As it was preparing to file for an initial public offering (IPO) of its stock in 2003, NitroMed estimated that there were approximately 750,000 African Americans who had been diagnosed with heart failure. One contemporary estimate placed the direct health-care costs of treating heart failure at between twenty and forty billion dollars annually. It is a complex condition and sometimes difficult to diagnose. Symptoms can include fatigue, weight gain, swollen legs or ankles, difficulty breathing, and a hacking cough, but in some cases the condition is asymptomatic. Unlike a heart attack, heart failure does not involve an immediate cessation of heart function but rather occurs when the heart functions improperly due to weakening by disease or defect. It is a progressive and ultimately fatal condition, with one in five persons dying within five years of onset. Guidelines current at the time of NitroMed's IPO specified that "most patients with heart failure should be routinely managed with a combination of four types of drugs: an angiotensin-converting enzyme (ACE) inhibitor, a beta-adrenergic blocker, a diuretic, and (usually) digitalis."[1] Adjunctive therapies, namely angiotensin II receptor blockers and spironolactone, further extended the therapeutic options within this scheme.[2]

BiDil is a combination of two potent vasodilators—hydralazine and isosorbide dinitrate (H/I). Vasodilators dilate blood vessels and so ease the strain put on the heart in pumping blood. BiDil, in particular, was believed to increase levels of nitric oxide in the blood, which was thought to greatly benefit individuals suffering from heart failure. Advocates of BiDil pointed to the widely cited statistic (featured prominently in NitroMed's press releases) that African Americans die from heart failure at a rate twice that of white Americans. They connected current research indicating the importance of nitric oxide in preventing heart failure to other research suggesting that blacks seemed to have lower levels of nitric oxide in their blood. They argued that the unique combination of drugs in BiDil might be particularly efficacious in black patients, because one of BiDil's components, isosorbide dinitrate, is a nitric oxide "donor" and its other component, hydralazine, is an antioxidant that may enhance the efficacy of nitrates.[3]

NitroMed's race-based A-HeFT trial was given the green light by the FDA in 2001. Writing several years after its completion, an A-HeFT investigator, cardiologist Keith Ferdinand, asserted that "the designers of A-HeFT understood that race was a limited surrogate marker for genetic differences between populations, and that there was no clear biologic marker for status as black or African American."[4] Such caveats did not seem to inform the approach of another A-HeFT investigator, Clyde Yancy, who argued at the time A-HeFT was being designed that heart failure in blacks was a "different disease."[5] Analyzing data published from the Studies of Left Ventricular Dysfunction (SOLVD) trials (examining racial differences in the natural history of left ventricular dysfunction), he asserted that socioeconomic factors could not account for the difference in mortality rates between African Americans and white Americans.[6] According to

Yancy, "all too frequently, there is an eagerness to impugn psychosocial factors, commonly known as socioeconomic status (SES), as the major explanation for any observed differences in cardiovascular disease seen in blacks."[7] As evidence, he pointed to a retrospective multivariate analysis of the SOLVD data controlled for educational level and "a history of financial distress."[8] Controlling for these limited socioeconomic factors, the data still showed a higher mortality rate in blacks. Without considering other possible social, economic, or environmental factors, Yancy concluded that this observation "seemingly supports the concept that physiologic explanations for disease expression might be present in this patient population."[9] This led Yancy to hypothesize that there is ultimately a basic genetic difference in blacks that accounts for the "unique epidemiology, worse prognosis, and potential variances in responses to pharmacological interventions in heart failure."[10]

The focus on locating differences at the molecular level is logically connected to the related search for a treatment that appears to work differentially well in blacks at this same level—hence BiDil. Further driving the case for BiDil were arguments made by some cardiologists that ACE inhibitors were less efficacious in black patients than in whites. Most prominent among these was a study published in 2001 in the *New England Journal of Medicine* that compared how blacks and whites responded to ACE inhibitor therapy. While making no claims as to mortality rates, the study found ACE inhibitor therapy to be associated with a significant reduction in risk of hospitalization for white patients but not for black patients. The authors argued that "on the basis of available physiological, pharmacologic, and clinical data, it seems appropriate to consider current therapeutic recommendations [concerning ACE inhibitors] as applying to white patients but not necessarily to black patients."[11]

Subsequent reporting on BiDil in major media—from the *Financial Times* and *Business Week* to ABC News and the BBC—consistently noted the differential response to ACE therapy between blacks and whites.[12] NitroMed's own website referred to such research, noting that the package insert for the ACE inhibitor enalapril states that "black patients receiving *the original case for BiDil*

ACE inhibitors have been reported to have a higher incidence of angioedema compared to non-blacks."[13]

Jay Cohn, who coauthored the ACE inhibitor study, followed up by arguing for a "unique strategy" for treatment of heart failure in African Americans. Cohn contrasted results from previous heart failure trials indicating that blacks did not respond as well as whites to ACE inhibitors with results seen with BiDil, which he argued actually provided a greater benefit to blacks than to whites.[14] The dual message was clear: ACE inhibitors did not work as well in blacks; BiDil worked better in blacks. The original case for BiDil can thus be roughly summarized as follows: 1) blacks die from heart failure at a rate twice that of whites; 2) given this great disparity it seems that there must be some underlying biological or genetic (as opposed to "merely" social or environmental) factor accounting for the difference; 3) supporting this hypothesis are studies that control for socioeconomic factors and still show racial differentials in outcome; 4) moreover, additional studies indicate that blacks do not respond as well as whites to certain first-line heart failure therapies; 5) therefore, a response is called for that addresses this different biology; 6) enter BiDil, a pharmaceutical response to the statistical disparity that appears to have a differentially beneficial effect on blacks at the molecular level.[15]

DECONSTRUCTING THE CASE FOR BIDIL

How did we get to this point? If we go back to its origins, we find that BiDil did not begin as a racial drug. Rather, it became racial over time and through a complex array of legal, commercial, and medical circumstances that transformed the drug's identity but not its chemical composition.

Over the previous twenty years, a revolution had occurred in heart failure treatment with the development of a wide array of pharmaceutical interventions that improved both the quality of life and the longevity of people suffering from heart failure. One of the earliest breakthroughs came

transformation in BiDil's identity but not its composition

in the 1980s with the first Vasodilator Heart Failure Trial (V-HeFT I). This trial was designed in the 1970s and lasted from 1980 to 1985. It involved cardiologists from around the country working together with the U.S. Veterans Administration. It took patients who were already on a background regimen of digoxin and a diuretic and randomized them into three groups, one receiving a placebo, one receiving an alpha-adrenergic blocker called prazosin, and one receiving a combination of hydralazine and isosorbide dinitrate, or H/I—the two drugs that comprise BiDil. The V-HeFT investigators found that prazosin proved no better than the placebo in reducing mortality. Their results indicated, however, that the H/I combination seemed to have a beneficial impact on mortality, though the difference was only of "borderline statistical significance."[16]

The V-HeFT I trial was soon followed by V-HeFT II, which lasted from 1986 to 1991. This trial compared the efficacy of the H/I combination against the drug enalapril, an ACE inhibitor. It found an even more pronounced beneficial effect on mortality in the enalapril group, confirming ACE inhibitors as a frontline therapy for heart failure.[17] ACE inhibitors, however, did not totally supplant H/I, because not everyone responds well to them and some cannot tolerate the side effects. One news report estimated that 20 to 30 percent of congestive heart failure patients do not respond favorably to standard therapies of "diuretics, digitalis or ACE inhibitors . . . particularly ACE inhibitors."[18] Given estimates that nearly five million Americans suffered from heart failure, that group potentially represented 1.5 million patients annually. The American College of Cardiology and the American Heart Association issued guidelines shortly after the V-HeFT trials that recommended considering the use of H/I for these patients. These guidelines made no reference to race.[19]

The V-HeFT investigators did not build the trials around race or ethnicity. They enrolled both black and white patients, and in the published reports of the trials' successes they did not break down the data by race. Rather, they presented H/I—BiDil's components—as generally efficacious in the population at large, without regard to race.[20] In 1987, one year after the results of V-HeFT I were published, Cohn, as one of the trials'

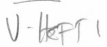

principal investigating cardiologists, applied for a patent on a "method of reducing mortality associated with congestive heart failure using hydralazine and isosorbide dinitrate."[21] The methods patent would not actually cover the drug itself (since it was merely a combination of two generics) but it would give the holder a monopoly on the marketing of the combination therapy for a particular purpose—treating heart failure. It would not, however, prevent doctors from substituting the generic equivalents on their own. The U.S. PTO issued the patent to Cohn in 1989. Referring to V-HeFT I and II in the patent description, Cohn asserted that it had been "surprisingly and unexpectedly discovered that . . . a combination of hydralazine hydrochloride and isosorbide dinitrate has been [found] to substantially and significantly reduce the incidence of mortality in [congestive heart failure] patients."[22] Cohn's patent application did not mention race. He clearly conceived of this as a method to treat all people suffering from heart failure.

Hydralazine and isosorbide dinitrate are generic drugs. Cohn and others later combined them into a single pill for easier administration. In 1992, a trademark application was filed for this new pill as BiDil. The mark was formally registered in 1995 to Medco Research, Inc.,[23] a biotech corporation in North Carolina's Research Triangle Park, which had earlier acquired the intellectual property rights to BiDil from Cohn. One report from 1997 estimated a potential market of up to sixty million dollars in annual sales for BiDil.[24]

By 1994, Medco had begun clinical testing of BiDil to establish its bioavailability and bioequivalence to the coadministration of the two H/I drugs separately—a critical precursor to approaching the FDA with a New Drug Application (NDA) to get approval for marketing BiDil.[25] By 1996, the completed study found BiDil to be bioequivalent, and Medco prepared to approach the FDA with its NDA. Cohn noted at the time that "the BiDil® formulation represents a very convenient dosage form that, once approved [by the FDA], should lead to increased usage of this effective therapy."[26] Later that year, Medco submitted an NDA to the FDA.[27] The following February, the Cardiovascular and Renal Drugs Advisory

Committee of the FDA's Center for Drug Evaluation and Research held a meeting to consider Medco's BiDil application. Medco sent Cohn and three other representatives to the meeting to make the case for BiDil.

Arguing for the bioequivalence of BiDil to the H/I formulations used in the prior trials, Cohn recommended approval of BiDil for congestive heart failure on the basis of a survival benefit in V-HeFT I and trends for increased exercise tolerance and long-term ejection fraction in both trials.[28] Ultimately, however, the Advisory Committee voted against approving BiDil.[29] The next day, Medco's stock plunged by 25 percent.[30]

The Advisory Committee's recommendation appeared to fly in the face of the extensive findings published in highly respected peer-reviewed journals that seemed to support Cohn's confident patent application claim that the H/I combination "substantially and significantly reduced the incidence of mortality"[31] in congestive heart failure patients. Moreover, as Cohn emphasized before the committee, the American Heart Association, the American College of Cardiology, and the World Health Organization had all included H/I as a recommended therapy for patients who did not tolerate ACE inhibitors.[32]

Why was the extensive data from V-HeFT I and II inadequate? Cohn and Medco had some intimation of these problems before the hearing. Cohn had actually first brought the V-HeFT data to the FDA back in 1988 to discuss adding its results to the labeling for H/I. After waiting almost a year to obtain the necessary data from the VA, the FDA statistician concluded in 1990 that there were "numerous problems with the study and the analysis."[33] Then two months before the 1997 hearing, Medco met with the FDA to explain that some of the statistical data might seem weak because "both the V-HeFT I and II trials had to be stopped prematurely due to funding problems. They therefore did not have sufficient power for their planned [statistical] analyses."[34] At the hearing, Cohn urged the committee to recall the age and the context of the study:

Keep in mind that this is a study designed 20 years ago. This was a VA cooperative study. This was not designed really as a regulatory study so that careful selection of criteria for endpoint were not as precise as one would see in a protocol designed today with the goal to come to this committee and ask for approval. So, one has to look at this a little differently than one might at a more recently organized mega-trial in which p values are clearly defined as the goals for the trial.[35]

The Advisory Committee agreed with Cohn as to the shortcomings of the dated study, but did not follow his suggestion that they look at its data "a little differently." Instead, the committee followed the recommendations of their biostatisticians, who found that "there were too many variables specified in the protocols as primary endpoints" for them to interpret the V-HeFT data "with any degree of certainty."[36] Therefore, the Advisory Committee voted nine to three against recommending that BiDil be approved for use in congestive heart failure.[37]

It is important to emphasize here that the committee did *not* find that H/I failed to work in a general population. Rather, it found that because V-HeFT I and II were not designed as new drug trials, the statistics they generated simply did not meet FDA regulatory criteria for new drug approval. The committee nonetheless believed the data to be promising and suggested a properly controlled follow-up trial might yield positive results. Such trials, however, cost a lot of money. One of the great appeals of bringing BiDil to the FDA had no doubt been the fact that the underlying clinical trials had already occurred and been paid for—largely with federal funds. And so rather than spend the millions of dollars required to conduct a new clinical trial, Medco got out of the BiDil business and let the intellectual property rights revert to Cohn.

BIDIL'S ETHNIC REBIRTH

At this point, BiDil appeared to be dead in the water. However, in the transcript of the FDA meeting, there is a hint of BiDil's road to resurrection. Early in his presentation before the Advisory Committee, Cohn noted:

The majority of the patients [in both V-Heft I and II] were Caucasian. That is, about seventy percent of them in both trials, but there was a fairly sizeable number of African Americans in the trial. We won't go into that, but we have much data comparing the Caucasian and African-American responses.[38]

The V-HeFT investigators had been tracking data by race from the outset. The investigators, however, clearly had not conceptualized BiDil as a race-specific therapy. To the contrary, Cohn chose quite deliberately not to "go into that" before the FDA.[39] Cohn's mention of race before the FDA review panel actually marks its first public mention in relation to BiDil. None of the numerous articles published on V-HeFT to that point had mentioned anything about any perceived racial difference in response to the H/I drug combination. It was only after the Advisory Committee recommended against approving BiDil for use in a general population that the V-HeFT investigators went back one more time to their data—data that Cohn himself reminded the Advisory Committee had been generated by a trial designed nearly twenty years earlier—and produced the first published study analyzing the differential effects of H/I and enalapril by race.[40]

This race-based study was completed in a broader context of rising political attention to the importance of addressing race and gender disparities in health policy and administration. In 1997, the federal government passed the FDMA, which, among other things, required the Secretary of Health and Human Services "in consultation with the Director of the National Institutes of Health and the representatives of the drug manufacturing industry, [to] review and develop guidance, as appropriate, on the inclusion of women and minorities in clinical trials."[41] That same year, President Clinton delivered a much publicized apology for the federal government's role in the notorious Tuskegee Syphilis Study, which exploited black men for decades in the name of medical research. The BiDil investigators, then, were not the only ones closely considering race in medicine.[42]

Against this backdrop, Cohn, together with Peter Carson, M.D., Susan Zeische, R.N., and Gary Johnson, M.S., published a paper in September 1999 titled "Racial Differences in Response to Therapy for Heart

Failure: Analysis of the Vasodilator-Heart Failure Trials."[43] The retro-spective analysis of data from V-HeFT I and II compared a total of 395 black patients with 1,024 white patients with similar baseline variables and characteristics (including age, history of coronary heart disease, hypertension, blood pressure, heart rate). It found that "the H-I combination appears to be particularly effective in prolonging survival in black patients and is as effective as enalapril in this subgroup. In contrast, enalapril shows its more favorable effect on survival, particularly in the white population."[44] Following a caveat about the limits of its data, the paper concluded that "the consistency of observations of a racial difference in response in V-HeFT I and V-HeFT II . . . lend credence to the suggestion that therapy for heart failure might appropriately be *racially tailored*."[45]

The paper argued that H/I (the BiDil drugs) appeared to work better in blacks than in whites. More importantly, though not explicitly stated in the paper, the statistics on H/I's impact on black mortality might be sufficiently powerful to meet the FDA's threshold criteria for regulatory significance.[46] Just before the article was published, Cohn and Carson (the lead author of the article on racial differences in the V-HeFT data) applied for a patent on "methods for treating and preventing mortality associated with heart failure in an *African American* [italics added] patient" with H/I or mononitrate. That same month, NitroMed, which specialized in the development and commercialization of nitric oxide–enhanced medicines, announced it had acquired the NDA for BiDil and related intellectual property rights from Cohn. NitroMed also revealed its plans to amend the NDA to seek an indication specifically for African American patients. Thus was BiDil reborn as an "ethnic" drug.[47]

Yet the actual impetus for this critical turn to ethnicity still remains somewhat clouded. Cohn later stated, "We studied an African-American population in this trial because that was the signal that we identified in our previous trials."[48] This certainly would comport with his statement to the FDA that he had data broken down by race from the V-HeFT studies. And yet, that was data he deliberately chose not to go into at the time. Moreover, the signal from the data itself was weak at best. As the studies and the subsequent review of them by the FDA made clear, the only distinct signal of

But. unsound afidence fuel Sample size, & for my

race difference in the V-HeFT trials came from V-HeFT I, where only 49 African Americans were actually placed on the H/I combination. Additionally, after the FDA approved BiDil, Cohn repeatedly maintained that he always believed that BiDil would work in people regardless of race. With such a firm belief, why turn to race with such a weak "signal"? Indeed, why turn to race at all, for this drug at this time? By the time the Carson article came out, Cohn had authored or coauthored 376 medical articles, not one of which discussed race.[49]

Perhaps the answer may be found in subsequent filings with the Securities and Exchange Commission revealing that NitroMed acquired the rights to BiDil in January 1999, nine months before the publication of the race-specific paper by Carson and Cohn.[50] The filing describes the sequence of events leading to its acquisition of these rights as follows:

In 1999, *we* [italics added] re-analyzed the results of the two prior BiDil mortality studies by ethnicity. Following this re-analysis and extensive discussions with the FDA, in 1999 we acquired the new drug application and a license to the BiDil intellectual property from Dr. Jay Cohn, Professor in the Department of Medicine at the University of Minnesota, who had acquired the new drug application and intellectual property from Medco Research.[51]

This characterization raises questions as to just who brought race into the analysis of the V-HeFT results and when. NitroMed said "we" conducted the studies. Indeed, NitroMed also provided a rationale for its turn toward ethnicity, stating:

Our extensive work in the field of nitric oxide-enhancing medicines led us to believe that BiDil might be particularly well-suited to enhance in-vivo nitric oxide levels and to protect the nitric oxide after it is formed. As such, we postulated that BiDil might provide preferential survival advantages to African-American heart failure patients suffering from a deficiency of nitric oxide. In 1999, *we re-analyzed V-HeFT I and II by ethnicity* [italics added].[52]

In this telling, NitroMed turned to ethnicity not because of any "signal" from the V-HeFT trials per se, but because of their specialized knowledge "in the field of nitric-oxide enhancing medicines." Cohn, on the other hand, originally thought the efficacy of BiDil would be due to its vasodilating capacities. NitroMed then states, "We reanalyzed V-HeFT I and II by ethnicity." But, it was Carson and Cohn who ultimately published the relevant paper that provided the basis for approaching the FDA for approval of a race-specific clinical trial. This opens the question of whether Cohn and Carson conducted the study at NitroMed's behest—that is, if they were part of the "we" who reanalyzed the data—or whether NitroMed conducted the study on its own and then farmed it out to Cohn and Carson to publish under their name. There is no direct evidence to resolve this question. Cohn and Carson had actually published a one-paragraph abstract on possible racial differences in response to ACE inhibitors in 1994 in the *Journal of the American College of Cardiology*.[53] Doubtless, this was the racial data Cohn referred to before the FDA. But this data lay fallow until after NitroMed acquired the intellectual property rights from Cohn and subsequently claimed credit for itself having reanalyzed the V-HeFT data by race. Carson himself, however, was not part of the deal assigning patent rights to NitroMed, nor did he ever receive royalties from later BiDil sales.

By 2000, NitroMed was well-positioned to introduce BiDil. In consultation with the FDA, NitroMed developed the protocols for its race-specific trial to produce race-specific results that would support the commercial value of its race-specific patent. The following year, NitroMed announced its plans to initiate A-HeFT, and the drive to develop and market the world's first "ethnic" drug was on.

THE ROLE OF LAW IN RACE-ING BIDIL

The role of law as player in the emergence of BiDil as an ethnic drug began in 1980, more or less coincidentally with the initiation of V-HeFT I.

*ı*hat year, President Carter signed into law two pieces of legislation that would transform relations between industry and academic researchers. The first, the Stevenson-Wydler Technology Innovation Act of 1980 (15 U.S.C. § 3701), encouraged interaction and cooperation among government laboratories, universities, big industries, and small businesses. The second, the Patent and Trademark Laws Amendment Act of 1980, commonly known as the "Bayh-Dole" Act (35 U.S.C. § 200–212), allowed institutions conducting research with federal funds, such as universities, to retain the intellectual property rights to their discoveries. It is in this context that the research findings of V-HeFT, produced in cooperation with the U.S. Veterans Administration, could be commercialized through patent and trademark law. Cohn and Carson were therefore able to obtain intellectual property rights in BiDil-related patents and to enter into deals with the likes of Medco and NitroMed to commercialize the discoveries made through the V-HeFT trials.[54]

The first intervention of patent law in the development of BiDil, however, was negative and restrictive, rather than productive. Following the successful completion of V-HeFT II in 1989, the next logical step would have been to conduct a trial that explored the combined effects of ACE inhibitors with H/I. Cohn pushed for such a trial and openly bemoaned the lack of corporate support to enable him and other cardiologists to go forward.[55] The key reason, as Cohn later noted, was because hydralazine and isosorbide dinitrate were both generic drugs.[56] In the absence of intellectual property rights to the therapeutic compound, corporate support for further tests involving the components of BiDil would not be forthcoming. Thus, years before BiDil was ever presented to the FDA, the lack of relevant intellectual property value seemed likely to condemn H/I to obscurity as treatments for heart failure. Not only did further trials of H/I in combination with other drugs seem unlikely, but there would be no money to push publicity and marketing of the H/I therapy as it was then understood.[57]

Cohn revived the commercial prospects for BiDil by patenting the *method of* combining hydralazine and isosorbide dinitrate to treat congestive heart failure, and then by developing BiDil as a new drug—being a combination of H/I in single-dose form. BiDil was a breakthrough of convenience: it made it easier to dispense and to use the H/I combination but was not itself a new therapy. With BiDil, a doctor only had to write one prescription and the patient only had to take a total of six pills (two pills three times a day) instead of sixteen for the separate generics (four pills four times a day).[58]

Yet the measure of convenience of BiDil alone was insufficient to drive its development. A consultant to the FDA panel that ultimately rejected BiDil's NDA in 1997 noted that the two generic component drugs of BiDil were available for anyone to use for heart failure. The FDA's denial of the BiDil NDA would not change that. Rather, he observed that "the practical impact of the FDA not approving this combination today is that there won't be an economic incentive for the sponsor to get out and provide educational material for a lot of doctors to know how to use the drugs best."[59]

The true breakthrough for BiDil, therefore, was not simply the combination of two generic drugs into one; it was the development of new intellectual property rights. With patent protection in hand, it would become advantageous for a drug company to develop and market BiDil aggressively to doctors and patients. For this reason, Medco acquired the rights to BiDil in the early 1990s and started investing time and money in conducting tests and developing marketing strategies in preparation for submitting its NDA to the FDA. Patent law, and to a lesser extent trademark law, which allowed for added brand name value in the marketing of BiDil®, thus provided a critical impetus toward the creation of BiDil. On the one hand, this comports well with the classic justification of patent law as providing a spur to invention. On the other hand, it indicates how patent law may also distort a market, potentially obscuring less expensive generic alternatives that have the same therapeutic value.

The intervention of the federal regulatory system in denying the initial NDA in 1997 marks a critical turning point on BiDil's journey toward ethnicity. The regulatory action taken by the FDA Advisory Committee led the BiDil researchers to reconceptualize their drug along racial lines in order to get a "second bite" at the apple of FDA approval. By 1999, the value of the intellectual property rights to BiDil rebounded—not because of any changes to the underlying molecular structure or biological effects of BiDil as a drug, but because of the reanalysis of the old V-HeFT data along racial lines.

In the hands of its new corporate handlers and their public relations consultants, BiDil soon was reborn as an ethnic drug. The subsequent spate of publicity attending the inauguration of A-HeFT demonstrated how the renewed value of the patent to BiDil provided an incentive for NitroMed to educate doctors and the public about the nature and value of this "new" drug for African Americans.

In the next logical extension of patent rights into the process of creating an ethnic drug, Cohn and Carson jointly filed for a new BiDil-related patent on September 8, 1999. With the title "Methods of Treating and Preventing Congestive Heart Failure with Hydralazine Compounds and Isosorbide Dinitrate or Isosorbide Mononitrate," the 1999 patent appears much the same as Cohn's original 1989 patent. Upon closer inspection, however, the abstract to the patent specifies that the "present invention provides methods for treating and preventing mortality associated with heart failure in an *African American* [italics added] patient."[60]

A typical patent is divided into several sections. The claims section presents a primary focus for investigation, because it is the legal heart of a patent. The abstract is the basic summary presentation of the central purpose of the patent. Other sections include the background or description of invention, plus drawings or other technical support data. When a patent application is filed with the PTO, it is assigned to a patent examiner and proceeds through a process known as "patent prosecution," during which the examiner and parties representing the patent applicant (generally attorneys) interact over the substance and procedure of the filing. This often involves a push and pull between the applicant and the examiner over such issues as the proper scope of the claims, whether the information in the written description section adequately supports the claims, and more basically, whether the patent as a whole satisfies the core requirements of patentability: utility, novelty, non-obviousness, and specification (or a written description sufficient to enable a person skilled in the particular art covered by the patent to make the claimed invention).[61]

The road to BiDil's second, race-specific, patent was not straight or smooth. Originally, the patent examiner rejected the new application as being an "obvious" extension of the original BiDil patent. In the language of patent review, the examiner found that "the patentee teaches patients in general and thus would have included all race populations."[62] The examiner's entirely reasonable logic here was that since the original patent covered all humans, it would also cover all racial subsets of the category "human."

In response, Cohn (or rather his patent attorney) asserted that the claim was not obvious because the administration of the H/I combination "produces unexpectedly superior results in the treatment of black patients when compared to white patients," which was not anticipated by any evidence (or in patent terminology, "teachings") in the prior patent.[63] It is the surprise of "unexpected results" that is claimed to make the new invention non-obvious. The comparative difference from the white norm is essential here, but it would only be relevant if claimed efficacy in whites were an attribute of the original patent. This could only be the case if Cohn and the patent examiner each accepted the idea that a white patient was the unstated norm behind the earlier patent. And indeed, in response, the patent examiner accepted Cohn's argument, agreeing that "applicants have established that unexpected results do occur when the active agents are administered to a black population," and finding therefore that the disputed claims "are deemed to be in condition for allowance."[64] The "unexpectedness" of the purported racial difference in response was critical to validating BiDil's turn toward race and paved the way for the ultimate granting of the patent in 2002.

The centrality of the trope of unexpectedness also points up an irony embedded in previous efforts by social and natural scientists to recharacterize race as a social construct: the only way that a race-based difference in drug response could be "unexpected" would be if the underlying assumption of the original studies (and patent) had been that there were no meaningful inherent biological differences among the races. Only then could the subsequent discovery of purported biological differences that correlated with race be understood as unexpected. (If the difference in response had been tied to environmental or other social factors that corr with race, then the patent claims would have had to focus on them, not race.)

The issuance of the new patent was commercially important, because the original patent was set to expire in 2007. In an SEC filing for its IPO, NitroMed highlighted the fact that the PTO had found the Cohn application's race-specific method of treatment to be a "non-obvious" extension of the earlier concept and hence patentable. Patent law is supposed to promote the invention of new and useful products. In the case of BiDil, patent law did not spur the invention of a new drug, but rather the recharacterization of an existing therapy for a particular segment of society—in short, the repackaging of the drug as ethnic.[65]

Perhaps the ultimate indication that NitroMed chose to exploit race strategically to gain added patent protection is to be found in a patent application it filed on September 22, 2009.[66] Titled "Composition for Treating Vascular Diseases Characterized by Nitric Oxide Insufficiency," the application covered a "sustained release" version of BiDil that could reduce its administration from three times a day to once a day. Developing a sustained-release version of BiDil was central to NitroMed's ongoing strategy to revive the drug's prospects by improving patient compliance and distinguishing it from substitute generics that would still have to be taken three times a day. The claims section of this application, however, made *no mention of race.* To be clear, this patent application simply covered "a method of treating a cardiovascular disease in a patient"—*any* patient, regardless of race. All references to the "surprising" and "unexpected" results in African Americans were gone. Because generics could not be readily substituted for a sustained-release version of BiDil, NitroMed would have nothing to fear from an FDA approval of the new drug for the general population without regard to race. When NitroMed did not need race to extend patent protection, it discarded it in favor of seeking a larger, nonracialized market for their product.[67]

Nonetheless, with the issuance of NitroMed's original race-specific patent on October 15, 2002, race entered the world of patent law in a new and explicit way. Previous associations of race and property have generally involved a devaluing of property associated with racial minorities. Certain more recent legal classifications of race, as in affirmative action, have the potential to offer challenges to exclusionary conceptions of racialized property rights.[68] The racialization of BiDil's patent appeared to be more in line with such assertedly "benign" uses of racial categories and actually added value to the drug, resulting in the readiness of such groups as the Association of Black Cardiologists and the Congressional Black Caucus to support A-HeFT.[69] In this regard, BiDil gained cultural capital by being characterized as a means to redress an important health disparity in a historically underserved population.

But there is something very different about race-specific drugs, which distinguishes them from other well-intentioned attempts to use racial categories to overcome past social, political, and economic injustices: they legitimize the use of race as a genetic category. The major civil rights struggles of the past several decades have focused around issues of desegregation, voting, affirmative action, and discrimination in such areas as housing, public accommodations, and employment.[70] To identify and address discrimination in these areas, it is necessary to collect and categorize data by race. Indeed, the current racial and ethnic categories used in the U.S. Census emerged largely in response to needs and pressures created by the civil rights movement and the legislation emerging from it. To track violations of voting rights or employment discrimination claims, it is essential to aggregate data by race. While highly problematic for an array of social and political reasons, the use of racial and ethnic categories in such contexts does not directly implicate them as biological or genetic constructs.

Over the past three decades, however, the movement for civil rights has continued, for very good reasons, to broaden its focus to encompass a much more explicit concern for health rights. From the creation of the Office of Minority Health in 1986 to the Minority Health and Health Disparities Research and Education Act of 2000 and the establishment of the Center for Research on Genomics and Global Health in 2008, major federal initiatives have been undertaken to identify and address racial disparities in health care.[71]

Insofar as these initiatives engage social, economic, and political influences on disparate health *outcomes*, they implicate racial and ethnic categories as social, economic, and political constructs. Such concerns mark a natural progression of civil rights activism from political and economic rights into the realm of health. However, when racial and ethnic categories are used to guide initiatives to uncover the underlying *causes* of disease, the implication arises that these categories may serve as biological and/or genetic concepts. This marks a fundamental difference between civil rights activism in the arena of health as opposed to political or economic rights.

Prominent among such otherwise well-intentioned federal mandates are the NIH Revitalization Act of 1993 and the FDMA of 1997. The former directs the NIH to develop guidelines for women and minorities in NIH-sponsored clinical research, and the latter directs the FDA to examine issues related to the inclusion of racial and ethnic groups in clinical trials of new drugs. Pursuant to these mandates, the NIH and FDA have issued detailed guidelines mandating certain procedures and practices concerning the inclusion of ethnic and racial minorities in clinical trials. While clinical trials and drug development may sometimes look at an array of factors, including social and economic variables, they also frequently look *only* at biomedical variables. This is especially true of drug development, which necessarily focuses primarily on establishing the biological safety and efficacy of chemical compounds to gain FDA approval. When a drug's efficacy or safety is correlated to racial or ethnic categories, it opens the door to reifying those categories as genetic.[72]

This, of course, brings us back to BiDil. The role of the federal legal and regulatory system in producing BiDil as an ethnic drug is especially important, because it lends the imprimatur of the state to the use of race as a biological category. Between the FDA's approval of BiDil as a race-specific drug and the PTO's issuance of the patent for using H/I in African American patients, powerful federal agencies legitimized the use of race as a marker for biological difference. To the extent that institutions of the state, such as the PTO or the FDA, come to mark certain biological conditions as "racial," race may become a surrogate not only for medical research, but also for a wide array of legally sanctioned discrimination.[73]

Perhaps sensitive to such dangers, many of the African American advocacy groups that supported BiDil, including the Association of Black Cardiologists and the Congressional Black Caucus, both of which had been instrumental in supporting A-HeFT, also urged that BiDil be approved without a race-specific indication.[74] Several of the A-HeFT investigators themselves declared that BiDil would work regardless of race. On the eve of the FDA approval of BiDil in June 2005, Cohn was reiterating that the V-HeFT results convinced him that BiDil would work in the general population: "Do I believe this drug should work in whites? Biology tells me it should."[75] He stated that he himself prescribed the generic combination to white patients who did not respond well to other drugs and concluded, "I actually think everybody should be using it."[76] The previous fall, Cohn had noted that "all the drugs the FDA has approved thus far resulted from studies in White people. But does the labeling say that this drug works in White people? No. But this time they're going to say this drug works in Black people. What's the matter with us? Why are we distinguishing?"[77] A reasonable question, yet it was Cohn who applied for and received the race-specific patent underlying BiDil, who helped drive the race-specific design of A-HeFT as a paid member of NitroMed's Board of Scientific Advisors, and who played a central role in NitroMed's presentation to the FDA Advisory Committee seeking race-specific labeling for the drug. All of this for a drug he believed should be prescribed without regard to race. Such extensive efforts to racialize BiDil to get it to market indicate a clear imbalance between medical and commercial rationales in directing drug development.

CONCLUSION

BiDil's peculiar history on the road to the market presents a wide array of troubling and important issues concerning the future status of race as a category for constructing and understanding health disparities in American society. Its development depended upon the strategic appropriation of the social category of race to justify patenting and regulatory approval of a drug that purports to act on a "true" biological basis of heart failure. The story of BiDil, however, is much more than an individualized account of how a particular drug became focused on a single, racial segment of the population. It is also part of a broader contest over classification systems and context—which variables matter, as well as how and when. Even as BiDil's proponents acknowledged race to be merely a crude marker for biology, they invoked race as biology to establish intellectual property rights, obtain regulatory approval, raise venture capital, and develop marketing campaigns. In the story of BiDil, race played the role of a valuable surrogate—i.e., it was presented as having no medical value in its own right but took on significance to the extent that researchers tie it to a "real" biological group through statistical correlations. The next chapter moves on to explore the power of misconstrued statistics to create a racial frame for BiDil that was critical to its ultimate approval by the FDA. As patent protection provided a key impetus toward BiDil's initial ethnic turn, statistics would provide a necessary added component to realize the value of the racial patent through regulatory approval of BiDil with a race-specific indication on its label.

3

STATISTICAL MISCHIEF AND RACIAL FRAMES FOR DRUG DEVELOPMENT AND MARKETING

N 2001, NITROMED FRAMED its announcement of the forthcoming A-HeFT trial for BiDil with a striking statistic: "Death rates from heart failure are more than twice as high in black patients than in white patients."[1] It heralded BiDil as presenting an opportunity to address "the disparity in outcomes for African American heart failure patients."[2] NitroMed posited that the disparity might be due to "a pathophysiology found primarily in black patients that may involve nitric oxide (NO) insufficiency."[3] A follow-up press release reiterated both the 2:1 statistic and the proposition that "observed racial disparities in mortality and therapeutic response rates in black heart failure patients may be due in part to ethnic differences in the underlying pathophysiology of heart failure."[4] This statistic would come to play a central role in framing NitroMed's drive to imbue its race-specific patent with commercial value by obtaining race-specific approval of BiDil from the FDA.

The statistic first emerged just months before Jay Cohn and Peter Carson published their article recasting BiDil as a racial drug. In February 1999, Carson was a coauthor on a study by Dries et al. on "Racial Differences in the Outcome of Left Ventricular Dysfunction"—a prime indication of congestive heart failure.[5] Based on retrospective analysis of data from the SOLVD prevention and treatment trials, the article suggested that "there may be differences in the natural history of . . . left ventricular dysfunction between black and white patients."[6] Significantly, the study purported to control for socioeconomic factors by analyzing "base-line data on educational level and the percentage of participants reporting 'major financial distress' (yes vs. no)" during the previous twelve months.[7] Framing the entire report was the assertion in the opening paragraph that "the population-based mortality rate from congestive heart failure is 1.8 times as high for black men as for white men and 2.4 times as high for black women as for white women"—an overall black-to-white ratio of heart failure mortality of approximately 2:1.[8]

The logic behind the study is clear: there is a 2:1 disparity in mortality rates between blacks and whites; it seems unlikely that socioeconomic status (SES) alone can account for such a large difference; therefore, conduct retrospective analysis of heart failure data that purports to control for SES, and see if there is any remaining disparity that can be attributed to biology. The 2:1 statistic thus shapes which questions get asked and how they are pursued. However, although the logic is consistent, there are two major problems with the study's premise. First, the study's conception of relevant socioeconomic influences on health is very thin. Second, the 2:1 statistic is not correct.

With regard to socioeconomic influences, the level of education and experience of financial distress certainly are relevant factors to consider in examining nongenetic environmental influences on the development and progression of heart failure. However, the implicit understanding that they are exhaustive of all nongenetic factors is puzzling, to say the least. As one letter in response to the article noted:

> Obviously, it is impossible to control perfectly for the complex and somewhat nebulous concept of socioeconomic status in any study, and Dries et al. appropriately advise caution in the interpretation of their results. By focusing, however, on biological factors as the fallback explanation for their findings, the authors pay inadequate attention to the environmental, psychosocial, and economic factors that are just as likely, if not more likely, explanations of racial differences in health.[9]

There is a vast array of medical and public health literature connecting racial differences in hypertension to social factors such as diet, environment, exercise, and stress. Many of these social factors correlate strongly with social categories of race. For example, one study has shown that the stress of experiencing racism seems to elevate blood pressure. The study by Dries et al. captures none of these variables. The thin conception of socioeconomic factors in the article by Dries et al. seems to indicate an underlying assumption that because hypertension is a biological condition, any disparities associated with its prevalence must similarly be biological.[10]

As for the 2:1 mortality statistic: the great problem with this is that the statistic is wrong—very wrong. In 2002, data obtained from the CDC and the National Center for Health Statistics placed the age-adjusted ratio of black-to-white mortality from heart failure at something under 1.1 to 1 for 1999—a far cry from the 2:1 statistic cited so prominently in both medical literature and popular media.[11]

This statistic had a curious life. It traveled the world, often in many guises, and appeared in multifarious public forums, both prominent and obscure. It was most commonly found in the company of another statistic, more of an estimate really, that somewhere around five million people in the United States suffer from heart failure, a serious, debilitating disease with a poor prognosis and a high cost of treatment. It proved to be a very powerful little statistic, invoked by medical researchers to guide the search for race-based drug development and therapy for heart failure; by biotech corporations and financial journals exploring the economic potential of such drugs; by professional associations seeking to advise their constituents; and, of course, by scholars and commentators of all stripes arguing over the appropriate use of racial categories in science and medicine.

The inaccuracy of the statistic is particularly problematic, first, because it may have distorted efforts to address the very real health problems associated with heart failure, and second, because it lent credence to those who argued that race can and should be used as a biological category. The medical literature is replete with well-documented health disparities that correlate with social categories of race. Addressing such disparities is not only legitimate, it is imperative.[12] But connecting these disparities to biological and/or

genetic differences is an enterprise fraught with peril. Certain genetic variations may well correlate with groups that are descended from populations
from particular regions of the world (e.g., the sickle cell trait correlates with
populations from areas of western Africa, the Mediterranean, and southeast India, where malaria has long been prevalent). These correlations can be
very helpful in identifying and treating diseases. Directly correlating genetic differences to social categories of race might even help to address certain health problems in the short run. In the long run, however, it opens the
door to a wide range of potentially devastating discriminatory practices—
some overt, others subtle and hard to anticipate.[13]

Such concerns are not merely hypothetical. In 2005, the European Patent Office granted a request by Myriad Genetics to modify its patent relating to general testing for the BRCA2 genetic mutation (which increases a
person's risk of breast cancer) to apply specifically to "diagnosing a predisposition to breast cancer in *Ashkenazi Jewish* women."[14] Myriad's broader
patent, covering the test in all people regardless of ethnicity, had been
successfully challenged in Europe, so they fell back to this narrower
ethnic-specific patent to salvage their commercial interest in testing for
BRCA2 mutations. Opponents of the patent noted that the test was available from other sources for all women regardless of ethnic or religious
background. As a practical matter, this new patent meant that individuals
identified as Ashkenazi Jews would either have to pay a premium for the
test or deny their identity. As with BiDil, Myriad apparently was marking
an ethnic group as genetically distinct not for scientific reasons but in order
to extend patent protection. Recent historical experiences of eugenics and
racial discrimination should give us pause when considering the potentially profound consequences of the geneticization of such socially marked
groups.[15]

I first encountered the 2:1 statistic in the summer of 2002, when I began
researching the origins and development of BiDil. In its first two press
releases announcing BiDil and A-HeFT, NitroMed foregrounded the 2:1
statistic.[16] From the outset, then, the statistical disparity played a central
role both in framing the racial disparity as biological—located in the bod-

Saving the patent
known to me (attment)

ies of black people—and in justifying the creation of a race-specific drug trial. Soon the word was out. The news of a new "ethnic drug" traveled far and wide with the distinctive speed and lack of nuance of any report that may possibly be (mis)construed as "proving" a biological difference among the races. A simple Google search revealed the issue had been taken up by websites ranging from the lunatic racist right to the Revolutionary Communist Progressive Labor Party. (It also put me onto a Cameroonian musician named "Bidil," who had quite an interesting website.) Of greater interest, however, was the extensive coverage by media in between the extremes. ABC, the BBC, the *Wall Street Journal*, the *New York Times*, *Business Week*, and the *Financial Times* were among the most prominent major media outlets reporting on the BiDil phenomenon and its companion mortality statistic. In an article about the use of racial categories in evaluating heart drugs, the *Chronicle of Higher Education* cited the 2:1 ratio and asserted, "Statistically, the higher rate of heart failure among black people is undeniable."[17] Of course, the author provided no citation for this undeniable fact. It had simply entered the commonsense realm of accepted reality—as one would not need to cite Copernicus for the proposition that the earth traveled around the sun.

Among publications with a more targeted expert audience, the journal *Science* and the newsletter of the American Academy for the Advancement of Science dutifully repeated the 2:1 statistic in brief reports about the announcement of A-HeFT, as did the newsletter of the American Medical Association, and *Today in Cardiology*. The Association of Black Cardiologists (ABC) reiterated the statistic the next year in a follow-up press release encouraging further enrollment in the A-HeFT.[18]

I began my search for the origins of the statistic with the most immediate source: the jointly issued press releases from NitroMed and the ABC that were quoted almost verbatim in many press accounts. In response to my queries, NitroMed provided a press kit that contained some news articles and press releases that cited the statistic, but nowhere was there any reference to an underlying source for the statistic. I then called the Association for Black Cardiologists and requested a citation to support the statistic. They did not have the source of the statistic ready to hand. Instead, they pointed me toward Feinstein Kean Healthcare, a subsidiary of Ogilvy PR Worldwide, one of the world's largest public relations firms. Feinstein and Kean, it turned out, was handling the publicity for the A-HeFT trials.

The people at Feinstein and Kean also did not have the statistic readily available, but assured me they would look for it. As days and then weeks went by, the firm was very good about letting me know that it was still working on my query and hoped to get back to me with the information shortly. Then, during one of my periodic follow-up calls, my contact at Feinstein and Kean was very pleased to have a citation for me. An article had just come out that week in the *New England Journal of Medicine* about a study in Cincinnati that considered race as a variable in heart failure. A *Wall Street Journal* article reporting about the study had cited the 2:1 mortality statistic. I thanked him and pushed no further for the time being. A week or so later, I left a message on his answering machine pointing out that while I appreciated the reference, it had come out just last week. What I was looking for was the reference that originally provided the basis for the press release eighteen months earlier. Indeed, it seemed more than a bit odd to me that the best a health-care public relations firm could do in supporting a statistical claim made in the course of announcing a breakthrough trial for an "ethnic" drug would be to refer me to a *Wall Street Journal* article published a year and a half after the fact.[19]

I then contacted the *Wall Street Journal* reporter who wrote the article with the statistic and asked where she had found it. She referred me to the website of the National Heart, Lung, and Blood Institute (NHLBI). One particular page, titled "Facts about Heart Failure," had the statistic. There the U.S. government told me: "Heart failure mortality is about twice as high for African Americans as whites for all age groups."[20] And yet, while providing ample justification for the *Wall Street Journal* reporter's use of the statistic, this was not quite the definitive resolution of the issue for which I had hoped. The NHLBI provided no citation to any underlying study to support its own use of this aggressive little statistic.

My next step was to contact the NHLBI and ask about their sources. It turns out the fact sheet was published in 1994 and was based on data from the National Health and Nutrition Examination Survey (NHANES), which was conducted from 1988 to 1991. This survey questioned thousands of Americans on a wide range of health and nutrition issues, including heart failure. It has provided a wealth of information to health researchers. There were two basic problems here. First, the data were old—over ten years old—and those intervening years had seen great strides made in the treatment of heart failure. Second, NHANES data provides information about the *prevalence* of disease in a population, not about mortality. These are two very different things. Prevalence is simply the number of persons with a particular disease at any given time. And, of course, while differences in prevalence are certainly important, using a study of prevalence to make claims about mortality rates is a statistical gaffe of the first order.

There was no reason for the *Wall Street Journal* reporter to know this. But one might have expected the NHLBI to know better. And, in fact, it did—sort of. After spending a little more time surfing around the NHLBI website, I found another page titled "Data Fact Sheet: Congestive Heart Failure in the United States: A New Epidemic." Here, citing the Vital Statistics of the United States (apparently from 1993), the page identified the ratio of black to white mortality as approximately 1.4:1; hardly 2:1, but still a significant disparity.[21] Nonetheless, the data were still old. I soon found a third page, a page citing recent data, a page nearly erasing the racial disparity. Titled "Morbidity and Mortality: 2002 Chartbook on Cardiovascular, Lung, and Blood Diseases," it stated: "In 1999, [age adjusted] death rates for CHF within sex groups were *slightly higher* [italics added] in blacks than in whites."[22] The underlying source for this claim was actually specified in the text of the document. It was the National Center for Health Statistics Compressed Mortality File, 1979–1999, CDC Wonder. I went to the CDC Wonder website, I typed in the relevant data, both for heart failure generally and more specifically for congestive heart failure mortality for 1999. Immediately I had the numbers before me: a black: white mortality ratio for both men and women of approximately 1.1:1. The

NHLBI website had provided statistics of race-based differentials in mortality that ranged from 2:1, to 1.4:1, to "slightly higher" (i.e., 1.1:1). As it turned out, the only statistic with a firm grounding in current mortality data from the CDC was the third.

The confusing profusion of web-based data available at the NHLBI appears to provide a modicum of cover for those in the public media who disseminated the incorrect 2:1 statistic. But what of the doctors and medical researchers who developed therapies and published papers in peer-reviewed journals? The first mention of the statistic in the medical literature related to the development of BiDil came in 1999: the *New England Journal of Medicine* article by Dries et al. presenting the retrospective analysis of data gathered largely in the 1980s from the SOLVD that purported to identify "racial differences in the outcome of left ventricular dysfunction."[23] The authors set their story against the backdrop of "population-based studies [that] have found that black patients with congestive heart failure have a higher mortality rate than white patients with the same condition."[24] This initially posited statistical disparity drove their hypothesis that "racial differences in the natural history of left ventricular dysfunction"[25] played a role in creating this disparity. Thus, from the outset, the statistic was being used to rationalize a search for race-based biological differences. It was paving the way for reconceptualizing race in biological terms.

The opening paragraph states: "The population-based mortality rate from congestive heart failure is 1.8 times as high for black men as for white men and 2.4 times as high for black women as for white women."[26] To their credit, the authors go on to note that "not all studies . . . have found a higher mortality among blacks than whites with heart failure."[27] Having acknowledged such studies, they simply dismissed them and let their initial citation of the high mortality differential drive the study. From whence did this particular rendition of the statistic come? Being a peer-reviewed study, published in one of the nation's preeminent medical journals, it naturally provided a citation—two, in fact. Both were editorials written by Richard Gillum, M.D., from the Office of Analysis and Epidemiology Program at the National Center for Health Statistics. The first, written in 1987, actually provides statistics on racial differentials in mortality from heart failure;[28] the second, written in 1996, although discussing heart failure in blacks, provides no new statistics.[29]

Gillum's 1987 editorial was based on examination of both published and unpublished data from the National Center for Health Statistics and does indeed present the statistic cited by Dries et al. in the *New England Journal of Medicine* study of racial disparities in the SOLVD trials. As Gillum states, "The ratio of age adjusted [mortality] rates in blacks and whites was 1.8 for men and 2.4 for women."[30] But this is not a complete reference. The whole sentence reads: "*For persons aged 35 to 74 years* [italics added], the ratio of age adjusted rates for blacks and whites was 1.8 for men and 2.4 for women."[31] Now let us add a little more context. First, this statistic refers to mortality rates from the year 1981 (that is, 18 years before the publication of the article by Dries et al.). Second, the editorial also noted that "the ratio of black-to-white rates [of mortality] was highest under age 65, approaching 1 [i.e., 1:1] in persons 75 years of age and older."[32] Third, by the numbers presented in Gillum's own table of statistics, this meant that the age group of 35 to 74 contained approximately 69 percent of black heart failure mortality but only 29 percent of white.[33] Thus, the 71 percent of whites who died from heart failure after age 74 were not captured in the age 34 to 74 statistic. By these statistics, blacks might have had *earlier* onset and mortality from heart failure, but this was not the same thing as a *higher* mortality rate. Earlier onset of heart failure certainly is significant, but it is very different from an absolute 2:1 mortality disparity. Indeed, if anything, it might point to environmental impacts, access to quality care, or other such nongenetic factors as a source of explanation for the disparity.

These fine distinctions, of course, pale in comparison to the glaring failure of Dries and coworkers to cite the initial statistic correctly. Their blithe conversion of an age-specific differential into one applicable to the entire population at issue is inexcusable. Moreover, the article by Dries et al. was published in 1999—when far more current data on mortality rates was readily available. Thus, for example, the CDC's *Morbidity and Mortality Weekly Report* the week of August 7, 1998 (six months before the article by Dries et al. was published) issued a study of "Changes in Mortality

(But: 5 years' survival...)

from Heart Failure—United States, 1980–1995."[34] Noting that approximately 94 percent of heart failure deaths occurred among adults aged 65 and older, the study found in this population that "because of greater declines in death rates for heart failure among black adults, from 1980 to 1995 the black:white ratio [of age-adjusted mortality rates] for men narrowed from 1.3:1 to 1.1:1 and for women from 1.4:1 to 1.1:1."[35] Either nongenetic social and environmental factors were primarily responsible for this observed change in heart failure mortality or these fifteen years witnessed the most dramatic incident of spontaneous genetic mutation in history.

All this was lost on the heart failure researchers. And so, later that same year (1999), Carson and Cohn's article on race-based differences in response to the BiDil combination cited the article by Dries et al. and noted that the racial differentials observed in the analysis of the SOLVD data buttressed its own findings and "lend credence to the suggestion that therapy for heart failure might appropriately be racially tailored."[36]

What happened to the racial framing of heart failure following the announcement of the A-HeFT trials? Clyde Yancy, a cardiologist involved in the trials, published several articles arguing, "Heart failure in blacks is likely to be a *different disease*."[37] Yancy posited that this "likely" difference was probably based on "physiological explanations." Specifically, he considered certain possible sites for genetic polymorphisms and asserted: "The emerging field of genomic medicine has provided insight into potential mechanisms to explain racial variability in disease expression and response to medical therapy."[38] Elsewhere, Yancy stated that the aims of A-HeFT include looking for a genetic pattern among the African American patients that may suggest a molecular basis for understanding differential outcomes in heart failure etiology and treatment.[39]

While surely motivated by a laudable desire to develop better therapies to serve African American communities, Yancy's articles effectively constructed race as a genetic category. Moreover, Yancy had a personal stake in framing racial differences in heart failure in a manner that supports the logic of BiDil's race specificity. Between 2000 and 2005, he received research support from NitroMed, served as a consultant to the company, and received honoraria as a member of NitroMed's speaker's bureau.[40] If pressed,

Yancy (like many in the field) might say that he was merely using race as a surrogate category to identify different degrees of prevalence among certain groups. But in practice, he recast the social category of race in genetic terms. Such a disjunction between a rhetorical acknowledgment of racial categories as social and continued practical use of such categories as, in effect, genetic is all too common in biomedical research.[41] Nonetheless, the logic seems reasonable enough at first blush: there was a major race-based health disparity; socioeconomic factors did not account for the disparity; therefore, the disparity must have a physiological (read "genetic") basis.

There are several problems with this. First, Yancy's own focus on hypertension as a key precursor to heart failure is particularly striking. Could he have been ignorant of the vast array of medical and public health literature connecting racial differences in hypertension to everything from diet, to environment, to exercise, to stress?[42] Many of these social factors correlate strongly with race; for example, a study suggests the stress of experiencing racism seems to elevate blood pressure.[43] In 2005, admittedly subsequent to Yancy's articles, Cooper et al. published a meta-analysis of international studies of hypertension that should lay to rest any claims for genetics as a primary contributor to racial differences in prevalence of hypertension. Using a standardized analysis strategy, Cooper and core-searchers examined hypertension prevalence estimates for 8 white and 3 black populations (a total of 85,000 individuals) around the world and found the range in hypertension prevalence was from 27 percent to 55 percent for whites and 14 percent to 44 percent for blacks. Most striking, perhaps, was their finding that the lowest level of hypertension was to be found in Nigeria (14 percent), while Germany had the highest level (55 percent). Certainly this flies in the face of arguments that people of African descent are genetically more predisposed to hypertension that those of European descent.[44]

Second, going back to the article by Dries et al., the more recent of the two editorials by Gillum cited in support of the 2:1 statistic (the one with no such statistic in it) actually argued that then current reports "indicate a real heterogeneity in the patterns of death from cardiovascular disease

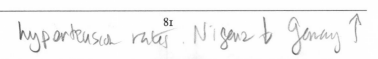

among black Americans" and suggested that "further research must now define the socioeconomic, cultural, behavioral, and ethnic determinants of these differences."[45]

Finally, it turns out that Dries and colleagues' idea of controlling for nonbiological variables that might affect differential rates of heart failure mortality involved ascertaining the participants' level of education and asking them to report "yes" or "no" on experiencing "major financial distress" at any time during the twelve months before enrollment.[46] As the numerous studies of hypertension and Gillum's own admonishment show, this represents a remarkably thin conception of the social, economic, and environmental factors that might influence heart failure.

The question then becomes how and why did Dries and his coauthors (and those who took up their misleading statistic) so readily come to biology as the "fallback explanation for their findings."[47] The first reason may simply be that these were cardiologists, trained to look inside the body to explain disease. They may have been aware that social, economic, and environmental factors affect "their" disease, but medical education and the incentives of biomedical research did not provide them with the tools or the inclination to explore such issues in depth. What they did was diagnose pathophysiological processes and deliver therapies to individual patients. Secondly, our statistic frames the entire analysis of the problem. Given the magnitude of a 2:1 difference in mortality rates, it simply seemed to make sense to look at biology as a major factor contributing to such a huge differential. Without the 2:1 statistic, the impetus toward a biological explanation of differences must dissipate.

In late 2003, I published an article detailing these problems with the 2:1 statistic in *Perspectives in Biology and Medicine*.[48] By mid-2004, NitroMed and the doctors around A-HeFT had changed their rhetoric somewhat to assert that African Americans had a "higher rate" of mortality than the "corresponding" white population.[49] It appeared that the article might have had some effect. The drive to perceive racial difference in the context of biology, however, is relentless.

So it was on January 11, 2005, that NitroMed, in a press release announcing that BiDil had been named to the American Heart Association's annual Top Ten Advances List, asserted that "African Americans between the ages of 45 and 64 are 2.5 times more likely to die from heart failure than Caucasians in the same age range."[50] NitroMed then repeated this statistic in a February press release announcing the FDA's acceptance of its amended NDA. It is perhaps testament to the power and importance of using statistics to create a racial frame for BiDil on its way to FDA approval that NitroMed decided to resurrect the race differential in heart failure with the old statistic in a new form.[51]

Unlike the previous 2 to 1 statistic, this new statistic was technically accurate. NitroMed failed to mention, however, that only about 6 percent of overall mortality from heart failure occurred in the 45-to-64 age range. About 93 percent of mortality occurred after age 65, and in that group there was almost no difference in age-adjusted mortality rates between blacks and whites. Indeed, the crude death rate for blacks is actually lower than that for whites.[52]

Why this investment in creating a major racial difference where none existed? One can only ask: If you have a medical interest in the underlying etiology of a disease do you look at a subgroup where 6 percent of mortality occurs or at one in which 93 percent of mortality occurs? If, however, you have a commercial interest in convincing the FDA and capital markets that there is a legitimate basis for approving a race-specific drug, then showing a huge difference becomes central to marketing your product, but, of course, you do not mention that your subgroup represents only 6 percent of the overall mortality rate.

STATISTICS + ACE = A RACIAL FRAME FOR BIDIL

A companion to the 2:1 statistic was the assertion that ACE inhibitors work less well in blacks than in whites. Derek Exner, with Cohn among his coauthors, made the assertion of racial difference in response to ACE inhibitors in an article published by the *New England Journal of Medicine* in May 2001—a mere two months after NitroMed's announcement of the commencement of A-HeFT. This assertion, when combined with the assertion that BiDil worked better in blacks, could be understood to imply that perhaps *all* African American heart failure patients should be taking BiDil—not merely those who could not tolerate ACE inhibitors—a substantial expansion of the potential market. Significantly, the entry for the ACE inhibitor Vasotec (enalapril) in the 2003 edition of the *Physicians' Desk Reference* (*PDR*), in apparent—but not explicit—reference to the article by Exner et al., states in the section on indications and usage that "in controlled clinical trials ACE inhibitors have an effect on blood pressure that is less in black patients than in non-blacks."[53] In 2005, the FDA issued a guidance for industry on the "Collection of Race and Ethnicity Data in Clinical Trials," which directly linked its recent approval of BiDil to the Exner et al. article to support its contention that "some differences in response to medical products have already been observed in racially and ethnically distinct subgroups of the U.S. population."[54] Within six weeks of the publication of Exner's call for racial medicines, NitroMed announced its plans to raise $31.4 million in private financing to develop BiDil.

Unlike the 2:1 statistic, the findings on ACE inhibitors did not go unchallenged. Surprisingly, one of the strongest critiques came from one of the coauthors of the original study, Daniel Dries—the very same Dries who was the lead author on the paper that gave life to the erroneous 2:1 mortality statistic. Dries published a paper in 2002 in which he took issue with the earlier *New England Journal of Medicine* piece and argued that "enalapril appears to be equally efficacious in black and white patients."[55] Another article found the retrospective analysis of the SOLVD data was too weak to provide any conclusions regarding the lack of benefit ACE inhibitors offer black patients.[56] Yet another article argued that the data on ACE inhibitors were insufficient to support a "unique strategy" for treating African American heart failure patients. A subsequent meta-analysis of major clinical trials found no evidence of racial differences in responses to ACE inhibitors.[57]

In 2010, long after the Exner study played a central role in driving BiDil toward FDA approval, Kaufman, Nguyen, and Cooper published a blistering critique of the paper by Exner et al. They noted that the framing of the article to highlight racial differences must be understood in relation to the emergence of BiDil, particularly the assertion that its findings "underscore[] the need for additional research on the efficacy of therapies for heart failure in black patients."[58] Kaufman, Nguyen, and Cooper noted that "even if a statistically significant difference existed between the two racial groups in the mean blood pressure response [to ACE inhibitors], it would not necessarily be a rational basis for individual therapeutic decisions, since an individual patient may fall far above or below the mean of their particular population."[59] As Ashwini Sehgal showed in his 2004 review of race differences in response to hypertensive drugs (including ACE inhibitors), the majority of whites and blacks have similar responses to commonly used antihypertensive drugs. Sehgal concluded that "race has little value in predicting antihypertensive drug response, because whites and blacks overlap greatly in their response to all categories of drugs. These findings are consistent with other work demonstrating that most genetic diversity exists within and not between races and that race is a poor predictor of drug-metabolizing enzymes (which in turn influence drug response)."[60]

In considering the implications of Sehgal's findings, sociologist Steven Epstein argues that "racial profiling poses the serious risk of improper medical treatment of a patient who doesn't conform to the stereotype that pertains to his or her group." Beyond the problems of racial definition, Epstein notes the additional issue of how to deal with a biracial or multiracial subject and concludes that "it is important to bear in mind that all claims of racial differences in diagnosis or treatment are statements about differences on average, not hard-and-fast differences between groups."[61]

The article by Exner et al. elided all such considerations. Yet, even taking the article on its own terms, Kaufman, Nguyen, and Cooper found significant shortcomings in its substantive arguments. Among their findings in the review of the Exner et al. data, "information on race is almost perfectly predicted by the medical [i.e., nonracial] covariates alone, making it essentially impossible to identify a race-specific effect, and making it clinically useless to attempt to do so (since a clinician could identity almost the exact same subsets of individuals by using clinical variables instead of race)."[62]

None of this mattered in the run-up to BiDil's FDA approval in 2005, as two sets of highly questionable data, the 2:1 mortality statistic and a purported race differential in response to ACE inhibitors, propelled the emergence of BiDil as an apparent means to redress a health disparity in an underserved population. Such slippage also allowed NitroMed to garner the support of the ABC and the Congressional Black Caucus (CBC) in its bid for approval of the racially repositioned BiDil. When NitroMed announced the initiation of A-HeFT at the annual meeting of the ABC, CEO Michael Loberg emphasized, "NitroMed looks forward to working closely with the ABC and other clinical thought leaders in the completion of this important trial."[63] B. Waine Kong, CEO of the ABC, declared, "It is in the name of science that we participate."[64]

4

CAPITALIZING [ON] RACE
IN DRUG DEVELOPMENT

T HE STORY OF BIDIL elucidates an alternative model to developing tailored therapies that promises to fill in the gap between the promise and reality of pharmacogenomic medicine. It is a model that exploits race to gain regulatory and commercial advantage, while ignoring its power to promote a regeneticization of racial categories in society at large.

The moment at which NitroMed succeeded in its strategy of creating a racial frame for the approval of BiDil is buried deep in the FDA medical review of its application. Dated May 12, 2005, section 1.2.6 of the review found, "The effect of BiDil in heart failure in this study was assessed solely in African American patients. The results of the A-HeFT study will not be generalizable to other ethnic groups."[1] The review followed this conclusion with an extensive discussion of racial difference in response to ACE inhibitors, demonstrating a complete acceptance of the contested racial frame presented by the paper by Exner et al. that purported to show that whites responded better than blacks to ACE inhibitors.[2] The assertion that the A-HeFT results were not "generalizable" marks another point at which the state cast race as biological. The only basis for denying generalizability to other "ethnic groups" was the idea that blacks were somehow a biologically distinct population.

Robert Temple, FDA associate director of medical policy, announced that BiDil "is a striking example of how a treatment can benefit some patients even if it does not help all patients."[3] The FDA support of BiDil can be understood as part of its rising emphasis both on more efficient drug review and on promoting the promise of personalized medicine. In fact, however, BiDil was not about personalizing medicine; it was about exploiting race to obtain cheaper, quicker FDA approval for a drug.

EXPLOITING RACE: BIDIL'S INTERIM MODEL OF PHARMACOGENOMICS

BiDil is the first time, the highest profile time, the model of "let's identify a target population and let's develop a drug for that population" has been pursued.

MICHAEL WERNER, FORMER REGULATORY AFFAIRS SPECIALIST
FOR THE BIOTECHNOLOGY INDUSTRY ORGANIZATION[4]

In addition to the medical promise of tailoring drugs to individual genetic profiles, pharmacogenomics also holds the commercial promise of greatly reducing the cost of bringing a new drug to market. While often contested by consumer advocates, industry estimates of the cost of bringing a drug to market at the time BiDil was approved ranged from $700 to $900 million, with time ranges of up to fifteen years;[5] by 2010, that estimate had risen to $1.3 billion.[6] Through identifying subgroups of people more likely to respond to and/or have fewer adverse side effects from a drug treatment, pharmacogenomic research aims to allow pharmaceutical corporations to design smaller, shorter, and cheaper clinical trials in order to develop the data necessary to present an NDA to the FDA for approval.

Yet, there lies a great tension at the heart of the commercial pursuit of pharmacogenomics. On the one hand, it is understood as the wave of the future, saving money and improving therapies.[7] On the other hand, it

involves narrowing the market for a drug down to smaller and smaller subgroups who show the best response. One of the little-known facts about
blockbuster drugs, such a Prozac or Lipitor, with annual sales in the billions
of dollars, is that most of them only work in a limited number of those actually taking the drug.[8] By identifying true responders, pharmacogenomics also threatens to reduce substantially (often by over 50 percent) the potential consumer base for any given drug. One study of data from the *PDR*
found "the percent of responders range from a low of 25% (oncology products) to a high of 80% (Cox2 inhibitors), with the majority of drugs having
a responder rate of 50–60%."[9] One professor of pharmacology characterized
pharmacogenomics like an arms race: big pharmaceutical corporations may
not want to develop targeted therapies that constrict their consumer base,
but they are afraid not to, lest the other guys get there first.[10] Fear of being
left behind has impelled some pharmaceutical corporations to move away
from a focus on major new multi-billion-dollar, blockbuster drugs to con-
centrate on developing drugs aimed at smaller groups of people that can be
developed quicker and more cheaply.[11]

A central irony of BiDil's presentation as the path-breaking example of
the coming of age of pharmacogenomics is that, strictly speaking, it is
not a pharmacogenomic drug. Indeed, the mechanism of action by which
it appears to have a beneficial effect on heart failure patients is unknown.[12]
The total absence of claims for a genetic basis to BiDil's efficacy, however,
did not stop Steven Nissen, chair of the FDA Advisory Committee reviewing BiDil, from confidently asserting that "we're using self-identified
race as a surrogate for genetic markers."[13] Nissen also explicitly cast BiDil
at the forefront of pharmacogenomics, stating, "It is very unusual; it is
precedent-setting. . . . But it is the case that we are moving forward to
genome-based medicine. It's going to happen."[14] Nor has the geneticization
of racial difference in the context of BiDil's success been limited to experts
on the FDA Advisory Committee. Thus, in addition to casual references to
a race-specific genetic basis for BiDil's efficacy in the popular media, articles
published in *Genome Biology* and the *British Medical Journal* also presumed
a genetic variation more prevalent in self-identified African Americans to
underlie BiDil's efficacy.[15]

The experience of BiDil indicates a strategic use of race to address a tension deep at the heart of tailored medicine: in an economic model driven by multi-billion-dollar sales of blockbuster drugs aimed at the general population, why should pharmaceutical corporations seek to develop drugs that are designed to narrow their potential market? In contrast with the hypothetical projection of possible future benefits to genetically tailored therapies, the overarching triumph of BiDil was to immediately exploit market demands created by the hype about the promise of truly individualized pharmacogenetic therapies to be realized at some undetermined time in the future. While truly individualized, genetically tailored medicines might threaten to narrow markets, NitroMed recognized that medicine by racial proxy presented a commercial opportunity.[16]

BiDil's exploitation of race had several related components that allowed it to take advantage of the cost-saving aspects of pharmacogenomics while subverting the pharmacogenomic logic that threatened to constrict potential markets. First, NitroMed used race to resurrect the fortunes of an apparently failed drug. Second, race allowed the sponsor to get FDA approval faster and more cheaply than the norm by conducting fewer, smaller, and more targeted trials. Third, once faster, less expensive approval had been obtained for a subpopulation, NitroMed could attempt to expand its potential market by informally promoting off-label use of the product to the general population at large.

RESURRECTING DRUGS

One of the many promises of pharmacogenomics is to resurrect failed drugs by finding narrower, genetically defined subpopulations in whom safety and efficacy can be established. BiDil exploited this model not by actually identifying genes, but by characterizing race as a surrogate marker for a genetically defined subpopulation. In its original FDA denial of the NDA for BiDil in 1997, the FDA requested additional clinical research—but with no mention of race. Most obviously, this could have meant conducting a new trial prospectively designed as a new drug trial with appropriate controls and statistical endpoints. Medco, however, was not interested, most likely because such trials are expensive—certainly far more expensive than retrospectively analyzing data from trials already conducted with federal money, as were V-HeFT I and II.[17]

Jay Cohn was then left with multiple avenues for further research, including looking at the causes of heart failure and the etiological importance of a history of hypertension.[18] NitroMed listed eighteen different baseline characteristics, including age, race, cardiovascular history, and clinical conditions (such as left ventricular ejection fraction), by which the data could have been broken down.[19] But they chose race. Based primarily on the forty-nine African Americans placed on H/I in V-HeFT I, Cohn and NitroMed argued that the data pointed toward a distinctive efficacy in African Americans.[20] This was done without the need to conduct any new trials, and it provided the basis for resurrecting the fortunes of BiDil on the cheap.

Another example of this strategy may be seen in the 2003 case in which VaxGen, a San Francisco–based pharmaceutical company, reached for race in an attempt to revive its commercial prospects by claiming that a retrospective analysis of the results of a failed AIDS vaccine trial seemed to indicate a beneficial impact on African Americans.[21] This story began in February 2003, when VaxGen claimed to have concluded the first-ever successful trial of an AIDS vaccine.[22] The overall findings from the trial, however, showed that the vaccine failed to protect against infection with the virus that caused the disease. The VaxGen researchers claimed to be surprised by the findings, but they were also undeterred. Like the BiDil researchers before them, they decided, post hoc, to break the results out by race and claimed that a retrospective analysis of the data revealed "significant efficacy in 66.8% of Blacks, Asians, and people of mixed race, and 78.3% in Blacks alone."[23] VaxGen's race-based claims, however, were quickly shot down by the medical and scientific communities as being a deeply flawed, even tortured, reading of the data, but not before VaxGen's stock value momentarily rallied—later giving rise to a spate of class action lawsuits for stock manipulation. As one HIV specialist at Emory University School of Medicine put it, "It was a desperate act by a company that was trying to save a failed product. . . . If they really cared about racial and ethnic differences, they would have structured a very different trial."[24] This was the BiDil model at work.

FASTER, CHEAPER APPROVAL

The original 1996 NDA for BiDil was submitted based on preexisting data produced by two government-sponsored studies in which Medco did not participate. This, of course, is the cheapest way to get a new drug approved. Failing that, Cohn and NitroMed used a race-based pseudo-pharmacogenomic model to take the next best route. That is, they argued that the data from A-HeFT, a single, relatively small trial in a targeted, racially identified subpopulation, when viewed in relation to the V-HeFT data, should be sufficient for FDA approval. Ultimately, the FDA accepted this logic and granted race-specific approval. In contrast to industry-estimated average costs of $700 to $900 million and fifteen years to bring a new drug to market, NitroMed spent only about $43 million on the A-HeFT trial and brought the drug to market within five years of obtaining its race-specific patent;[25] by any measure, this was certainly an appealing model of the savings possible through "tailored" drug development.

How did this happen? At the 2005 FDA Advisory Committee review of BiDil, one of NitroMed's own representatives acknowledged that the "conventional standard" for FDA approval was two clinical trials, not one. But he urged the committee to view the A-HeFT in relation to V-HeFT I and II and to find the "consistency" sufficient to support approval. "It is not a mathematical way of getting there," he admitted, "it is an intuitive way of getting there."[26] The Advisory Committee was receptive to NitroMed's plea to supplant mathematical rigor with intuition. Thomas Fleming, the lead biostatistician consultant to the committee, cautioned that "if a trial should stand alone, both FDA and European regulatory authorities have said, yes, single trials can be an adequate basis for approval. Results have to be robust and compelling, pristine trials, internal consistency, high quality conduct and, vaguely stated, stronger statistical evidence."[27] He later concluded that viewing A-HeFT in relation to the V-HeFT data was a "close call, but in my view it does meet the general fundamental principle." The only statistically powerful data from the V-HeFT trials directly relevant to A-HeFT came from V-HeFT I, in which only forty-nine African Americans were placed on the H/I drug combination.[28]

Shortly after the approval of BiDil, the two FDA administrators overseeing the review panel, Robert Temple and Norman Stockbridge, published a response to critics in the *Annals of Internal Medicine* further elaborating the reasoning behind the FDA's race-specific approval. They invoked the purported racial differences in heart failure mortality and response to ACE inhibitors as part of their defense. Then, referring to A-HeFT and the two V-HeFT trials, they asserted that "the mortality benefit of BiDil in black patients is . . . supported by 3 well-controlled studies."[29] This is quite striking, given the 1997 FDA review panel's conclusion that the data from the V-HeFT trials was essentially a statistical hash because those trials were designed as test-of-theory trials, not as new drug trials. The FDA's reliance on the 1980s V-HeFT studies in 2005 was particularly problematic, because it involved a retrospective post hoc subgroup analysis of this already questionable trial data. As Drs. Kirsten Bibbins-Domingo and Alicia Fernandez noted in response to the FDA's explanation of its race-specific approval of BiDil, "In general, post-hoc subgroup analyses should be interpreted with caution and should be used primarily for generating hypotheses—not for determining policy, which appears to be the case here."[30] Moreover, the claim by Temple and Stockbridge that a race-specific indication was justified by the "striking effects in black patients in A-HeFT and V-HeFT I"[31] does not stand up to scrutiny. Conducting an independent review of the statistical data, Ellison et al. found that "these claims are based on ambiguous *post hoc* subgroup analyses in which the only statistically significant difference observed between black and white patients was found without any adjustment for potential confounders in samples that were unlikely to be adequately balanced."[32]

Similar concerns were expressed at the FDA Advisory Committee review, but the committee chair, cardiologist Steven Nissen, had few such reservations about the data. "I am not as conflicted as several of you are," he stated toward the end of the meeting. "I find the evidence more compelling. Compelling doesn't necessarily mean statistical. Compelling to me means also clinical and, as a clinician, I find the evidence more than adequate to vote for approval."[33] Nissen went on to state "My job as a clinician on the panel is to adjust p values [measures of statistical significance] for clinical and I think societal considerations."[34] Nissen's readiness to address "societal considerations" is striking in light of the FDA's own repeated assertions that such considerations were irrelevant to its review of the data.

Memoranda of teleconferences between NitroMed and the FDA reveal that both parties agreed to bracket such considerations and keep the politics of race out of the review. Two months before the FDA hearing on BiDil, NitroMed and the FDA spoke about the "political ramifications of targeting one racial group."[35] NitroMed expressed concern that "the meeting may lead them to having to address the broader issue; race in medicine." The FDA representative, Norman Stockbridge, assured NitroMed "that is not the intent and that we want to stay focused on the drug."[36] The next month, NitroMed "expressed concerns" that "they are not the right people, nor is the CRAC [Cardio-Renal Advisory Committee] the right media for that discussion."[37] Again, Stockbridge agreed that NitroMed should "focus on presenting the developmental program for the drug," and concluded "there is no need to address race in medicine."[38] NitroMed and the FDA were concerned that the politics of race might present a barrier to BiDil's approval and so kept such considerations out of the review, generally dismissing them when they were raised by outside parties offering testimony at the hearing. Nissen, in contrast, saw race as a means to facilitate BiDil's approval and so incorporated it into his evaluation of the data.

Before the hearing, I had made a decision to enter BiDil's story more directly and to go to the hearing in Bethesda to offer testimony (limited to five minutes) before the panel, urging that BiDil be approved but without a race-specific label. Previous to this, I had e-mail correspondence with Robert Temple, who told me he had read my 2003 *Perspectives on Biology and Medicine* article on BiDil exploring the use and misuse of statistics in framing the drive toward marking it as a race-specific drug. Nissen, however, was singularly unimpressed. He dismissed all challenges to the statistical evidence underlying claims of a purported 2:1 disparity in heart failure mortality between blacks and whites, asserting, "I think this was a courageous thing to do, to try to develop a drug for this population which seems to have a disproportionate burden of disease. By the way, I did not agree with the speaker[39] who argued that there isn't a disproportionate burden. I am convinced that there is. That is important."[40] Here it seems that clinical expertise allowed Nissen not only to "modify" p values but also to disregard statistical evidence altogether if it did not comport appropriately with his world of individual clinical experience.

My goal had not been to question evidence of the efficacy of BiDil, merely to challenge its racial framing. Like many testifying before the review board that day, I had explicitly called for the approval of BiDil, but without a race-specific indication. Nissen, however, disagreed with this evidence. He found this disagreement "important." Indeed it was; together with his earlier affirmation of the notion that "ACE Inhibitors don't work so well in [African Americans],"[41] it was essential to maintaining his racial frame for reviewing and weighing the power of the statistical evidence.

Nissen's arguments stand in striking contrast to the discussion of the relation between clinical and statistical data that occurred during the first review of BiDil by the FDA in 1997. At that first review, BiDil was presented as a drug for the general population, without any reference to race. Committee members raised similar issues regarding striking the proper balance between statistical data and clinical experience. In presenting the V-HeFT data, Jay Cohn had urged Barry Massie, the committee chair,

> to go back to the mortality issue and ask the panel whether they think the mortality reduction is real, even if not statistically significant by nominal p values because that is clearly the question that is being proposed by the agency to find out. The p value question only can depend upon Lem [Moye] and Ralph [D'Agostino, the committee biostatisticians], but the implication of the reduction of mortality requires the *clinical judgment* [italics added] that Marvin [Konstam] has identified.[42]

In response, Robert Temple (who would later be present at the 2005 review of BiDil) urged caution:

Barry, I want to object. I'm sorry. We are dancing with words here and it is treacherous.

If the committee wants to tell us, yes, I sort of believe it, I can't quite tell you why, the p values are all over the map, that is not very helpful to us because that's information we can't use. *You can't approve a drug because someone has an emotional reaction to it* [italics added].[43]

Nonetheless, Ray Lipicky, also of the FDA, later added,

The question I want to ask the committee to address now with just a yes and a no vote, is, even though they think that [the statistics are weak], *what does their gut say* [italics added]? And I don't know that we'll pay attention to your gut, and probably should not, but because this discussion is going on, I would just like to know what the result of that vote would be.[44]

Following this discussion, the committee ultimately voted to reject the BiDil NDA. Jeffrey Borer, a committee consultant, expressed the belief that BiDil probably was efficacious as a treatment for heart failure but ultimately rejected the application, stating, "Yes clinical, no regulatory."[45] Similarly, Marvin Konstam framed his negative vote by stating, "I would readily use it in clinical practice. But am I convinced it's right? No."[46] In the end, then, the committee members generally believed that the V-HeFT data might well affect their practice as clinicians. But in making their final decisions, they carefully separated this role from their duties in the FDA regulatory process and followed Temple's admonition to avoid acting on "emotion."

This contrast between conceptions of clinical as opposed to regulatory significance is, in itself, noteworthy. It takes on heightened importance in light of the further contrast with how the 2005 Advisory Committee review of BiDil handled similar issues. As noted above, the committee biostatistician found the evidence to present a "close call." Committee chair Nissen repeatedly noted potential discrepancies between knowledge gained from clinical practice versus the statistical data. Yet, this second time around, the committee seemed far more willing to allow for clinical experience to modify interpretations of the statistics.

At least one member of the 2005 committee, Vivian Ota Wang of the NHGRI, expressed concern over what she perceived as

[the] thought that there is a notion that for some types of research, for some types of communities or populations we can actually lower the bar in terms of scientific integrity that we are using to evaluate the research.[47]

Committee chair Nissen's response to Ota Wang illuminates the dynamic at work in his support for BiDil:

I am going to answer that for myself and tell you that, you know, if you develop a drug and the people you can enroll in a clinical trial is the entirety of the population in the United States for the disease, let's say heart failure, it is a lot easier to study that population than it is a population that represents a relatively small fraction of the population. This is just a practical matter. We love to have trials that have more than enough power to answer the questions very, very well. That is hard to achieve when the population that you are trying to study—the FDA has recognized this in some of the policies related to orphan drugs where you have a small number of people that have a disease. *So, if you are developing a drug for a disease and there are not many people that have it, you get some points for doing that* [italics added]. I am arguing that it is not unreasonable public policy to make some adjustment for that.[48]

What accounts for this different attitude toward clinical and statistical data in BiDil trials? What allowed the common sense of clinical expertise to trump the equivocal conclusion of statistical expertise? Race, of course, made the difference. Here the review panel layered a *biological* meaning on

race derived from its "common sense" understandings of its *social* significance. Perhaps there are times when race should make a difference in evaluating social, economic, or environmental impacts on health outcomes. But
in this case, race was not being used to understand socioeconomic phenomena. Rather, Nissen argued for using race to "get points" as a matter of
"public policy."

Nissen compared the over 750,000 African Americans then suffering from heart failure to people having an orphan disease. The Orphan
Drug Act defines an orphan disease as a condition that affects fewer than
200,000 persons in the United States. The analogy to an orphan disease
could thus not be based directly on equivalent population sizes. Nissen
began with a rationale for special consideration based on a disease population defined by its small size (orphan disease groups) and transferred the
rationale to a population defined by its racial identity (African American).
Nissen, thus, was not saying that heart failure was like an orphan disease—
the number of African Americans with heart failure is too great to warrant
special consideration. It was race itself that he connected to disease—
people suffering from "African-American-ness" deserved the same special
consideration as those suffering from an orphan disease. As in the case of
an orphan disease, Nissen believed that public policy might justify making
allowances in the interpretation of the racialized clinical data. In his apparently well-meaning attempt to approve a drug for a group that he legitimately perceived to be woefully underserved by the current health-care
system, Nissen not only biologized race, he pathologized it. Race as pathology, it seems, was powerful enough to modify statistics. In the end,
with the exception of Ota Wang and one other member, the committee
followed Nissen's lead and voted for race-specific approval despite a total
lack of evidence from A-HeFT that BiDil worked differently in African
Americans than anyone else.[49]

Ultimately, the FDA framed its approval as "representing a step toward
the promise of personalized medicine."[50] The FDA had made a major
commitment to promoting the development of pharmacogenomic approaches to drug development, and had issued a special guidance to

industry on the collection of pharmacogenomic data. The lure of true pharmacogenomic medicines apparently led the agency to what can only be understood as a premature embrace of the relevance of race to understanding the efficacy of BiDil. Following the lead of Nissen and the Advisory Committee, it apparently made "public policy" allowances in construing the A-HeFT data, and so granted NitroMed's request for a race-specific label.[51]

Additional policy considerations were evident when the FDA's Robert Temple and Norman Stockbridge subsequently justified the BiDil approval by asserting, "We also would not want to stifle innovation and efficient studies and deprive the community of valuable treatments."[52] A perfectly reasonable assertion on the face of it, but efficiency is an economic concept that has nothing to do with safety or efficacy—and hence is supposedly beyond the FDA's mandate. Indeed, the FDA was quite selective in what policy consideration it deemed to be legitimately within its purview in reviewing the BiDil application. Thus, in response to my critique of their explanation of the FDA's approval, Temple and Stockbridge averred, "Dr. Kahn focuses mainly on commercial matters that are not pertinent to regulatory approval."[53] Apparently, patents are commercial, but efficiency is not. Ironically, the primary justification for the patent system is precisely to promote the sort of efficiency and innovation that Temple and Stockbridge asserted to be worthy of their consideration. Nonetheless, Temple and Stockbridge's disclaimer echoed those of many clinicians involved in the A-HeFT trials, who considered such "commercial matters" as how patents might drive the design of a clinical trial to be similarly beyond their purview.

To a certain extent, such convenient blindness merely reflects a broad social understanding and acceptance of the fact that drug development is a commercial enterprise. Of course, NitroMed or other companies are going to want to get drugs approved in order to make a profit. But recognizing an inevitable commercial context to drug development should not be allowed to slip into turning a blind eye to how those commercial interests may be shaping the presentation of data before regulatory agencies.

Off-label

OFF-LABEL PROMOTION

"Off-label" prescribing is a fairly common practice whereby doctors prescribe drugs for indications that are not formally specified on a drug's FDA-approved label. Such prescribing is often based on clinical studies conducted after the initial drug approval that show it efficacious for other indications. Since the initial publication of the V-HeFT data in the late 1980s and early 1990s, the generic components of BiDil (hydralazine and isosorbide dinitrate) have often been prescribed off-label to treat heart failure. The two drugs have been listed by the American Heart Association for over fifteen years as a treatment for heart failure in the general population without regard to race.[54]

The FDA technically prohibits pharmaceutical corporations from explicitly advertising or promoting off-label uses, but it does not regulate how doctors may prescribe or talk about the possible uses of particular drugs. Off-label use commonly develops through information published in professional journals and presented at "educational" seminars for medical practitioners. Pharmaceutical corporations have often skirted (and sometimes violated) FDA limitations on off-label marketing through such means as funding seminars, actually conducting in-house research on new uses and then soliciting doctors to sign on as authors, and paying hefty "consulting" fees to doctors responsible for setting formulary reimbursements or overseeing NIH-funded research. One of the most notorious examples involves the epilepsy drug Neurontin. Documents produced through a lawsuit indicate a massive corporate strategy to expand the market for Neurontin by promoting it for dozens of unapproved uses. In addition to paying academic experts to put their names on in-house research and sponsoring education meetings and conferences all over the country, Neurontin's promoter also paid a doctor at the University of Minnesota $300,000 to write a textbook on epilepsy.[55]

Within a month of FDA approval, NitroMed had sponsored a symposium titled "Examining the Evidence: Optimizing Heart Failure Management in African American Patients" at the annual meeting of the International Society on Hypertension in Blacks. In addition, the University of

Pittsburgh's School of Pharmacy announced a grant from NitroMed to begin Helpful Hands for Healthy Hearts, an educational program for minority communities in the Pittsburgh area. NitroMed, however, did not need to engage in such egregious behavior as Neurontin's sponsors to try to expand its market for BiDil beyond the 750,000 African Americans with heart failure to an estimated 4.25 million other Americans suffering from the condition. It had able surrogates on hand to do the job for it. Prominent among them were the ABC, the National Minority Health Month Foundation (NMHMF), and U.S. Representative Donna Christensen (D-Virgin Islands), who headed the Congressional Black Caucus "Health Braintrust." B. Waine Kong, CEO of the ABC, Gary Puckrein, director of the NMHMF, and Congresswoman Christensen all testified at the FDA Advisory Committee urging approval of BiDil. Kong noted that the ABC had received $200,000 from NitroMed, and Puckrein acknowledged that the NMHMF had received an unrestricted educational grant from NitroMed. Christensen failed to note that during a one-week period the previous fall, she had received $14,000 in campaign donations from individuals associated with NitroMed, its lobbyists (FoxKiser), and its public relations firm (Spectrum Science Communications). In 2004, Fox Kisser also provided its lobbying services pro bono to the ABC.[56]

Notably, the day before the FDA Advisory Committee meeting, the NMHMF staged a press conference with an array of African American–identified interest groups, including representatives from the Alliance of Minority Medical Associations, the ABC, the International Society on Hypertension in Blacks, the National Association for the Advancement of Colored People (NAACP), and the National Medical Association. These groups issued a joint press statement calling for FDA approval of BiDil. The announcement garnered much media attention. Less noticed, however, was the fact that the press release contained such statements as, "The assertion that this is a race drug is misguided," by Randall W. Maxey, president of the Alliance of Minority Medical Associations, and another by Gail Christopher, vice president of the Joint Center for Political and Economic Studies' Office of Health, Women and Families, stating, "It would be 'bad science' to label or market this drug as a 'Black' drug. More

nportantly, race-based claims are not credible in the face of modern genetic science." The press release was titled "Organizations Unite to Support BiDil's Approval for Heart Failure, Rebuff Designation as 'Race-
Only Drug.'"[57]

In obtaining such support from groups with a legitimate concern to
serve the health needs of their African American constituents, NitroMed
was able to have its pharmacogenomic cake and eat it too. Not to put too
fine a point on it, these groups enabled NitroMed to put a "black face" on
BiDil as it went before the FDA for race-specific approval. Moreover, in
rebuffing the designation as a race-specific drug, these groups also actually
helped NitroMed get out the message that doctors should be prescribing
BiDil off-label to the huge market of non-African American heart failure
patients. This brings us back to the A-HeFT investigators themselves, who,
like Jay Cohn, were free to make the point that BiDil should be prescribed
for everyone, regardless of race. As the beneficiary of royalty payments
from sales of BiDil, Cohn also had a clear financial interest in making
such statements.

What accounts for this strange duality of doctors lining up en masse
to support NitroMed's race-specific development of BiDil while arguing
that BiDil should be prescribed without regard to race? There was the pervasive refrain articulated by Clyde Yancy, an A-HeFT investigator involved in NitroMed's presentation of the data to the FDA, who declared
for a syndicated NBC news story that same day, "We can save lives based
on our data."[58] The trope of saving lives lies at the core of the doctor's self-
conception and was reiterated throughout the process by Yancy and others
as the rationale for their avid support of BiDil. It is hard to argue with
saving lives. But since there was no scientific evidence that BiDil worked
differently or better in African Americans, there was no basis for connecting saving lives to race. The relatively uncritical willingness of both doctors and large segments of the African American political and professional
establishment to rally behind BiDil as NitroMed's race-specific therapy
remains striking.

An explanation for the doctors' relatively uncritical support of BiDil
may perhaps be found in market research sponsored by NitroMed that

indicated doctors were ready and willing to embrace the concept of race-specific therapies. A national survey of 800 physicians, released to the public the same day as BiDil's FDA approval, found that 81 percent agreed with the FDA advisory panel's recommendation to approval the drug BiDil for use among African Americans. Moreover, 81 percent of physicians also believed that "race should be used as a biological basis for determining ailments or diseases."[59]

When confronted with questions regarding the larger social, political, or commercial implications of developing BiDil as a race-specific drug, Cohn's response was typical of many involved in A-HeFT: "There is richness in that diversity, and knowing about that diversity helps us to understand people. . . . Now, the fact that that distinction leads to social prejudice is completely outside of my arena."[60] Medical professionals' willful blindness to the larger implications of their work served NitroMed well for a time. It fueled the strategy of exploiting race to gain quick, cheap approval for BiDil in a race-specific manner that extended its patent protection to 2020. At the same time, it allowed NitroMed, with a wink and a nod, to expand its market potential fivefold to sixfold by acquiescing when the doctors put forth the message that BiDil should be prescribed to everyone with heart failure regardless of race. As early as October 2004, analysts at the investment firm S. G. Cowen Securities were saying that off-label prescriptions of BiDil could effectively drive NitroMed's "mid-term performance."[61]

PRICING

One week after the FDA approved BiDil, NitroMed found another way to expand its market opportunity: pricing. On June 6, 2005, ten days before the FDA Advisory Committee recommended approval for BiDil, NitroMed CEO Michael Loberg discussed BiDil pricing before an audience at the Pacific Growth Equities-Life Sciences Growth Conference. "We haven't established a pricing," he said, "but if you were to use [beta-blocker] Coreg pricing which is pretty much a pure heart failure play," it leads to about a "billion dollar market opportunity." In the same talk, Loberg priced Coreg at $3.56 per day. He also declared that NitroMed had the drug stock in place necessary to go forward with a full commercial launch in anticipation of FDA approval by June 23.[62] On June 27, in a conference call for NitroMed investors, Loberg continued to demur on giving a specific target price for BiDil, declaring that the corporation was taking the newly approved label to "payers" to discuss possible pricing.[63] Then, four days later (with the FDA approval firmly in its pocket), NitroMed announced its BiDil pricing at $1.80 per pill, with a target dose of six pills per day that amounts to $10.80 per day—three times the price of Coreg and more than seven times the estimated price of $0.25 for the combined generic equivalent.[64] Thus, less than a month after Loberg used Coreg as a guide to potential pricing, NitroMed presented a pricing structure that tripled its market opportunity from one to three billion dollars; and indeed, three months later at another investment conference, Loberg recharacterized the BiDil market opportunity from one billion dollars to "in the billions [plural] of dollars."[65]

NitroMed's pricing was based on what is known as "pharmacoeconomic" analysis. In this case, NitroMed calculated the price largely by considering the significantly reduced rates of hospitalization for heart failure expected to result from the use of BiDil. Hospitalization costs are among the highest expenses borne by health insurers. NitroMed expected these third-party payors would embrace the higher price for BiDil, because their expected savings from reduced hospitalization costs would more than offset the difference. In this calculation, the actual costs of developing and producing the drug played almost no role. It was all about what the NitroMed pharmacoeconomists thought the market would bear. In this context, the trope of "saving lives" receded before the less altruistic slogan of "reducing hospitalization costs."[66]

The markets were happy with the pricing announcement. NitroMed's stock rose significantly on the news. *Forbes* observed that NitroMed's market opportunity was "Substantially Improved" as the investment firm Friedman Billings Ramsey raised its price target on NitroMed from twenty-six dollars to thirty-two dollars after the pricing announcement.[67] A-HeFT investigator Flora Sam observed that the actual label approved by the FDA appeared to broaden the use of BiDil in two ways: by calling patients "black" and by not distinguishing how sick black patients have to be to receive BiDil. "You can use it for any heart failure patient," she stated, "which I think is the best-case scenario for the company."[68] One might think that the more closely the label reflected NitroMed's desires, the lower it would be able to price the drug. And yet, after taking this best of all possible labels to payers for discussion, NitroMed's pharmacoeconomic analysis led it to set BiDil's price at three times the model Loberg had mentioned less than a month earlier.

Flora Sam also noted, "We've actually had a lot of interest from patients. Non-African-American patients have asked about it. I think physicians will prescribe it as an off-label use."[69] Here again at work was the dynamic whereby NitroMed exploited race to facilitate acceptance of high pricing while at the same time individual doctors associated with A-HeFT discounted race in a manner that increased the potential for expanding the market to non-African Americans.

SURROGATE MARKERS AND
SURROGATE MARKETING

From the moment NitroMed acquired the rights to BiDil, it embarked on a strategy of framing the drug in a manner that enabled it literally to capitalize on race. The reinvention of BiDil as an ethnic drug enabled NitroMed to garner support beyond the ABC and the CBC. On June 14, 2001, NitroMed announced the completion of a private financing round raising $31.4 million from several venture capital firms to support the race-specific A-HeFT trials.[70] NitroMed's ability to raise such substantial funding in the aftermath of the "dot com" collapse in the stock market is a testament to the business appeal of developing a drug at the forefront of biological niche marketing. Where drugs such as Viagra targeted one sex or another, BiDil promised to lead the way in ethnic niche marketing of pharmaceuticals.

Branding has long been a central component of consumer marketing. In recent years, pharmaceutical manufacturers have developed the art of what is known as "branding a condition." In contrast to branding a product by granting it a unique identity that enables a consumer to distinguish it from competitors, the pharmaceutical marketers have developed the technique of actually branding a medical condition that a particular product is able to treat.[71] NitroMed took this strategy one step further by branding race as a medical condition and making it the dominant frame for developing and marketing BiDil.

On November 6, 2003, in a second round of fundraising to support the development and marketing of BiDil, NitroMed went public. The initial public offering was managed by Deutsche Bank Securities and J.P. Morgan. NitroMed offered six million common shares at a target price of eleven dollars per share with a proposed market cap of $305 million.[72] As drug companies were hoping to tailor therapies ever more closely to the genetic profile of individuals or groups of consumers, identifying racial/ethnic correlations with disease was becoming big business. One announcement for a 2004 conference on multicultural pharmaceutical marketing and public relations noted:

> Major U.S. drug manufacturers are making it a high priority area to cultivate relationships with ethnic consumers, physician groups, community networks and other key stakeholder groups to uncover new market growth. Disproportionately high incidence of diabetes, obesity, heart disease, cancer, HIV/AIDS, asthma and other health conditions among these segments require many strategic and tactical moves in pharmaceutical marketing and PR.[73]

To a significant degree, NitroMed's development of BiDil can be viewed as one such move.

Ironically, many of the BiDil researchers were among the first to caution that they were merely using race as a surrogate marker to identify underlying genetic variation that accounted for the differential response to BiDil. Cohn himself noted that "skin color is only a crude indication of underlying genetic differences."[74] He also cautioned in a co-authored article that "racial categorization is only a surrogate marker for genetic or other factors responsible for individual responses to therapy."[75] Yet race remained a primary category around which these researchers organized their efforts. They presented race as instrumental—a means to a larger end of more precisely tailored drug therapy, therapy that would be able to overlook race altogether. Sally Satel, a psychiatrist and author of a prominent *New York Times Magazine* article called "I Am a Racially Profiling Doctor,"[76] characterized the work on BiDil this way:

> The ultimate purpose of work like Cohn's and other biological realists is to identify factors that may be genetic in origin. First, researchers hope that identifying particular genetic markers with certain ethnic groups will yield insight into the genetic basis of disease and reveal why certain conditions are more prevalent in some groups. Second, the ultimate goal is to understand differences between *individuals*, not between races or ethnic groups.[77]

Satel here laid out an idealized progression of medical research and, by implication, of marketing, toward truly individualized pharmacogenomic approaches to therapy that focus on genetic variation independent of racial categories. On the road to this ideal, Satel and others characterized race as a useful category of medical analysis. For example, Cohn has explained that "it seems . . . absolutely ludicrous to suggest that this prominent characteristic [i.e., race] that we all recognize when we look at people should not be looked at."[78] Such relatively straightforward and apparently benign invocations of race obscure the critical fact that the real issue is not *whether* to use race in medical research or practice, but *how* to use it.

Satel, Cohn, and others who embrace such "racial profiling" in medicine move from social group to biological group to individual genome. They begin with the assumption that it is useful and legitimate to use social categories of race as "crude markers" to get at biological groups of people who share a common genetic predisposition to a particular disease. After a group is identified, the goal is to proceed to the level of the individual genome to explain disease. Once it is possible to scan individual genomes for genetic variations, the need to refer to the biological group fades away. Without the biological group, the initial surrogate social group—in this case a racial group—is erased as irrelevant to understanding the disease. Here race is cast as epiphenomenal. True difference is located at the material level of the molecule.

This logical progression was captured by Clyde Yancy in an article titled "Does Race Matter in Heart Failure?" Answering his title's question in the affirmative, Yancy went on to assert that

> a group of patients do exist that appear to be at a particular risk for less good outcomes. Currently this group shares the same racial designation, a grouping that is overtly crude and completely arbitrary. What will hopefully emerge, however, are the exact clinical and *genetic descriptors of race* [italics added] that will supercede something as nebulous as skin color and address the more compelling and appropriate physiological traits that put all persons at risk for heart failure.[79]

Yancy's use of the term "genetic descriptors of race" alongside his recognition of racial groupings as crude and arbitrary markers attests to how biomedical researchers may at once acknowledge concerns about the use of race as a biomedical category, while in practice affirming race as an objective genetic classification. Furthermore, his reduction of race to "skin color" evidences a strikingly simplistic conception of the term, given social scientists' longstanding critique of it as unstable, historically contingent, and generally difficult to define in a concrete way.[80]

When a drug such as BiDil gets produced, researchers understand that it works at the molecular level, affecting, for example, levels of nitric oxide in the blood. Nonetheless, a drug company cannot effectively market BiDil to the biological group of individuals who have a particular genetic polymorphism that may lead to lower levels of nitric oxide. Rather, NitroMed marketed BiDil to the social group known as African Americans, because at this point we currently lack the resources or technology to scan every individual's genetic profile. (Even were such technology widely available, no specific genes have been identified to account for BiDil's efficacy.) Furthermore, although many individuals identifying with non-African American racial groups might have some relevant, though as yet unknown, genetic variation, BiDil researchers simply hypothesized that on average, a higher proportion of African Americans had it.

It was far easier for NitroMed to target African Americans than to identify a market of particular individuals who happened to respond well to BiDil because of their genetic makeup and regardless of race. Indeed, the very lack of knowledge about specific genes actually served to create a larger market opportunity for NitroMed. Capitalizing on this "unknown" aspect of BiDil's mechanism of action, NitroMed was able to frame BiDil as a drug for the African American market. A little bit of knowledge might be a dangerous thing, but for NitroMed, it was an opening to create a commercial opportunity. The corporation used the fact of an identified but nonspecific biological difference to create a market based on a social group. BiDil thus illuminates a dynamic whereby *medical researchers might use race as a surrogate to get at biology in drug development, but corporations use biology as a surrogate to get at race in drug marketing.* Thus does the slippage enabled by casual treatment of race as a surrogate for purportedly unknown genetic variation enable corporate strategies for exploiting race in the marketplace.

BIDIL AT THE FOREFRONT OF ETHNIC DRUG MARKETING

The entire marketing model for BiDil, including its presentation to the FDA for approval, was framed by the appeal of personalized medicines tailored to particular individuals or groups. NitroMed capitalized on the wave of enthusiasm for "personally tailored" pharmacogenomic therapies to position its product within a matrix of biomedical discourses and practices.

Its success here was evident in the FDA press release announcing the approval of BiDil, which characterized the drug as "representing a step toward the promise of personalized medicine."[81]

In the emerging field of pharmacogenomics, in which drug companies are hoping to tailor therapies ever more closely to the genetic profile of individuals or groups of consumers, identifying racial or ethnic correlations with disease is becoming big business. The drive to develop race-specific therapies was not subtle, and NitroMed's A-HeFT model of race-specific trials was on its way to becoming a new market paradigm.[82]

B. Waine Kong, CEO of the ABC, was one of four featured "thought leaders" who gave a keynote address on BiDil to a 2005 Multicultural Pharmaceutical Marketing conference.[83] The sponsoring website urged attendees to "find out how NitroMed partnered with the Black Cardiologists Association [sic] to conduct this study [A-HeFT] and understand the opportunities and implications for drug manufacturers, disease management, clinical trials and health care companies."[84] Similarly, NitroMed's chief medical officer, Manuel Worcel, was a featured speaker at the 2005 Bio-IT World Conference and Expo in Boston, where he gave a presentation on A-HeFT as part of the section on "Advances in Genomic Medicine."[85] Additionally, a report on "Cardiovascular Marketing: Budgets, Staffing and Strategy," from Cutting Edge Information, which bills itself as "The World's Largest Market Research Resource," featured BiDil as a teaser to sell the report, which retails for $5,995.[86] As one senior analyst at Cutting Edge put it: "If trials prove successful, and drug responses prove different based on ethnicity, drug companies will certainly have new avenues for the discovery, development, and marketing of medications."[87]

In webcast presentations to the J. P. Morgan 23rd Annual Healthcare Conference and the UBS Global Life Sciences Conference, NitroMed CEO Michael Loberg discussed the company's marketing strategy for BiDil. As part of the rollout for BiDil, the company hired 195 sales representatives through the multinational public relations firm Publicis exclusively to sell NitroMed products. NitroMed used this sales force to focus on those doctors who were providing cardiovascular and metabolic care to

African Americans and was especially interested in "specializing in the African American cardiovascular marketplace."[88]

Even if a distinctive genetic component to BiDil's efficacy were identified (which it has *not*), NitroMed could not effectively market BiDil to the biological group of individuals who have a particular genetic polymorphism that may lead to lower levels of nitric oxide. Rather, NitroMed hired Vigilante, a subsidiary of Publicis, to help market BiDil to African Americans. NitroMed's vice president of marketing, B. J. Jones, described Vigilante as "a leader in the field of advertising and marketing to the African American, minority, and urban communities."[89] The firm also handled the publicity for the noted giveaway of a fleet of Pontiac automobiles to audience members on the *Oprah Winfrey Show*.[90]

Other firms have attempted to emulate the BiDil model in creating distinctive racialized branding for their pharmaceutical products, particularly as a means to distinguish their products (and patents) from similar products in crowded markets.[91] For example, deCODE Genetics explicitly invoked BiDil as a precedent in its pursuit of a race-specific patent. On December 7, 2007, deCODE filed a patent application titled "Susceptibility gene for myocardial infarction, stroke, and PAOD; methods of treatment." Its first claim specified: "A method of prophylaxis therapy for myocardial infarction (MI) in a human, comprising: selecting a human subject having a race that includes *black African* [italics added] ancestry, and administering to the subject a composition comprising a therapeutically effective amount of an MI therapeutic agent that inhibits leukotriene synthesis in vivo."[92] This application was a continuation of an earlier one, filed in 2005. That first application, however, was not race-specific. Its first claim was almost identical to that in the 2007 application, except for the fact that it did not have the phrase "having a race that includes black African ancestry."[93] In the time between the two applications, deCODE published a purported finding of a gene variant that "confers [an] ethnicity-specific risk of myocardial infarction."[94] The study examined variants of the gene *ALOX5AP* (also known as *FLAP*) that encodes a protein known to be associated with risk of myocardial infarction. deCODE also had purchased the rights to a drug, known as Veliflapon (or DG-031) from Bayer, that showed promise in addressing this risk. To test this theory, deCODE began enrolling African Americans for a race-specific clinical trial of Veliflapon in 2006. The trial itself was subsequently suspended due to a combination of technical difficulties with the drug tablet formulation and severe financial problems faced by deCODE as world financial markets collapsed in 2008.[95] Nonetheless, in its patent application, deCODE explicitly invoked BiDil as a model for its race-specific approach both to studying the *FLAP* gene and to developing related biomedical products. Citing the BiDil patent, deCODE's application asserted, "Race-based therapeutics are emerging to treat populations of human patients that are at a high risk based on their race. For example, BiDil (isosorbide dinitrate hydralazine hydrochloride) is currently approved for treatment of heart failure in self-identified black patients to improve survival, to prolong time to hospitalization for heart failure, and to improve patient-reported functional status."[96] The application again cited BiDil as precedent for race-specific diagnostics, also a component of deCODE's product portfolio: "It is well established that different racial and ethnic groups show greater or lesser susceptibility to certain diseases and conditions, and there is at least one drug (BiDil™) that is FDA-approved for race-specific administration. A need exists for improved materials and methods for diagnosing racial or ethnic ancestry using genetic techniques."[97] deCODE was directly attempting to leverage BiDil as a precedent for gaining race-specific patent protection for its products.

A particularly striking example of using race to differentiate a product in a crowded marketplace is the beta-blocker nebivolol, marketed as Bystolic by Forest Laboratories. Beta-blockers are one of the most widely used classes of drugs in the United States. Doctors have prescribed them for decades to treat hypertension and other cardiovascular conditions, such as heart failure.[98] The cardiovascular disease pharmaceutical market is vast and presents great commercial opportunities. Sales of beta-blockers amounted to $2 billion in 2004. In 2009, there were over 128 million beta-blocker prescriptions dispensed in the United States—the fifth largest amount of any class of drugs.[99]

Product differentiation presented Forest with a challenge, because there were already at least eighteen beta-blockers on the market, several available as low-cost generics.[100] In such a market, it might seem unusual for Forest Laboratories to take the time and money to bring yet another beta-blocker to the FDA for approval in 2007. Yet this is exactly what it did with nebivolol, a beta-blocker that had been used in Europe for over a decade but whose original patent holder, Janssen Pharmaceutica, had never sought to bring it to the American market. Forest received approval for nebivolol in December 2007, and began marketing it as Bystolic shortly thereafter. In numerous press releases and discussions of funded clinical research, Forest and its surrogates (including the doctors conducting Forest-sponsored clinical trials) emphasized two key aspects of Bystolic's profile in order to differentiate it from the other eighteen beta-blockers on the market. First, it had fewer side effects—in particular fewer incidences of erectile dysfunction; and second, it worked well in African Americans.[101] This latter claim was particularly significant, because there had been ongoing debate in the medical literature about the relative efficacy of beta-blockers in self-identified African American patient populations.[102] Being able to make affirmative claims about the efficacy of Bystolic in African Americans thus immediately distinguished it from the pack of other beta-blockers.

Forest Laboratories made this claim based on a race-specific drug trial, mimicking in many respects the A-HeFT trial for BiDil, that tested Bystolic exclusively in self-identified African Americans.[103] Drawing another example from NitroMed's playbook, Forest was also able to enlist the support of a prominent African American health organization when it presented the first results of its race-specific trial in 2005 at a meeting of the International Society for Hypertension in Blacks (ISHIB). Following the presentation, the ISHIB issued a press release hailing nebivolol as "just what the doctor orders to control high blood pressure, especially among African Americans."[104]

In reporting the results of this race-specific study, Dr. Elijah Saunders stated, "There is a perception that beta blockers are not effective in blacks. But this study refutes that idea."[105] Paul Underwood, a Phoenix cardiologist and then president of the ABC, praised the study, stating, "We're excited to add another therapeutic tool to the armamentarium in the treatment of high blood pressure in African-Americans."[106] An article on the study in the web-based journal *MedScape Today* quoted Saunders as stating that "The findings of this study are important considering the excessive burden of high blood pressure in African Americans and the need for new treatment options. Advances like this in the beta blocker class are *particularly important because African Americans have a historically poor response to beta blocker therapy for hypertension* [italics added]."[107] The article went on to note that "data suggesting that beta-blockers as a class are less effective than other agents in black patients, as well as the association with poor tolerability and adverse metabolic effects, have *led to underuse of traditional beta-blockers in black patients* [italics added]."[108] Saunders's juxtaposition of efficacy and underuse implies that more blacks should be using beta-blockers but do not. The tension here is that if blacks "have a historically poor response to beta blockers," then lower usage is not "underuse." As framed here, the advance seems to be as much about opening up the beta-blocker market to greater use by blacks as to finding a distinctive new therapy—or rather the distinctiveness of the therapy opens up the market. In this regard, the purportedly poor response of blacks to beta-blockers became a market opportunity.

With its race-specific trial results, Forest was also able to obtain a race-specific mention in its FDA-approved label. Specifically, the clinical studies section of the label states, "Effectiveness was established in Blacks."[109] This distinguished Bystolic from other beta-blockers. So pleased was Forest, that CFO Frank Perier highlighted the race-specific labeling in a presentation to investors at the 2009 UBS Global Specialty Pharmaceuticals Conference, noting that "Bystolic has also in the label been proven as effective in difficult to treat populations such as African-Americans."[110] This distinction, however, was one of labeling, not of established clinical difference. This for the simple reason that other, older beta-blockers were never prospectively tested in race-specific trials that were then presented to the FDA as a basis for labeling. Nonetheless, the race-specific information on the label enabled the dissemination of race-specific information in 1 context of marketing Bystolic.

Commenting on the potential place of race in Forest's marketing strategy, *Medical Marketing & Media* asked, "Does the world need another beta blocker?" It went on to note that "Forest Labs and Mylan say their newly approved ß-blockade drug, Bystolic, is different. According to Charles Triano, Forest vice president of investor relations, setting the new drug apart from traditional beta blockers are its greater tolerability, vasodilating qualities and efficacy in a broader group of patients, including blacks. Those insights are likely to feature in promotions."[111]

Thus, for example, in February of 2008, Saunders gave a presentation to pharmacists in Pennsylvania titled "The Treatment of Hypertension in the Very Tough to Treat Patient (Obese, Diabetic, African-American)."[112] The promotional material emphasized that "Bystolic is a *totally unique and novel* [italics added] Beta-Blocker that is cardio selective and is a vasodilator."[113] Here the promoters of Bystolic linked novelty, difficulty, and race. The presentation frames African Americans as a problem, akin to such undesirable physical states as obesity and diabetes. This critical move associated race with disease. This was different from grouping together African Americans as a population with a high prevalence of diabetes. The latter characterization leaves open the consideration of a wide variety of socioeconomic and environmental factors affecting the etiology of the disease. In contrast, Saunders's grouping marked race itself as akin to the biological condition of disease. Similarly, in 2008, the American Pharmacists Association issued a new product bulletin on Bystolic. After noting that "blacks typically have a poorer BP response to . . . β-blockers," the bulletin highlighted Bystolic's "demonstrated efficacy in black and elderly patients."[114] Such bulletins are used to educate pharmacists on the proper use of new drugs. From the race-specific clinical trial, to the FDA-approved label, to presentations such as the one given by Saunders, to the bulletin, we see a racial frame radiating outward to carve out a market niche for this new drug.

Race was essential to making Bystolic stand out, especially given its much higher cost. Just as BiDil used a racial frame to support its pricing at nearly six times the generic equivalents, so too has Forest relied, at least in part, on race to establish a beachhead for Bystolic, which, at a monthly per-patient drug cost of $30.90, was priced anywhere from 1.5 to 200 times as much as various other beta-blockers, depending on the particular drug and the condition being treated.[115] All this marketing seemed to pay off, as Bystolic had just over $70 million of sales in the first year of launch; this rose to $264 million in sales for the 2011 fiscal year.[116]

In 2008, on a list of the top pharmaceutical advertisers in the country, Forest moved up from number eight to number two. As the trade journal *Medical Marketing & Media* noted, Bystolic, at $8.4 million, was the most heavily advertised drug in the country during the first half of 2008.[117] As Forest rolled out Bystolic, reports of its race-specific efficacy served as a critical adjunct to its general advertising efforts as it was seeking to gain a foothold in the crowded beta-blocker market.

Beyond these examples, a 2008 article in the *Pharmacogenomics Journal* reported on nine clinical trials then underway around the world that were "enriched for race, gender, or both."[118] That same year, officials from the FDA published an article identifying seventeen "currently marketed drugs with labeling that includes specific racial or genetic information intended to facilitate the optimal use of medications in various population groups."[119]

BEST LAID PLANS: THE COMMERCIAL FAILURE OF NITROMED

For NitroMed, BiDil appeared to be a marketer's dream. As the first FDA-approved drug with a race-specific indication, BiDil garnered un-told millions of dollars worth of free publicity as media outlets around the world devoted extensive coverage to its rollout.[120] This promise was real-ized early on, as NitroMed's stock prices more than tripled from about $6.90 per share to over $21 in the week after NitroMed announced the early successful termination of A-HeFT in 2004. The stock price would go on to crest at nearly $29 per share in early 2005 on the run-up to FDA approval.

Following a slight slump, the stock surged again to around $27 in the month after FDA approval when NitroMed announced its pricing scheme for BiDil. From then on, however, it was all downhill, as the actual rollout of the product produced consistently disappointing sales numbers. By the end of 2006, NitroMed's share price was back down in the $6 per share range. In January 2008, as part of a general retrenchment, NitroMed shut down active efforts to market BiDil, while still making it available to patients who sought it out. At the time, the *Wall Street Journal* noted, "BiDil has never come close to initial sales projections. Analysts predicted sales of $130 million in 2006, but actual sales came in at $12.1 million."[121] On September 18, 2008, NitroMed received a letter from the NASDAQ warning that its stock might be delisted from the exchange because it had been trading under $1 for the past thirty days.[122] Later that fall, NitroMed began looking for a buy-out partner to help salvage its business. After a couple of aborted deals, NitroMed announced in January 2009 that it had agreed to be acquired by the private equity firm Deerfield Capital for roughly $36 million. Deerfield planned to continue development of an extended-release form of BiDil, which would make it commercially more appealing by reducing dosages from three times a day to once a day.[123]

What accounts for this meteoric rise and subsequent plunge into obscurity? Many were ready with explanations, all of which were necessarily speculative but also probably captured some of the varied factors that must have contributed to NitroMed's decline. Linda Moussatos, an analyst with Pacific Growth Equities in San Francisco and an early, avid booster of NitroMed, opined in 2008 that the product mostly was hurt by competition from generic components that were readily available at a fraction of the cost.[124] Analyst Robert Uhl, of Friedman Billings Ramsey, suggested that the $15 to $30 co-pay for BiDil "may still represent a financial barrier to patients with heart failure, who are likely suffering from multiple concomitant conditions and taking many medications."[125] As early as June 2006, Kenneth Bate, then CFO of NitroMed, noted that prescriptions were significantly below expectations because NitroMed was having trouble getting "large payers" (i.e., prescription benefit management corporations or PBMs) to put BiDil in the preferred Tier 2 level of coverage, which would lower co-pays. He also identified a need to work more directly with hospitals to get them to place BiDil directly on their own formularies.[126]

The "tier" of coverage granted by formularies was particularly important, because it determined the amount of co-pay the patient would have to bear. A typical formulary tier structure ranges from the most preferred Tier 1 status, which requires little or no co-pay for generic drugs, up through Tier 6 for "specialty non-preferred/non-formulary brand-names," for which the PBM might offer no coverage at all. The Tier 2 status sought by Kenneth Bate covered "preferred/formulary brand name" drugs and carried a significantly lower co-pay than Tier 3 "non-preferred/non-formulary brand name" drugs.[127] One PBM, RegenceRx, rejected Tier 2 status for BiDil after reviewing it in November 2005, finding that "there is not sufficient evidence to conclude isosorbide dinitrate/hydralazine (BiDil) provides superior health outcomes in comparison to currently available forms of isosorbide dinitrate and hydralazine on the Regence preferred medication list/formulary."[128] The availability of generic substitutes combined with the significantly higher price of BiDil similarly led the Veterans Health Administration (VHA) to deny preferred Tier 2 status to BiDil. The VHA also directly challenged NitroMed's claims of cost-effectiveness. Noting that the annual cost of BiDil would range from $1,382 to $2,765 per patient, while the annual cost of comparable generics would range from $45 to $63 per patient, the VHA concluded that if BiDil saved money from hospitalization costs, then the lower-priced generic substitutes would save even more money. In this regard, NitroMed's aggressive pricing strategy for BiDil seemed to have backfired badly. Where NitroMed thought that saved hospitalization costs would support the higher price for BiDil, third-party payors saw even greater savings from substituting generics.[129]

To address such concerns, NitroMed embarked on an aggressive campaign to undermine the perception that generic hydralazine and isosorbide dinitrate could be substituted for BiDil. On April 26, 2006, NitroMed's public relations firm, FoxKiser, petitioned the FDA, asking for a declaration that it had not found any other drugs to be "bioequivalent" to BiDil.[130] A week later the FDA obliged with a letter stating:

FDA has not approved any drug product under Section 505 of the Federal Food, Drug, and Cosmetic Act that is designated as therapeutically equivalent (i.e. substitutable) to BiDil. In addition, neither approved labeling for isosorbide dinitrate drug products nor approved labeling for hydralazine hydrochloride drug products contains information regarding the use of these drug products for the treatment of heart failure.[131]

NitroMed seized on this information in its marketing strategy, posting on its website an entire PowerPoint presentation for doctors titled "There Are No Generic Equivalents for BiDil—the Evidence."[132] NitroMed subsequently conducted a follow-up study to establish that the two different generic combinations of hydralazine and isosorbide dinitrate used in V-HeFT I and II were not bioequivalent to the fixed-dose combination of BiDil used in A-HeFT and approved by the FDA.[133] This was not too surprising, given that the FDA had found much the same in its original 1997 review of BiDil.[134]

What was surprising, or at least inconsistent, in NitroMed's renewed interest in the lack of bioequivalence between the V-HeFT trials and A-HeFT, was the fact that it had avidly touted the data from V-HeFT I and II to the FDA as sufficient to support the approval of BiDil. The gold standard for FDA approval of a new drug is two well-controlled confirmatory studies in which a statistically significant difference has been shown on the primary endpoint in both studies.[135] When NitroMed went before the FDA for approval, they had solid data from A-HeFT, but that was only a single prospectively designed, well-controlled clinical trial. The V-HeFT data on its own had been insufficient to support approval when Medco first went to the FDA in 1997. Nonetheless, NitroMed was able to recharacterize the V-HeFT data—particularly the data from V-HeFT I— as sufficient to constitute the equivalent of a second clinical trial to support BiDil's approval. The FDA signed on to this recharacterization, with Robert Temple later referring to the V-HeFT I and II as "two well-controlled VA studies."[136] One of the great ironies of NitroMed's focus on bioequivalence was that it actually denigrated the data from V-HeFT I, asserting that "the retrospective analysis of black patients in V-HeFT I vas] not directly comparable to A-HeFT," because the improvement seen in V-HeFT I "was based on only 49 . . . patients."[137] Yet, before the FDA, NitroMed had argued that it was precisely these same forty-nine patients who provided the "signal" to look at race in the first place. One might argue that either bioequivalence matters, in which case the "signal" from the V-HeFT trials showing efficacy in African Americans dissolves into insignificance, or bioequivalence does not matter, and generics can be substituted. Again, the logic behind NitroMed's have-your-cake-and-eat-it-too distinction seems to have been a product more of commercial than medical considerations. Less charitably, one might argue it shows how commercial considerations actively skewed the production, interpretation, and presentation of scientific data.

Beyond generic substitution, a study by Frank et al. found a high level of skepticism among medical professionals about the motivations behind BiDil that may also have contributed to low levels of prescriptions. Despite earlier studies showing a general receptiveness among doctors to the idea of race-specific therapies, this study of specific attitudes toward BiDil found that "physicians overwhelmingly voiced concern that commercial considerations shaped the development" of BiDil, and "expressed dismay at what they perceived to be the primary aim of race-specific pharmaceutical trials, namely to get physicians' attention for marketing purposes."[138]

More anecdotally, I have spoken with some physicians who chose not to prescribe BiDil because it was an adjunctive therapy, layered onto a regimen in which their patients might already be taking three or four other drugs. If their patients were stable, the idea of adding an additional drug that must be taken three times a day struck them as a recipe for increasing problems with compliance. Add to this the fact that most believed the much cheaper generic equivalents were valid substitutes, and there was very little incentive to prescribe BiDil.

Then there was NitroMed's own questionable marketing strategy for the drug. Shortly after BiDil's approval, NitroMed's director of marketing, B. J. Jones, spoke to investors about the "buzz" behind BiDil. "I have never seen in all my experience the type of excitement from physicians" over a new drug, Jones effused, noting that studies showed a 96 percent awareness of BiDil among cardiologists. Clearly, Jones believed the "buzz" of free publicity surrounding BiDil would lead the drug to practically sell itself. Jones went on to describe a strategy for working with patient advocates and interested professional associations, such as the ABC, the National Medical Association, the CBC, and the NMHMF, to help promote the drug.[139]

NitroMed also focused on direct-to-consumer grassroots marketing, distributing pamphlets and providing health services at churches in African American communities. One report of early marketing efforts noted that in the first nine months following approval, NitroMed had "been sticking with narrowly targeted, homespun-style pitches." But it also noted that it was trying "to turn around disappointing initial sales that led two top executives to resign."[140] NitroMed suggested that, ironically, part of the problem was that BiDil was approved faster than anticipated. As a result, NitroMed was unprepared to market the drug by itself and had to turn to a contract sales force, which was "not ideal."[141]

Finally, there was the problem of patient trust. Business analysts have noted that "marketing to the black community in the US posed an even greater challenge as the community, in general, was perceived as having distrust toward the healthcare system."[142] One marketing executive noted that "when it comes to addressing the African American community, drug companies and doctors face a steep, uphill battle, and have to be particularly innovative to overcome the well-documented, deeply rooted distrust for the medical establishment that is shared by many blacks within the U.S."[143] Business analysts were not the only ones to raise the issue of trust. While most of the publicity "buzz" for BiDil was positive, an episode of the popular television series *House, M.D.* (about a brilliant but misanthropic doctor) showed an elderly African American man refusing to take a BiDil-like drug because of suspicion that a drug designed for black people could be harmful. "I'm not buying into no racist drug," the character declares. "My heart's red, your heart's red. And it don't make no sense to give us different drugs."[144]

Despite such concerns, in 2004 at least one A-HeFT investigator, Clyde Yancy, explicitly dismissed such history, declaring the infamous U.S. Public Health Service experiments on African American men at Tuskegee, Alabama, as "almost irrelevant now, especially with more blacks and others sensitive to ethical issues and having a voice in 'investigative medicine.'"[145] This casual dismissal of one of the most infamous examples of racist exploitation of African Americans by the United States health-care establishment was framed by the assertion that in the context of BiDil, "health benefits . . . outweigh racial politics."[146] Yancy seemed to be implying that the mere awareness of Tuskegee was enough to transcend its legacy. Memory, here, paradoxically leads to oblivion. He also posited a false dichotomy between health and politics—as if the mere fact that BiDil showed efficacy were enough to trump any concerns about how, whether, or why it was being framed as a race-specific drug.[147] Yet, following BiDil's approval, the FDA committee chair, Steven Nissen, echoed Yancy, asserting, "We were putting [Tuskegee] . . . to rest."[148] Similarly, NitroMed's vice president for marketing told a reporter that BiDil was the antithesis of Tuskegee.[149]

In place of the social history of Tuskegee implicated by the racial politics of BiDil, Yancy, Nissen, and NitroMed would have substituted a natural history of biological difference; the former being "irrelevant," the latter transcending historical patterns of racial subjugation. Yet, as historian Susan Reverby has noted, the basic approach of both Tuskegee and the A-HeFT study shared an underlying logic. Just as Yancy had posited that heart failure was a "different disease" in African Americans, so too had Joseph Earle Moore of Johns Hopkins told a Tuskegee Study physician in 1932 that "syphilis in the negro [sic] is in many respects almost a different disease from syphilis in the white."[150]

The subsequent experience of BiDil and the controversy it engendered seemed to chasten Yancy somewhat. In 2008, he explicitly stepped back from his earlier assertions that heart failure was a "different disease" in blacks, noting that recent studies had shown "when patients with heart failure are treated similarly, African Americans do similarly and perhaps even better [compared with whites]."[151] Reflecting specifically on the experience of BiDil, he also concluded, "My sense surprisingly is that we should not again do a race-based clinical trial."[152] By 2009, Yancy, then president-elect of the American Heart Association, simply asserted, "We need to move away from race quickly."[153]

In the end, all that can be known for sure is that NitroMed failed to realize its dream of dominating the "African American cardiovascular marketplace."[154] BiDil is still available, though not actively marketed, and its commercial prospects could potentially be revived if Deerfield Capital were able successfully to complete development of an extended-release version of the drug.

5

RACE-ING PATENTS/
PATENTING RACE

An Emerging Political Geography
of Intellectual Property in Biotechnology

E MERGING WITH THE rise of racial branding in drug marketing is a powerful new legal and commercial phenomenon that has led to a far more focused and instrumental capitalization of race in biomedicine: the strategic use of race as a genetic category to obtain patent protection. Patent law is supposed to promote the invention of new and useful products.[1] In recent biotechnology patents, race and ethnicity are being exploited in new ways that do not spur the invention of new products, but rather the reinvention or recharacterization of existing products as racial or ethnic. In so doing, patent law racializes intellectual property, transforming it into a terrain for the renaturalization of race as some sort of objective biological category. It also commodifies race as a good to be patented and subject to the dictates of market forces.

BiDil is a clear example of this, but more broadly, a dramatic rise in the use of race in biotechnology and related patents since the completion of the first draft of the human genome in 2000 indicates that researchers and affiliated commercial enterprises are coming to see social categories of race as presenting opportunities for gaining, extending, or protecting monopoly market protection for an array of biotechnological products and services. Racialized patents are also providing the basis for similarly race-based clinical trial designs, drug development, capital-raising, and marketing strategies that extend the implications of constructing race as genetic to ever-widening and consequential segments of society.

Race has long played a role in patents. Legal scholar Shubha Ghosh has documented numerous patents dating back as far as the early nineteenth century that used negative racial stereotypes as part of an invention, often in the form of games or displays. Since World War II, patents with race-specific attributes have been particularly present in the field of cosmetics (e.g., skin depigmentation) and hair care (e.g., hair straightening). Such patents, however, generally did not employ racial categories in the legally operative claims section of the patent, nor were they premised on marking genetic distinctions among races. Rather, they invoked race descriptively in the body of the patent when elaborating upon the claimed invention.[2]

Racialized biotechnology products are also different from other attempts at so-called "ethnic" or "multicultural" niche marketing, which simply aim to sell a variety of products to socially identified racial groups, because they are premised on unsubstantiated understandings of race as genetic. When the federal government grants a patent to an invention that is based on an asserted or implied genetic basis for a particular racial group, it gives the imprimatur of the federal government to the construction of race as genetic. Such an imprimatur opens the door to new forms of discrimination based on genetically reductive conceptions of racial difference.[3]

INTELLECTUAL PROPERTY AS
A SITE FOR RACIALIZATION

Intellectual property law is fully engaged in the pervasive management of genetic material and information. The rush to patent genetic material has implicated existing patent law to a much greater degree than most other areas of law. While many ethical, legal, and commercial implications of patenting human genetic material have been explored at length, little attention has been given to the ways in which social categories of race and ethnicity are increasingly being mobilized in the context of biotechnology patents.[4]

American law has a long tradition of characterizing property and physical spaces in racial terms—often to devastating effect. Whether in the most egregious and obvious form of race-based slavery or in subtler identifications of neighborhoods or even names making it more difficult to obtain mortgages or jobs because of their association with a certain race, the nature and value of property has long been profoundly influenced in and through its association with race.[5] Previous associations of race and property have generally involved a devaluing of associations with racial minorities, while investing whiteness with added value. George Lipsitz has identified what he terms a "possessive investment" in whiteness, which, for much of American history, has provided racially conditioned access to power and resources.[6] In contrast, more recent legal classifications of race, as in affirmative action, have the potential to challenge exclusionary conceptions of racialized property rights.[7] Indeed, since the 1960s, new civil rights and fair-housing laws, combined with the ebb and flow of affirmative action initiatives, have provided American minorities a substantial, if tenuous, "possessive investment in blackness."[8]

BiDil gained cultural capital by its characterization as a means to redress an important health disparity in a historically underserved population. Unlike similar efforts at affirmative action, however, the underlying patents and commercial-market value of BiDil gave new meaning to a concept of a possessive investment in blackness. The health of black people (and others) may ultimately benefit from the drug, but not because of their racial identity. Rather, it was NitroMed, the corporate sponsor of BiDil, that "invested" the drug with race, and it was also NitroMed that aimed to reap the commercial benefits of thirteen additional years of patent protection provided from appropriating race to mark its product.

PATENT LAW BASICS

A patent grants the owner the *right to exclude* others from making, using, or selling the invention for a period of twenty years.[9] This authority derives

Phosita

RACE-ING PATENTS/PATENTING RACE

from the U.S. Constitution, Article 1, Section 8, which states: "The Congress shall have power to . . . promote the progress of science and useful arts, by securing for limited times to authors and inventors the exclusive rights to their respective writings and discoveries." All patent applications must meet several statutory requirements. The most prominent of these are known as "useful[ness]" (or utility),[10] "novelty,"[11] "non-obvious[ness],"[12] and "specification."[13]

The usefulness (or utility) requirement can be met by a showing that the claimed invention has a specific, substantial, and credible utility.[14] Specificity requires the use to be specific to the character of the claimed subject matter.[15] A use is substantial if it involves a real-world use that represents an end in itself.[16] A credible utility is one that would be believable by a person skilled in the field of the invention.[17] The novelty requirement is met if a single reference of "prior art" (e.g., another patent or a published scholarly paper) does not "anticipate" (describe in its relevant particulars) the invention.[18] An invention meets the non-obviousness requirement if "the differences between the subject matter sought to be patented and the prior art are such that the subject matter as a whole" would not be perceived as obvious to a person having ordinary skill in the art (known in patent lingo as a PHOSITA).[19] Specification requires a written description of the invention that is adequate to enable a PHOSITA to make and use the invention.[20]

INTELLECTUAL PROPERTY, IDENTITY, AND THE NATURE/CULTURE DIVIDE

A "product of nature" cannot be patented. The patenting and subsequent commodification of genes (racialized or otherwise) is enabled, in part, by the way in which intellectual property law divorces physical genetic material from its human subject or source in nature. This divorce demarcates the legal boundary between "natural" and "man-made" objects, allowing for the free alienation of genetic material otherwise designated by science

NB

127

patently genes

as constitutive of individual identity. As boundaries between nature and culture are central to ongoing debates about the use of race in biomedicine, considering how legal regimes of intellectual property construct and manage this separation may provide a useful background for approaching broader issues at the intersection of race, law, and medicine.[21]

A gene unencumbered by its original human associations is a patentable gene. It is genetic material that has been stripped of its identity as natural through a powerful combination of legal and scientific interventions. Patent law depends from the outset on marking a product as "made by man," thus demarcating and separating it from the world of nature. In the famous 1980 case of *Diamond v. Chakrabarty*,[22] the U.S. Supreme Court upheld the patentability of a "live, human-made micro-organism" (a genetically engineered, living bacterium useful in cleaning up oil spills). In support of its decision, the court asserted that "anything under the sun that is made by man" may be patented.[23] In contrast, nature is where patents cannot go. The presence of nature in a product may be conceived as a sort of legal pollution. It taints the product and obstructs the entry of patents, and by extension, of the market.

In the realm of biotechnology, engineered organisms or molecules are separated from nature through the concepts of isolation and purification. While clearly scientific and technical in origin, isolation and purification are distinctively legal concepts when it comes to granting a patent. Thus, in response to numerous comments arguing that genes were nonpatentable products of nature, the PTO asserted that "the inventor's discovery of a gene can be the basis for a patent of the genetic composition *isolated from its natural state* [italics added] and processed through *purifying* [italics added] steps that *separate* [italics added] the gene from other molecules *naturally associated* [italics added] with it."[24] The technical process to which the PTO alludes here involves the creation of cDNA molecules. In contrast with DNA found "in nature," which contains large nucleotide sequences that apparently do not code for specific proteins (introns), cDNA is synthesized in vitro by using an enzyme (reverse transcriptase) that produces a molecule containing only those nucleotide sequences from the original DNA that code for proteins (exons).[25]

Sheila Jasanoff observes that "biotechnology . . . renders continually problematic the boundary between the natural and the unnatural."[26] The authoritative discourses of science and law, however, are rendered precarious by such uncertainty. Therefore, those seeking the legal recognition of patentability for biotechnological achievements work hard to resolidify and naturalize the boundary between natural and unnatural. Thus, the PTO recognizes arguments that scientific intervention creates a patentable object by severing it from its natural associations. The PTO constructs cDNA as isolated, not only in the sense of separating exons from introns, but more powerfully, in the sense of separating the genetic material itself from nature. *This is not a scientific process but a legal one.* The scientist may create cDNA, but the PTO draws the line between nature and artifice. Similarly, purification involves stripping the genetic material of its identity as a part of nature—purifying it of its natural associations. Thus stripped of its identity as natural, the unencumbered gene becomes readily susceptible to the creation and layering upon it of a new legal identity as man-made through scientific interventions.

When it comes to biotechnology, the patent process thus does not simply recognize inventions; it plays an active role in constructing and characterizing the substantive identity of those inventions. When it comes to race, this can involve taking social categories of race and according legal status in a patent in a manner that effectively recharacterizes (or "refines") them into genetic categories.

Race enters the world of biotechnology as a social construct, often in the form of OMB Directive 15 classifications. It serves as a surrogate for presumed underlying genetic variations in particular populations. The patent process, however, implicitly recodes race as a genetic category by according it legal force as a component of a biotechnological invention. In cases such as BiDil, the patent and drug approval process produce a transformed understanding of race as genetic when the end product is marketed to the public. BiDil obtained its commodity value from the re-biologization of race in the regulatory process. In the context of gene patents, genetic race literally became a commodity, as the race-specific patent allowed NitroMed to raise venture capital and develop a marketing strategy that ultimately led to the commercial launch of BiDil in June 2005, after FDA approval. In the course of its strategic commodification of race, NitroMed presented a reified conception of African American-ness as genetic to doctors, regulators, and the public at large.

THE RISE OF RACIAL PATENTS

A review of the claims and abstract sections of gene-related patents and patent applications filed since 1976 indicates a significant trend toward using race in gene-related patents with a marked increase in just the past few years (Table 5.1). This rise coincides with both an increase in genetic information being produced through the federally sponsored Human Genome and HapMap projects, and the rising federal emphasis on requiring the use of racial and ethnic categories in the collection of data relating to clinical trials and drug applications.[27]

A typical patent is divided into several sections. The claims section presents a primary focus for investigation, because it is the legal heart of a patent.[28] The claims specify the legally operative scope of the patent, defining the formal, legal "metes and bounds" of the territory covered by an invention.[29] The abstract is the basic summary presentation of the central purpose of the patent. Other sections include the background or description of the invention, plus drawings or other technical support data.[30] A review of the claims or abstract sections of patents that employ OMB Directive 15 categories of race and ethnicity in a manner implying or asserting a genetic component to race is summarized in Table 5.1.[31]

The results indicate a remarkable trend toward the increased use of racial and ethnic categories in relation to patenting gene-related biomedical innovations. The number of references to racial and ethnic categories in gene-related patent applications from 2001 to 2007 is more than five times the number found in issued patents between 1976 and 2007. While there are some overlapping references (e.g., patents that use more than one OMB category), the trend remains strong and tracks the availability of vast new

TABLE 5.1 THE RISE OF RACIAL PATENTS (1976–2007)

CATEGORY	ISSUED PATENTS		PATENT APPLICATIONS FILED 2001–2007
	1976–1997	1998–2007	
Race	0	2	15
Ethnic	0	9	39
African American/black	0	7	14
Alaska Native	0	0	0
Asian	0	1	17
Caucasian/white	0	6	44
Hispanic/Latino	0	3	7
Native American	0	1	14
Pacific Islander	0	0	1
Total	0	29	151

amounts of genetic information being produced and classified in federally sponsored databases. This rise does not reflect that race was not previously used in biomedical research, but rather that it was taking on increasing significance in the commercial world of biotechnology patenting.

A comparison of the use of race in patent applications between 2005 and 2007 (Table 5.2) indicates a dramatic rise in the use of the terms "ethnic" (from two to thirty-nine) and "Caucasian" or "white" (from eighteen to forty-four) that is suggestive of certain emerging conceptualizations of race at work in biotechnology patenting. First, the embracing of the term "ethnic" seems to reflect a broader social move to replace the politically charged terminology of race with the purportedly more neutral concept of ethnicity. Second, as discussed below, the rising use of the terms Caucasian and white may reflect a dawning recognition among researchers (and patent attorneys) that the hitherto largely taken for granted category of white actually constitutes a race that can be made the subject of a patent claim.

TABLE 5.2 THE RISE OF RACIAL PATENTS (2001–2007)

CATEGORY	PATENT APPLICATIONS FILED 2001–2005	PATENT APPLICATIONS FILED 2001–2007
Race	15	15
Ethnic	2	39
African American/black	11	14
Alaska Native	0	0
Asian	13	17
Caucasian/white	18	44
Hispanic/Latino	3	7
Native American	2	14
Pacific Islander	1	1
Total	65	151

THE USE OF RACE IN BIOTECHNOLOGY PATENTS

How exactly is race used in these patents? At the most pragmatic level, patent applicants appear to be invoking race in a strategically defensive manner to provide added protection against possible patent challenges. The structure of a typical claims section of a patent begins with a preliminary claim that is as broad as possible.[32] Successive claims increasingly narrow the patent's focus.[33] Accordingly, if the broadest claim is struck down by the patent examiner or on a subsequent challenge, the narrower claims may still survive. Patent claims are thus structured something like a medieval castle, with an outer ring encompassing the most territory, and successively smaller rings providing additional layers of protection back to the core area of the castle keep.

A patent application for "detection of susceptibility to autoimmune diseases," filed on July 1, 2004, exemplifies the use of concentric rings of race to provide maximum protection for its claims. Its first three claims provide the following:

1. A method for determining an individual's risk for type 1 diabetes comprising: detecting the presence of a type 1 diabetes-associated class

I HLA-C allele in a nucleic acid sample of the individual, wherein the presence of said allele indicates the *individual's* [italics added] risk for type I diabetes.

2. The method of claim 1, wherein the individual is of *Asian* [italics added] descent.

3. The method of claim 1, wherein the individual is of *Filipino* [italics added] descent.[34]

Claim 1 is not race-specific, referring only to an "individual's" risk. Claim 2 takes a smaller subset of humanity, which it marks as "Asian." Claim 3 takes yet a smaller subset of the group "Asian," which it marks as "Filipino." In each case, the applicant clearly links the categories to the HLA-C allele specified in claim 1, forcefully implying a genetic basis to the specific racial groups.[35]

The logic of connecting race and genetics in this context, however, is not driven by science so much as by the commercial imperatives of patent law. The body of this patent application, which generally describes the invention and its background, reviews the scientific literature underlying the claims. In this portion of the patent, which is of less legal significance, the applicant invokes the terms "Asian" and "Filipino" to reference variable distributions of HLA allele frequency across populations. The description section of the patent, for example, compares the incidence of type I diabetes in populations in Japan and China to populations in the United States and Europe. It goes on to discuss the frequency in the Philippines as well. In this context, the boundaries of the racial or national categories are not hard and fast. It is not that "Asians" per se have different genes from "Europeans." Rather, the application notes that there appear to be variable allele frequency and disease incidences across certain populations. Such uses of population categories may remain problematic, but they are not genetically reductive, because they deal with relative allele frequencies that are acknowledged to exist across populations.[36]

By contrast, in the summary of the invention section, the patent states: "The individual can belong to any race or population. In one embodiment, the individual is an Asian, preferably a Filipino."[37] An embodiment refers to the formal metes and bounds of the patent delineated by the claims. Like the claims themselves, the summary sets forth definitively bounded categories that mark specified races as (genetically) distinct.[38] Here, the legal and commercial imperatives of effective patenting have promoted the transmutation of variable genetic frequencies across populations, that nonetheless all share common alleles, into bounded genetic categories that are marked as distinct and functionally different.

Also of note in this patent application is that the category "Asian" is apparently derived from studies only of Japanese and Chinese subjects,[39] thus conflating two national populations with an entire continent. Moreover, there are separate claims regarding Asians and Filipinos, which implies that Filipinos have some distinctive genetic basis that distinguishes them from other populations encompassed by the larger category "Asian."[40] This separate claim was apparently based on a study of ninety Filipinos discussed in the body of the patent.[41]

THE UNSTATED WHITE NORM IN BIOMEDICINE

Many of these patents invoke race when the inventors construct a perceived departure from an unstated white norm (e.g., of disease or allele prevalence) in a nonwhite group. In such contexts, the term "individual" or "human" implicitly stands for "white" in the claims.[42] As legal scholar Rene Bowser notes:

In nearly all racialized research published in the United States, the comparison group has been the majority (White) population. Far from being a neutral category, this approach consolidates Whites as the group with which all "others" should be compared; it also disregards research that demonstrates the value of studying variations in health among, say, Blacks, as opposed to always comparing them with White Americans. The norm in racialized research is and has always been an unspoken but taken-for-granted White norm.[43]

The use of a white norm is particularly evident in one of the BiDil patents. Issued on October 15, 2002, the patent refers in claim 1 to "a method of reducing mortality associated with heart failure . . . in a black patient."[44] Claim 2 goes on to specify "the method of claim 1, wherein the black patient has a less active renin-angiotensin system relative to a white patient."[45] Here, white is the norm from which black deviates. As elaborated in the background of the invention, the patent goes on to assert that "heart failure in black patients has been associated with a poorer prognosis than in white patients. In diseases such as hypertension, blacks exhibit pathophysiologic differences and respond differently to some therapies than whites."[46] Beyond deviation from a white norm, the body of the patent pathologizes blackness as both biologically distinct and less healthy.

Another typical example of the white norm may be seen in a patent application for a "method of identifying a polymorphism in CYP2D6," filed June 5, 2002.[47] The first claim specifies "a method of determining a cytochrome P-450 2D6 genotype of an individual. . . ."[48] Claim 12 specifies "the method, as claimed in claim 1, wherein said individual is Asian."[49] The focus on an Asian individual is explained in the background to the invention, which says "Differences between Caucasians and Asians are explained by an unequal distribution of CYP2D6 alleles."[50] The application asserted different population-based allelic frequencies between Caucasians and Asians; but this is a two-sided difference—that is, each differs from the other. However, it is only Asians that are specified in the claims as a subset of the broader term "individual." Caucasians logically could be put here, but are not similarly marked out. On the one hand, this appears to be a failure of legal imagination to take advantage of an additional defensive claim. On the other hand, it seems to indicate an uncritical assumption that the categories "Caucasian" and "individual" in the first claim were coextensive and that only nonwhite races counted as distinct subgroups to be marked out as the basis for defensive claims.

This patent, like many others, constructed a broad racial category, Asian, out of much smaller subgroups. Further examination of the background section quoted above reveals that the category "Asian" is actually based on a study of allelic frequencies in what the application terms "the Chinese population."[51] Several paragraphs later, it turns out that the Asian-specific claim is based on an analysis of "77 Asian samples."[52] This indicates that samples from seventy-seven individual Chinese people came to stand for the entire population of China, which in turn came to stand for Asia. This sort of extended extrapolation from such limited samples to huge racially marked populations is quite common both in patents and the underlying studies upon which they are based. It appears to be an artifact not only of the dynamics of patent law but also of the tendency to conflate more specific population designators into the broader racial categories defined by OMB Directive 15.

WHAT DOES RACE ADD TO A PATENT?

Racializing patents changes the concepts and dynamics of claims that can be made for, about, or on behalf of race. To assess what race adds, we begin with a consideration of how race interacts with the basic criteria of patent validity: utility, novelty, non-obviousness, and specification.

UTILITY

The requirement of utility is generally regarded as fairly de minimis, demanding only that the invention achieve some sort of pragmatic result.[53] Often, the concept of utility is conflated with marketability—the idea that if someone is willing to pay for it, it must be useful.[54] Nonetheless, it is apparent that invoking race is deemed "useful" by patent applicants, in both the colloquial and formal legal sense of the term. Race is most commonly useful as a defensive claim, adding another ring to the battlements of patent protection. But race can only stand if it is deemed relevant to the invention. It should be contributing some utility to the invention—making it somehow different than it otherwise would be absent race. In many instances, race is not being used as an end in itself, but as a proxy or surrogate for identifying populations that are deemed relevant targets for a particular invention.

A racialized biotechnology patent typically links race to presumed group-based genetic differences underlying different responses to drugs or disease susceptibility. While the patent constructs race as useful, it also invariably constructs it as genetic. Absent the patent advantages it conveys, however, there is often little reason to otherwise use race in a claim. Race is patentable because it is reified as genetic, and it is reified as genetic in order to render it patentable. In a curious tautology, race becomes useful precisely because it is patentable. The primary utility of race, however, is legal and commercial, providing extra layers of patent protection. The tenuousness of race's scientific or medical utility is evident in the more extensive discussions of racial categories in the less legally potent description sections of patents, in which racial categories are often acknowledged to be only rough surrogates for differing allelic frequencies that exist across all populations. To meet the requirement of utility, race must be constructed, at least implicitly, as fixed and stable—as genetic. But, if more appropriately understood as, at best, a tenuous surrogate category ultimately grounded in complex and mutable social understandings, race would not add clear utility to these patents.

NOVELTY

To meet the requirement of novelty, an invention must not be "anticipated" in a single prior art disclosure that contains every element of the claimed invention.[55] Almost any biotechnology invention can be made novel through the simple addition of race. This is apparently what happened in the case of BiDil, where one might well ask how the addition of race, specifically being black, could mark the method of administering the drug as new, when the previous patent for essentially the same method covered all of humanity. The answer seems to be that the previous non-race-specific patent was premised on an unstated white norm that excluded nonwhites.[56] The implication is that identified and articulated blackness is novel because it is not white. More troubling still is the further implication that blackness is somehow not encompassed by a general non-race-specific patent that presumably covers all human beings. Indeed, this was the tacit message sent by the FDA's approval of BiDil for use only by African Americans. The rationale for such approval was that the A-HeFT trials tested the drug only in self-identified African American subjects. This marks the logical extension of the rationale for the underlying patent that drove the design of A-HeFT, which presumes that adding race marked the invention as somehow new and different. Without the implicit logic supplied by the unstated white norm, the BiDil patent, and others like it, would fail to meet the requirement of novelty.

NON-OBVIOUSNESS

The non-obviousness requirement is met if "the differences between the subject matter sought to be patented and the prior art are such that the subject matter as a whole" would not be perceived as obvious to a "person having ordinary skill in the art."[57] Explicitly marked race similarly becomes non-obvious when the unstated norm is white—it being non-obvious that unmarked population groups would contain nonwhites; or rather, it being assumed in retrospect that the unstated white norm did not contain nonwhites. Ironically, this dynamic works in the context of biotechnology patents, in part because of the hard work done by social scientists to mark race as a social category.[58] It is precisely because patent applicants and PTO examiners are willing to accept the obviousness of race as a social construct that race as genetic can be construed as non-obvious, and hence a relevant, patentable use of race in biotechnology inventions. Social race alone is deemed too obvious to be of use to the patent applicant. The description sections of biotechnology patents thus commonly treat race as a social category that acts as a surrogate for genetic variations in particular populations. In contrast, the salient claims sections make more definitive associations between race and genes and are presented as so scientifically sophisticated and distinctive as to be useful, novel, and non-obvious.

To mark out the metes and bounds of a biotechnology patent, surrogate markers and correlations become naturalized into fixed racial categories, thereby producing a previously unarticulated, purportedly genetic component to race. Yet race is not a coherent genetic category; therefore, such uses of race should be insufficient to meet the requirement of non-obviousness.

The patents' implicit construction of social race as obvious is further evidenced by their general failure to provide any substantive definition of the terms "race" or "ethnicity" or to define any of the specific racial categories they use. This stands in marked contrast to the care that is taken in defining certain scientific terms regarding specific chemical compounds or genetic terms employed in the body of the patent.

SPECIFICATION

The concept of "enablement" is at the heart of the requirement of specification. The written description of the invention must be sufficient to enable a person skilled in the art to make and use the invention.[59] Where nonobviousness relies on a previously unseen purported genetic basis for race, enablement relies on the presumed obviousness of race as a social category to facilitate the later use of the invention by other PHOSITAs. For example, a reference to "Asians" or "blacks" or "Caucasians" may be deemed enabling only if those categories are not seen as problematic. They are implicitly cast as merely social and therefore obvious. Social scientific constructions of race as complex, difficult, and problematic categories cannot be allowed to enter this realm, because they would challenge the assumptions underlying the patent's racial enablement.[60]

In so-called "unpredictable arts," such as biotechnology or some branches of chemistry, courts are often stricter in reviewing whether a particular written description of an invention is sufficiently enabling, because small changes to the structure of the invention may lead to vastly different behaviors.[61] For this reason, patent specifications within unpredictable arts must be particularly detailed.[62] Patent applicants must therefore render references to social categories of race as predictable and unproblematic—not a difficult task, given the apparently low level of scrutiny given to racial claims in biotechnology patents.

Yet given the contingent, socially constructed, and temporally variable nature of race, one might argue that race itself should be considered a type of "unpredictable art." Biotechnology, of course, is not an "art" per se. It is a technology whose complexity currently renders it less predictable than more basic mechanical technologies. Thus, the PTO training materials for patent examiners note that a claim covering DNA that codes for a particular protein might require great specificity, because a small change in the amino acid sequence of a protein could result in a very large change in the actual functioning of the resulting protein.[63] The training materials further note that

> before any analysis of enablement can occur, it is necessary for the examiner to construe the claims. For terms that are not well-known in the art, *or for terms that could have more than one meaning*, it is absolutely necessary that the examiner select the definition that he/she intends to use when examining the application, based on his/her understanding of what applicant intends it to mean, and explicitly set forth the meaning of the term and the scope of the claim when writing an Office action.[64]

Racialized biotechnology patents use race, in effect, as a technology of classification. It becomes an essential component of defining the scope of the claimed invention. But it is clear that patent applicants and examiners alike have failed to appreciate the fact that race, too, is uncertain or unpredictable or can "have more than one meaning."

As the Federal Circuit Court of Appeals stated in *Amgen v. Chugai Pharmaceuticals,* "When the meaning of claims is in doubt . . . they are properly held invalid."[65] Neither the examiners nor the patent applicants have taken the trouble to define the racial terms they use, much less consider the highly problematic and uncertain nature of claiming correlations between historically unstable and shifting racial categories and specific genetic or biological structures or processes. In short, both the patents and the examiners generally fail to adequately "specify" race as mandated by 35 U.S.C. section 112.

Proponents of using race in biotechnology patents may invoke commonsense social understandings of race to argue that functionally everybody "knows" what is meant by particular racial categories, and that such categories are therefore enabling. When discussing claims to cDNA sequences in *Regents of the University of California v. Eli Lilly*, however, the Federal Circuit Court of Appeals clearly stated that "a definition by function . . . does not suffice to define the genus because it is only an indication of what the gene does, rather than what it is. . . . Accordingly, naming a type of material generally known to exist, in the absence of knowledge as to what that material consists of, is not a description of that material."[66] As with genes, so too with race: merely naming a race generally known to exist (socially) is not an enabling description of that race. Scientists wishing to claim race in biotechnology patents should be required to exercise the same care and expertise in elaborating definitions of race as they do in elaborating definitions of DNA sequences.

ENABLING GENETIC RACE: THE PTO STANDS UNPREDICTABILITY ON ITS HEAD

Such has often not been the case in practice, as a review of recent patent prosecutions before the PTO indicates its examiners are actually requiring applicants to include racial categories in the claims sections of some of their biotechnology patent submissions. Such claims not only reify race as genetic, they may also form the basis for subsequent research, development, and marketing of products developed from the patent.

The general contours of this phenomenon first came to light in December 2008, at a quarterly meeting of the PTO's Biotechnology, Chemical, and Pharmaceuticals (BCP) technology groups' Customer Partnership. Among the presentations was one by PTO Quality Assurance Specialist Kathleen Bragdon titled "A Look at Personalized Medicine,"[67] which focused on the concept of "enablement." To meet this requirement, the "full scope" of the patent claim must be enabled. The presentation noted that this requirement demands that an examiner reject a patent application if it fails to teach how to make and use the invention as broadly as claimed without undue experimentation. All this is fairly routine knowledge in the world of patents. The presentation, however, moved on to explore its application in the field of personalized medicine by using an example that explicitly implicated race as a requirement for patent approval. As reported by John Aquino of the *Life Sciences Law & Industry Report*, Bragdon went on to present a PowerPoint slide with the claim:

A method for treating a human subject having breast cancer, said method comprising: a) obtaining a nucleic acid sample from said human subject; b) subjecting the sample to PCR and identifying the nucleotide present at position 101 of SEQ ID NO:1; and c) treating the human subject with "breast cancer drug X" when a cytosine is detected at position 101 of SEQ ID NO:1.[68]

The specification in this example did not distinguish the race in the patients tested; it simply assumed "human" to be the relevant category for the invention. The next slide, however, began with the statement, "Prior art teaches that ethnicity is an *unpredictable* factor in single nucleotide polymorphism (SNP) correlation studies," and that studies published after the filing of the patent application indicated that "breast cancer drug X" was ineffective for African Americans. The analysis concluded that because effectiveness for all races was not established, "a scope of enablement rejection *must* be considered."[69] There was a measure of push-back against this conclusion during the question and answer period following the presentation. Some noted that "African American" was a social not biological category and hence an inappropriate basis for rejection, particularly given the increasingly multiracial nature of American society. Another questioner pushed the logic of the conclusion to ask, "What if the data had said that the treatment was ineffective in left-handed Eskimos?"[70]

Following the controversy elicited by the race-specific example, the slides were replaced on the PTO conference website with slides using the phrase "patient populations" instead of race- or ethnic-specific terms. Also, the statement that a "scope of enablement rejection *must* be considered" was modified to "the appropriateness of making any enablement rejection *should* be considered based on the foregoing facts."[71] The use of "population" to replace a racial signifier evidences the first step in the dynamic of recursion, whereby an actor tries to replace a politically charged

racial term with some other more neutral designation that acts as a defini-
tional fig leaf to cover up what persists and later re-emerges as a reinvigo-
rated, biologized conception of race.

Kathleen Bragdon's BCP presentation indicates that race has been entering biotechnology patents not only as a defensive measure or, à la BiDil,
as a means to capture a particular market, but as a response to affirmative
demands placed upon the applicant by the PTO itself. In these cases we
see agents of the federal government themselves requiring the introduction of race into biotechnology patents. The presentation itself involved
only a hypothetical, but a review of some recent patent cases indicates that
in actual practice, PTO examiners are requiring inventors to add race to
their biotechnology patents.

For example, while Bragdon was making her presentation, a case was
pending before the Board of Patent Appeals and Interferences (BPAI) contesting a patent examiner's race-based rejection of an application covering a
method of screening for a gene mutation that indicates an increased risk for
prostate cancer. In that case, the examiner had rejected an application, inter
alia, for failure to enable the full scope of the claimed method because it
"has not [been] shown that the correlation between the claimed mutations
and the risk of both sporadic and hereditary prostate cancers is significant
in all populations."[72] This finding, in turn, was apparently based on the application's disclosure that one of the relevant mutations was found in Caucasians, while another was found in African Americans. For the examiner,
this meant that the same level of risk was not present in all racial populations, hence a lack of enablement. The examiner rejected the patent claims
because they did not differentiate risk by racial group but simply covered
"a method of screening a subject."[73] This is a real-life example of the exact
same logic evident in Bragdon's presentation. The examiner here was denying a patent application for its failure to use race as a genetic construct. In
order to succeed, the applicants would either have to add race in a manner
they did not think valid, or take the time and money to appeal the decision.
In this case, they appealed—and won.

In its March 2009 decision reversing the examiner's rejection of the application, the BPAI found that "it is unnecessary for Appellants to prove

with 100% certainty that a correlation exists between the . . . mutations and an increased prostate cancer risk. It is sufficient that the evidence is 'reasonably indicative' that a correlation is present."[74] It concluded that "it is unnecessary for the claims to exclude all inoperative embodiments as long as the generic invention is enabled,"[75] meaning that the same degree of risk need not be present in all races in order to make a claim to cover the method for use in a generic human subject.

One might hope that this common sense result would send a message to PTO examiners to reconsider their understandings of the place of race in biotechnology patents. Unfortunately, this has not been the case. In April 2010, a similar application rejection was also appealed. In this case, the application claimed a method of screening "a human individual" for genetic polymorphisms that might indicate a "predisposition to atopy" (an allergic hypersensitivity, including such conditions as eczema and asthma). The patent examiner rejected the broad claim to cover a "human individual," primarily because the studies underlying the patent application had been conducted in "Caucasians" and "Asians." The examiner concluded, therefore, that the claim was only enabled as to these specific racial groups and not to humans in general. On June 18, 2010, the BPAI reversed the examiner's decision, noting that the fact that some of the claims "encompass other ethnic groups than Caucasian or Asian does not necessarily render these claims lacking in enablement," and finding that "a claim may encompass inoperative embodiments and still meet the enabling requirement."[76]

Between Bragdon's presentation and the multiple appeals, it is evident that the practice of requiring patent applicants to introduce race into their biotechnology patents has become routinized at the PTO. We might take solace in the apparent readiness of the BPAI to correct this errant behavior. But corrections will only take place if applicants have the wherewithal to continue the prosecution of their patent up through the appeals process. The BPAI opinions, therefore, are just the tip of the iceberg. One must ask how many applicants simply accede to the examiners' demands and incorporate racial categories into their patents in order to avoid the long, drawn-out process of appeal? In this regard, patent number 6,716,581, which presents a method to screen for a genetic polymorphism to help determine susceptibility to colorectal cancer, offers a cautionary tale.[77]

The patent was issued in April 2004, long before Bragdon's BCP presentation. In the original application, filed in April 2001, the first claim read: "A kit for determining whether a subject has, or is at risk of developing, colorectal cancer wherein said kit is used to amplify and/or determine the molecular structure of at least a portion of the MnSOD gene." The application went on to enumerate a total of 35 claims, the very last of which introduced ethnicity, reading: "The method of claim 29; wherein the ethnicity of the subject is Hispanic." (Claim 29 covered individuals under 35 years old.)[78] In this original form, the patent used Hispanic ethnicity, but in a defensive manner, much as the patent discussed previously used the categories of Asian and Filipino. Here, ethnicity seems to have been almost an afterthought, thrown in as the very last claim.

Yet, by the time the application had gone through the prosecution process, the examiner had effectively forced the applicants to reconfigure the patent to foreground ethnicity. As ultimately issued, the first claim of the patent begins: "A method of determining relative age-related risk of colorectal cancer in a Hispanic subject, comprising . . ."[79] The examiner's objections to the early iterations of this application were much the same as those stated by the examiners in the two later applications discussed above, which were successfully appealed. The application was based on a study conducted in self-identified Hispanic men under 35. The examiner rejected several earlier claims, stating that the specification, "while being enabling for methods for identifying increased risk of colon cancer in Hispanic subjects under the age of 35 . . . does not reasonably provide enablement for methods wherein . . . the subjects [sic] is not Hispanic or is over 35."[80] Stating an argument that clearly foreshadowed the logic of the Bragdon presentation, the examiner concluded, "Given the unpredictability in the art of genetic diagnosis, one cannot extrapolate the findings obtained with a single ethnic group to the general population."[81]

Most striking here in the examiner's logic is how she interpreted the issue of "unpredictability" as exactly the opposite of how it should be understood with respect to race or ethnicity. Patent law holds that in the "unpredictable arts," such as genetics, greater specificity is required in the characterization of an invention in order to render it fully enabled.[82] The examiner's idea was that genetic diagnosis is unpredictable and its characterization in an application must therefore be limited to the specific ethnic groups in which it has been tested. This echoes the claim in Bragdon's slide that "ethnicity is an unpredictable factor in [SNP] correlation studies," which meant that correlations varied by ethnicity. But correlations vary across all sorts of categories.

What both Bragdon and the examiner failed to consider is that race and ethnicity are more than just unpredictable "factors" in the realm of genetics; they are, in effect, "unpredictable arts"—that is, technologies of classification—which themselves require specific definition if they are to be enabling. This is because race is not a coherent genetic concept. At best, it is, as NIH Director Francis Collins has noted, a "weak and imperfect proxy" for genetic variation.[83] The examiner's focus on the category "Hispanic" is particularly striking in this context, for, as the eminent biologists Richard Lewontin and Daniel Hartl have noted, it "is a biological hodgepodge. It includes people of Mexican, Puerto Rican, Guatemalan, Cuban, Spanish, and other ancestries."[84] As such, "Hispanic" would probably top any list of population categories deemed "unpredictable" in their genetic implications. Bragdon and the patent examiners operationalize race as itself enabling in biotechnology. They do not construct race as a mere surrogate or proxy for underlying genetic variation; they make race itself the salient basis for constructing material biological difference.

Moreover, the PTO training materials state that when considering a scope of enablement rejection, the burden is firmly on the examiner to "provide evidence or technical reasoning" supporting his or her decision. In the case of race, Bragdon and the other patent examiners simply asserted that in situations in which a study underlying a patent claim was conducted in one racial group, the results could not be extrapolated to cover other racial groups. They provided no evidence or technical reasoning to support this assertion. To the contrary, the assertion was based on a tacit understanding of races as biologically bounded and distinct entities. Perhaps not surprisingly, this sort of flawed reasoning echoes that provided by the FDA in granting a race-specific approval for BiDil: a drug tested in one self-identified race should only be approved for that race. The difference is that in this case, instead of commercial imperatives, federal mandates drove the reductive rendering of race as an unproblematic, fixed, and predictable biological construct.

The applicants for the 2004 patent indicated a sense of these problems when they argued to the examiner that "there is no plausible scientific evidence to support any assertion that Hispanics differ from other groups" with respect to the substance covered by the application.[85] They tried to resist the imposition of ethnicity onto their patent, noting that their choice "to perform their study in Hispanics, an underserved population whose involvement in medical studies should be encouraged, not used to impair Applicants' patent rights." Ultimately, however, they acceded to the examiner's demands rather than go through the appeals process.

The truly chilling aspect of this story is the questions it raises as to how many other applicants have given in to examiners' demands that they include race in their biotechnology patents? How many others have gone against their better scientific judgment to appease an examiner? The implications go far beyond the mere issuance of narrower patents, as such patents can subsequently influence the design of clinical trials, the interpretations of results, and the marketing of end products.

This is not to say that race cannot necessarily be used at all in biotechnology patents, but its use should require genetically relevant specificity of definition and application, something more than mere self-identification—which is a social, not a genetic, definition of race. If race is to have a place in biotechnology patents, it must not be casually imported as a social construct into biological contexts. It could be that the age and ethnicity of Hispanic men under 35 were somehow relevant to identifying the risk of colon cancer, but absent any evidence, this should not be presumed—just as it should not be presumed that because a study of genetic correlations with some other cancer did not include "left-handed Eskimos" its results do not apply to that group. The question is which categories the researchers (or examiners) are choosing to make matter for what purposes. It is quite possible that the BiDil researchers did not enroll anyone in A-HeFT who was under five feet tall. Height is one of the phenotypes most strongly correlated with genotype. But this does not mean that the PTO or FDA should have recognized BiDil only for people over five feet tall. If race (or height) are not appropriately controlled and compared variables, they cannot legitimately be used to make scientific claims—or claims for patenting and drug approval. Rather, to be the basis for any scientific claim, the use of race—by applicant or examiner—must be rigorously defined and must clearly articulate and justify any purported relationship to underlying genetic attributes.

This is much the approach taken by the examiners in the European Patent Office (EPO), who recently rejected an application for a patent covering "Treatment of Hepatitis C in the Asian Population with Subcutaneous InterferonBeta," on the grounds that it "does not clearly define 'Asian race.' Therefore, . . . no meaningful examination of novelty and inventive step appears possible."[86] In coming to this conclusion, the examiner cited recent work by Lewontin along with critiques from social scientists, bioethicists, and lawyers recognizing that "a heated debate on the legal and scientific value of the concept of race and the meaning of race-specific medication was going on."[87] Additionally, the examiner noted that "self identification of a patient as belonging to (one or more?) specific 'race' or not has to be considered vague, since it is highly influenced by specific (and sometimes temporally very contradicting) emotional, social and/or political situation and pressure, as history has shown on several occasions."[88] The EPO's recognition of the complexities of using racial categories in biotechnology patents presents a stark contrast to the U.S. PTO's approach, but it also indicates the legitimate possibility of applying a more nuanced approach to race in the review of racialized patent applications.

SEGREGATED GENOMES AND THE RACIAL GEOGRAPHY OF INTELLECTUAL PROPERTY IN BIOTECHNOLOGY

The introduction of race to the field of patent law as an adjunct to biotechnological inventions is producing a new political geography of intellectual property in which the very metes and bounds of the territory covered by patents are becoming racially marked.[89] As patents are racialized, racial identity itself is becoming a patentable commodity, the value of which is being appropriated to expand market control and extend the market life of products. Generally speaking, however, those capitalizing on race are not necessarily those who belong to the racially identified groups, but rather corporations that are literally "investing" their patents and products with race to gain commercial advantage in the research, development, and marketing of new biotechnology products.

Of course, race has a long history of being commodified in this country.[90] Beyond the most egregious form of chattel slavery, race was also implicitly constructed as a form of property to buttress the Jim Crow laws of the late nineteenth century until *Brown v. Board of Education* struck down the doctrine of separate but equal in 1954.[91] The Supreme Court's decision in *Plessy v. Ferguson* laid the constitutional foundation for decades of Jim Crow laws by upholding an 1890 Louisiana statute "providing for separate railway carriages for the white and colored races."[92] Homer Plessy, a resident of New Orleans, was seven-eighths white and one-eighth black. On June 7, 1892, Plessy bought a first-class ticket on the East Louisiana Railway for passage from New Orleans to Covington, Louisiana, and took a seat reserved for white passengers. He was arrested for violating the separate-car law. As historian Charles Lofgren notes, the arrest "was surely arranged," because, as his counsel later asserted, "'the mixture of colored blood [was] not discernible'" in him—that is, he "appeared" to be white.[93]

Cheryl Harris persuasively argues that a central component of *Plessy* was a dispute over the plaintiff's claim to a property interest in his reputation as a white person.[94] A brief filed by Plessy's attorneys asserted that "reputation is a species of property . . . and is valuable in proportion as it entails rights and privileges, whether social or political."[95] Justice Brown rejected this argument, largely on procedural grounds, asserting that any such claims could be asserted as a matter of civil tort independent of a challenge to the constitutionality of the law and were therefore not the concern of the Supreme Court in this case. Specifically, Brown asserted that

> if [Plessy] be a white man, and assigned to a colored coach, he may have his action for damages against the company for being deprived of his so-called "property." Upon the other hand, if he be a colored man, and be so assigned, he has been deprived of no property, since he is not lawfully entitled to the reputation of being a white man.[96]

This rhetorical gesture, argues Harris, implicitly recognized and protected a property value in "whiteness."[97]

Justice Brown's opinion effectively denied Plessy's claim to property in a reputation as white. If Plessy "be a colored man," he could not claim injury to reputation, because it did not accord with the Court's implicit understanding of the "reality" of race as something fixed and determinable. Nonetheless, the same if-then structure of Brown's qualification of Plessy's claim also raised the specter of racial indeterminacy—that Plessy's racial identity might not be immediately obvious. Thus, in the very act of trying definitively to locate the right to claim possession of whiteness, the majority opinion in *Plessy* underlined the problematic nature of the state's project of forced racial identification.

In a similar dynamic, the background and description sections of racialized patents often acknowledge the indeterminacy of race, a social construct, when used as a surrogate for uncovering underlying genetic differences. But in the legally operative claims sections, such indeterminacy is effaced, and race is naturalized as a fixed genetic category as the patent applicant tries to draw a clear and unequivocal ring of race to defend the metes and bounds of a patent. Such legally sanctioned, reified racial categories draw additional strength from the underlying premise that patents have the power to mark boundaries between the worlds of nature and culture. As a patent legitimizes the use of race as a fixed genetic category, it constructs race as natural and objective. Patentability here is premised on a falsely constructed "discovery" of a mischaracterized connection between two purportedly "natural" phenomena—race and genetics.

As corporations and markets come to attach commercial value to race as a genetic commodity, there will be increased incentives to produce more examples of race as genetic in a commercial context. It is almost as if social categories of race are being used as seed money to produce genetic race as a commodity. Alternatively, social race may here be viewed as analogous to a sort of raw material that the patent process refines—that is, purifies and strips of its *"social associations"*—into a "novel" and "useful" manufactured product composed of genetic race. In patenting race, biotechnological inventions actually produce (or reproduce) race as genetic.

Much recent genetic research on population structure across populations literally identifies and segregates distinct blocks of genetic material on chromosomes with particular ancestral groups. These studies generally share the common tendency in biomedical studies of population to fall back onto traditionally racialized population groups, such as European, African, and Asian. The chart of chromosome admixture from an article on "Mapping Genes That Predict Treatment Outcome in Admixed Populations" in the *Pharmacogenomics Journal* is fairly typical of the technology and approach (Figure 5.1).[98]

The chart itself refers genetically to chromosomes from "ancestral populations," but the body of the article discusses, for example, "the admixture between geographically isolated populations such as Europeans, Africans and Native Americans." The framing of Europeans and Africans as "geographically isolated" is particularly striking, given common and fairly extensive contacts between the continents since antiquity, and outright colonization dating back to the seventeenth century. Nonetheless, the chart presumes "pure" and distinct racially marked ancestral chromosomes at some time in the past that became mixed over the generations, yet are susceptible to being disaggregated (or segregated) by original racial identity through analysis of ancestry informative markers. Unlike many such articles, the authors here actually provided a definition of race—a genetic definition: "The term race (often used to imply geographic or genetic ancestry) reflects population clusters based on genetic differences due to evolutionary pressure."[99]

The article is also an example of the problem of racial recursion, as it derives much of its data from the HapMap project, which it describes as "an important resource in the selection of markers for the characterization of complex traits such as drug outcome."[100] It will be remembered that the

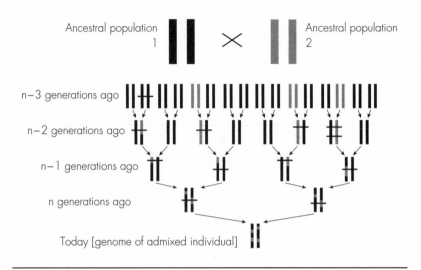

FIGURE 5.1 Chart of genetic admixture.

HapMap project itself took great care to characterize its samples with great local specificity (such as 90 Yoruba from Ibadan, Nigeria) so as to avoid the improper racialization of its genetic database. Yet the authors of the *Pharmacogenomics Journal* article not only racialized the samples, they used them as a basis for racially segregating genomic territory at the molecular level.

The segregated genome of biotechnology patents may be compared to the legally managed production of racially identified neighborhoods in residential communities. Legal scholar John Calmore refers to the "racialization of space" as "the process by which residential location and community are carried and placed on racial identity."[101] Through a series of legal and regulatory interventions, ranging from racially restrictive covenants to zoning laws and sanctioned red-lining, specific social and residential spaces have become racially marked and segregated over time.[102] Calmore hypothesizes that for whites, "the compoundness of race and space . . . is taken for granted; white space is not problematic and black space is somewhere else. For whites, the broad notion of housing simply does not present the problems that it has for blacks."[103] In a similar manner, those who submit racialized patents to the government for approval are using the legal system to inscribe portions of the genome (usually identified as areas of differing al-

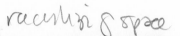

lelic frequency) with distinct racial identities. Thus, for example, while the description section of a patent may assert that a particular allelic frequency is lower or higher in Asians, the claims section will definitively mark that segment of the genome as Asian. Such inscription, in effect, creates a segregated genome with black, white, Asian, Hispanic, etc., neighborhoods.

Patents exploit such racialized neighborhoods of the genome to literally capitalize on race. Unlike residential segregation, biotechnology patents have the added convenience of being able to make use of racially marked genes without having to deal with the troubling presence of actual human bodies. Living individuals who share the racial identities being exploited in biotechnology patents would likely have no more success in challenging such patents than individuals who have objected more broadly to patents covering any human genetic material as an affront to human dignity or as an impermissible commodification of the common heritage of humankind. This is for the simple reason that, like other human gene patents, the actual personal DNA of such concerned individuals would not be at issue, and the patent system is unlikely to acknowledge a more amorphous claim to appropriation of racial identity in the context of biotechnology patents.

In the political geography of biotechnology patents, race becomes a statistical concept based on molecular correlations and frequencies—not on the embodied experiences of actual people walking in real time through physical space. Traditional legal schemes of embodied segregation in the United States were based on the concept of "hypodescent," in which "one drop of blood" was sufficient to consign a living person to the marked racial category of "black."[104] In the new, statistically informed legal schemes of biotechnology patents, it is "one drop of correlation" that provides the basis for making claims that segregate the genome into racially identified neighborhoods—the slightest correlation of variable allelic frequencies with particular racial groups racializes the alleles, which in turn geneticizes race. Some of these racial neighborhoods may be marked as genomic ghettos, areas associated with blight, disease, or weakness. But, as with contemporary dynamics of urban gentrification,[105] a blighted neighborhood may also present a distinctive opportunity for development—as NitroMed discovered with BiDil.

Genomic segregation thus keeps races separate in order to develop and market products. It manages relations among haplotype blocks and SNP frequencies, rather than housing patterns or school enrollments. The racialized patent divorces race from the body, reducing it to a function of correlation and allelic frequencies. Thus molecularized, race is more readily susceptible to scientific and commercial manipulations to appropriate its value in a manner that both naturalizes it as genetic and inhibits interference from living individuals who represent embodied claims to a particular racial identity.

We may take the racial characterization of neighborhoods for granted, just as we take the social meaning of race for granted. Bureaucrats at the PTO and the FDA generally cast themselves as mere transparent reviewers of the information provided to them by applicants. Their acts are largely viewed as reactive and constructed as autonomous of independent political significance. The applicants, in turn, use the legal regime of intellectual property to, in effect, zone the genome into racially identified neighborhoods in a manner that goes unchallenged and, indeed, unnoticed.

Legal scholar Richard Thompson Ford, however, argues that the perception of space as neutral rather than as political maintains and perpetuates segregation. He argues in particular that "political space does the work of maintaining racially identified spaces, while reified political boundaries obscure the role of political space and represent it either as the delegation of state power and therefore inconsequential, or as natural and therefore inevitable."[106] In the context of biotechnology patents, race itself is also viewed as either opaque or transparent. Opaque race is genetic race. It is reified as complex, pre-political, and natural. Transparent race is social race. It is implicitly devalued as obvious and hence constructed as irrelevant or at most instrumental to the assertion of a racialized patent claim. Such a construction of race creates and perpetuates the genomic segregation necessary for pseudo-pharmacogenomic, race-specific product development emerging in the gap between today's biomedical realities and tomorrow's promise of truly individualized medicine.

The racialized spaces of biotechnology patents provide a basis for directing the flow of capital to the patent holders. In cases such as BiDil, racial marking made the neighborhood of the patented biotechnology more valuable. Significantly, however, the added value provided by race is appropriated by the patent holder—the landlord, so to speak—rather than by the community whose race has been commandeered into the service of producing the relevant product. Indeed, to the extent that a patent is conceived of as a right to *exclude* others from use of a particular invention, a racialized patent gives the patent holder the right to exclude members of the identified races from access to or control over the terms through which the patent process appropriates and commodifies their racial identity. Patents place the refinement of race from a social into a genetic category, beyond the reach of the implicated racial communities.[107]

CONCLUSION

The implications of the striking rise of race in biotechnology patents have yet to fully develop. Federal mandates and intellectual property law have played a central role in shaping the production, classification, and circulation both of genetic data and racial categories in biotechnology research and product development. Racialized patents are coming to play a central role in biotechnology research, development, and marketing. Adding race to the patents does not change the technology, so much as it provides an added incentive to market and extend monopoly control for the product. These examples provide a model for transforming what may have initially been a defensive use of race in patent protection to affirmative projections of race as a central component of product development and marketing.

Cases like BiDil are paving the way for a proliferation of applications producing new, highly problematic understandings of race as genetic. BiDil obtained its commodity value from the re-biologization of race in the regulatory process. Additional racial patents, for products not yet as prominent as BiDil, have secured regulatory imprimatur for using race as a genetic category. Like more traditional extractive industries, biotechnology corporations are mining the raw material of race as a social category and using the patent process to refine it into a natural construct, lending legal utility and novelty to their inventions. The patents are in place and proliferating, ready to be invoked to protect a product or extend a market. In the context of gene patents, genetic race is becoming a commodity, as race-specific patents allow biotechnology corporations to raise venture capital and develop marketing strategies that present a reified conception of race as genetic to doctors, regulators, and the public at large. In the process, racialized biotechnology patents are also marking neighborhoods of the genome with racial identities as they both produce and appropriate a new genetic commodity value in race.

6

NOT FADE AWAY

The Persistence of Race and the Politics of the
"Meantime" in Pharmacogenomics

N 1878, Friedrich Engels famously wrote that on the road to realizing
the communist utopia, "the state is not abolished, it withers away."[1] In a
similar manner, biomedical researchers tell us that come the promised
land of individualized genomic medicine, the need for using race will also
"wither away" in the face of scientific progress. Such millennial hopes are,
no doubt, sincere, but they enable the continued casual proliferation of racial
categories throughout biomedical research, product development, marketing, and clinical practice. My contrasting quotation to frame this chapter is
drawn from the twentieth-century pioneer of rock and roll, Buddy Holly,
whose 1957 hit "Not Fade Away" begins with the line, "I'm a-gonna tell you
how it's gonna be";[2] the point being that far from withering away, race is
persisting, even as genomic milestones are being reached and passed. In
short, despite biomedicine's promises to the contrary, race will "not fade
away" of its own accord, even as the science of genetics progresses.

This chapter is concerned with what may be happening to race and
medicine in the "meantime" between today's clinical realities and the
promised land of pharmacogenomics. It argues that previous debates over
the use of race in medicine are being sidestepped as race is being reconfigured from a "crude surrogate" for genetic variation into a purportedly viable placeholder for variable drug response—to be used here and now until

the specific genetic underpinnings of drug response are more fully understood. Embracing the trope of "promise" in pharmacogenomics alongside the idea of using race as a useful interim proxy for genetic variation raises concerns that new diagnostic and therapeutic interventions may reflect or be mapped upon existing social categories of race, class, gender, and ethnicity in a harmful or dangerous manner.[3]

Race is gaining renewed legitimacy as an interim measure on the road to individualized medicine. I begin with a brief general examination of how race is persisting in biomedical research, giving particular consideration to how the concept of the "unknown" is used to create a space for race as a genetic construct. After marking the power of the concept of race as a stepping-stone in biomedical research, I move on to explore the case of the widely prescribed blood-thinning drug warfarin (marketed by Bristol-Myers Squibb under the trade name Coumadin), which involves the persistence of race, even as specific genetic variations directly tied to warfarin response are being identified.

Following upon my earlier discussions of the influence of legal mandates on the use of race in biomedical research and product development, I argue here that race is persisting for an additional three reasons. First, race is evolving into a "residual category" that is being used to explain any variation in drug response not captured by specifically identified genetic or social factors. Genetics will never explain 100 percent of variable drug response, because many complex environmental, dietary, and behavioral factors also affect drug response. There will always be an unknown aspect to drug response, therefore there will always be a potential use for race as a category to catch this residuum of unexplained variation. The problem comes with the tendency of researchers to geneticize this racial residuum simply because they cannot locate specific nongenetic factors to account for variation. Second, as is particularly evident in the case of warfarin, there is an inertial force to race in biomedicine. Once introduced into a conceptual system for evaluating biological difference, race is very difficult to dislodge. It becomes part of the common sense of biomedical practice and continues to be used almost reflexively—not least because the array of federal mandates requires biomedical research to gather and classify data by race. Third, beyond the case of BiDil, race continues to have a commercial value both as a means to differentiate products in a crowded market and in contexts in which it is more viable to market products to racial and ethnic groups than to individuals with particular genetic profiles.

"WHY RACIAL PROFILING PERSISTS IN MEDICAL RESEARCH"

Aug 2009 Time

In August 2009, *Time* magazine published a story titled "Why Racial Profiling Persists in Medical Research."[4] The article is not remarkable for any particularly new insights but stands as a prominent example of a type of reasoning that typifies a powerful strand of current discourse about race, medicine, and genetics. Curiously, the article began with a reference to Harvard professor Henry Louis Gates Jr., who had been arrested on his front porch the previous month by a Cambridge police officer. Gates is one of the country's most prominent African American intellectuals. The officer had responded to a call from a passerby who had seen Gates and another black man seeming to force their way into the house. It later turned out that Gates had just returned from a trip to China, found the front door to be stuck, and asked the driver to help him force it open. The officer arrived on the scene after Gates had gained entry. Gates showed the officer his identification and explained that it was his home. Gates took umbrage at being questioned in his home, allegedly shouting, "This is what happens to black men in America." A loud argument ensued, which continued onto the front porch, and finally the officer arrested Gates for disorderly conduct. Shortly thereafter, President Obama caused a furor when he referred to the Cambridge Police Department's handling of the affair as "stupid." The famed "beer summit" ensued, with President Obama, together with Vice President Biden, hosting Gates and the arresting officer for a reconciliatory beer at the White House.[5]

The article's brief reference to this event was used to juxtapose racial profiling as a "social" practice versus racial profiling as a "scientific" practice. The former was clearly understood as "bad," while the latter was presented ematic but potentially useful. This established the frame for the ...ιc article, which focused on the publication that July of a study by Kathy Albain et al. in the *Journal of the National Cancer Institute* (*JNCI*) involving a meta-analysis of data from more than 19,000 patients who participated in clinical trials involving treatments for a variety of cancers.[6] As presented by *Time*, the major finding of the study was "that *all other factors being equal* [italics added], black patients had on average a significantly lower cancer survival rate than whites."[7] The article took this finding as emblematic of a strain of biomedical research whose use of racial categories was "borne out in studies that attribute health disparities between blacks and whites not to socioeconomics or access to health care alone but also to genetic differences between the races—a concept that implies that a biological category of race exists." The article went on to compare this study to the sorts of race-specific claims made in relation to BiDil.[8]

The article is premised on the idea that when "all other factors" are held equal, observed racial differences in cancer are likely due to genetics. Being genetic, these "differences" are not "disparities" implicating socioeconomic forces. By implication, such purported genetic differences require biomedical interventions at the molecular level but do not require policy interventions to address questions of equity or social justice.

What, then, are these "other factors"? If we look at the actual article published by Albain et al., we see that its conception of "other factors" is encompassed by "estimates . . . derived from education category and income level as assessed by the linkage between patient zip code and the US census data."[9] This is different from, but perhaps even more flawed than, the limited controls for socioeconomic status in the Exner et al. study of racial difference in response to ACE inhibitors that framed the rollout of BiDil. As subsequent critical letters to the *JNCI* pointed out, Albain et al. presented a remarkably thin and fundamentally flawed approach to controlling for nongenetic factors. One joint letter from epidemiologists at the CDC, Duke University, and McGill University pointed out several particularly glaring flaws "rendering [Albain et al.'s] adjustments inadequate and their conclusions therefore unsupported." First, they noted that as long ago as 1998, a study had shown that using "zip code–level socioeconomic status proxies . . . for individual-level socioeconomic status" was inappropriate and misleading (essentially conflating group statistics with individual attributes); second, the article Albain et al. cited as a source for using such census data actually "proposes that aggregated statistics be used for monitoring disease trends and not that they be used for individual-level control in racial disparity studies"; and third, even by Albain and colleagues' own account, "the socioeconomic status data were missing for between 27% and 79% of subjects depending on the clinical trial."[10] Another letter to the editors noted that "Albain et al. provide no information about how they measured the central variable: race. This omission makes it impossible to disentangle the many behavioral, environmental, or genetic influences on cancer mortality that may be associated with race."[11]

Albain and coworkers' flawed approach to controlling for "all other things" was essential to creating the space for genetics to enter into the characterization of racial difference. As Albain told *Time*, "something big is going on among people who are getting equal care"; that something, the authors concluded, "must be some unknown biological or genetic factor that differs by race."[12] The "unknown" was central to the dynamic of geneticizing racial difference. The logic here is similar to that invoked on the road to BiDil's race-specific approval by the FDA: first, observe a biomedical racial difference (response to a drug or experience of a disease); second, "control" for nongenetic factors (conveniently reducing these to income and education or some even more flawed identification with census data); third, attribute any residual racial difference to genetics (even though you have no specific genes identified). Voila! A genetic basis for race.[13]

Albain, however, claimed that race was merely a surrogate for unknown genes. "When we find out what the [genetic] 'it' is," she asserted, "we will be able to test everyone for 'it' and we will find some Caucasians who have it and some blacks who don't and we won't be talking about black and white anymore." Albain here adopted the familiar trope of race as merely an interim measure, to be used as a proxy for genetics in the "meantime" until we reach the promised land of genomic medicine, where race will "wither away." In this approach, however, rather than questioning their limited use of socioeconomic controls, the authors used race as a residual category to capture and geneticize all "unknown" causes of racial difference. As epidemiologist Jay Kaufman noted in criticizing the *JNCI* study, "If you are trying to make the argument that [different health outcomes] must be genetic by exhausting other possibilities and saying what is left over must be genes, well, that's never going to work. There are a million things that affect people's lives. If you think it's genes, then measure genes."[14]

Albain and colleagues' approach is all too common. Many studies dismiss sociocultural and environmental variables in a similarly offhand way.[15] Given the complexity of interactions among human biology, behavior, history, society, and the environment, there will always be some causes of biomedical differences correlating with race that remain "unknown" and susceptible to being geneticized. As long as biomedical researchers give short shrift to sociocultural variables, there will continue to be a place for a flawed genetic concept of race long after the promised land of individualized pharmacogenomic medicine is reached.

STEPPING-STONES AND THE UNKNOWN

The productive power of the unknown to create a space for race is clearly evident in a 2008 article published by Robert Temple, Director of the Office of Medical Policy at the FDA's Center for Drug Evaluation and Research, and his colleague, Shiew-Mei Huang, of the Office of Clinical Pharmacology. Discussing the role of genes and race in predicting drug response, they cited a range of currently marketed drugs that included race-specific or genetic information on their labels and noted,

> Some of the observed racial differences may be explained by the *genetic* differences listed in the labeling (e.g., warfarin and carbamazepine). Possible mechanisms for others either have not yet been included in labeling (e.g. rosuvastatin and tacrolimus) or are as yet *unknown* (e.g. isosorbide dinitrate-hydralazine [H/I], which is effective in heart failure in *black* patients [italics added]).[16]

Temple and Huang bind together race, genes, and drugs through the concept of the unknown. In the examples of warfarin and carbamazepine, race was being used to identify differing allelic frequencies across population groups. Yet in the case of H/I, race was simply being used to account for an otherwise unexplained observation of purported difference in drug response across racial groups. All were deemed legitimate references by the FDA. As long as there is an unknown, there will be a space for race, or so it seems here.[17]

The H/I combination referred to by Temple and Huang is, of course, BiDil. Steven Nissen, the chair of the FDA panel reviewing BiDil, directly cast race as an acceptable surrogate for genetics,

> What we are doing is we are using self-identified race as a surrogate for genomic-based medicine and I don't think that is unreasonable. I wish we had the gene chip. I wish we could do it on a genetic basis. But, in the absence of that, we have some information that suggests that African Americans—we know that African Americans, self-identified, get a pretty robust response to the drug.[18]

Nissen related race to "some information," but its true justification came from its purported ability to stand in for the unknown underlying genetics of drug response. Until adequate genetic technology came along, Nissen deemed race sufficient and therefore to be embraced.

Similarly, on the eve of BiDil's approval, Lawrence Lesko, Director of the Office of Clinical Pharmacology at the FDA, and a point man in the FDA's efforts to integrate genomics into the drug-approval process, asserted that race-based medicine could be a "stepping stone" to the higher goal of "target treatment."[19] As one news report put it: "Lesko and other advocates of this approach envision treatment tailored to people according to the results of genetic tests. They say that race-based medicine is just a first step toward discerning people's genetic makeup for the sake of better individual treatments."[20]

Lesko defused myriad controversies surrounding BiDil by casting race-based therapies as mere stepping-stones. Any problems created by using race in a biological context (e.g., the reification of race as genetic, the perpetuation of racial stereotypes that cast one race as more biologically "fit" than another, or concerns about the misallocation of scarce health-care dollars) were minimized as temporary and a small price to pay for the ultimate goal of "better individual treatments."

The advocates of race-based medicine might even concede the point that race is a crude surrogate for genetic or other biological variability and yet still use it. Thus, Temple and his FDA colleague, Norman Stockbridge (both involved in the approval of BiDil) declared, "Race or ethnicity is clearly a highly imperfect description of the genomic and other physiologic characteristics that cause people to differ, but it can be a useful proxy for those characteristics until the pathophysiologic bases for observed racial differences are better understood."[21]

Similarly, the year after BiDil's approval, the *Journal of Clinical Pharmacology* published an article on "Race and Ethnicity in the Era of Emerging Pharmacogenomics" asserting, "As the science of pharmacogenomics develops more accurate tools to identify the molecular underpinnings of drug response, the need for classification by race will be replaced by more accurate and specific identification of each individual person's likelihood of responding to a particular drug therapy."[22]

Such instrumental characterizations construct race as a useful fiction, a means to an end that is to be discarded once its temporary utility has faded. As a "meantime" solution, race is presented as only temporarily genetic. Genes are layered onto race (or race is layered onto genes), "just for now," until something better comes along. Then, presumably, the two will be disentangled, each allowed to go its own separate way. No provision, however, is made for such disentanglement; rather, in this grand march forward to pharmacogenomics, race, like Friedrich Engels's state, is supposed to "wither away."

Some biomedical professionals take issue with this approach. One recent study by Yen-Revollo, Aumen, and McLeod specifically considering the legitimacy of using race as an interim surrogate for genetic variation found that "racial generalizations for treatment recommendations are not valid,"[23] and concluded that "race should not be used as a predictive substitute for individual patient genotyping."[24] Significantly, even as it debunked the legitimacy of using race as a surrogate, the study also considered its appeal:

> The promise of personalized medicine has not been realized as of yet because personal genotyping is *cost prohibitive* and most drug-genotype interactions remain *unknown*. Since individual causative alleles usually have distinct frequencies across the "Old World" populations, *there is potential utility in using race labels as a surrogate for genetic information, as a means to the ultimate goal of individualized therapy* [italics added].[25]

In this scheme, cost and the unknown are the operative factors leading toward the use of race "as a means to the ultimate goal of individualized therapy." Theoretically, as costs come down and knowledge grows, the need for race will diminish. Yet means have a curious way of devolving into ends, and stepping-stones may somehow remain underfoot long after a particular destination has been reached. So it appears to be with the unfolding case of warfarin in pharmacogenomics.

WARFARIN: THE POSTER CHILD

In 2009, the FDA declared warfarin to be a "pharmacogenomic opportunity."[26] As one leading warfarin researcher had recently noted, "Warfarin is the ideal drug to test the hypothesis that pharmacogenetics can reduce drug toxicity: it is commonly prescribed, has a narrow therapeutic/toxic ratio, and is affected by common genetic polymorphisms."[27] Similarly, in January 2009, after he stepped down from his post as director of the NHGRI under President George W. Bush and before his later elevation to director of the NIH by President Barack Obama, Francis Collins noted that warfarin "has become a poster child for the future of pharmacogenomics."[28]

Warfarin, an anticoagulant, is among the most widely prescribed drugs in modern medicine. In 2004, more than 30 million prescriptions were written for the drug in the United States alone.[29] Sales of warfarin in the

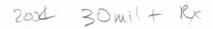

United States were approximately $500 million in 2002.[30] There was a 1.5-fold increase in warfarin prescriptions between 1999 and 2005, perhaps reflecting the demographic shift toward an aging population, which is typically a primary target of warfarin therapy.[31] It is commonly prescribed to patients who are at risk of developing blood clots, such as persons with atrial fibrillation, recurrent strokes, deep venous thrombosis, or pulmonary embolism, or those who have received heart valve replacements. It is difficult to calibrate the right dose for an individual patient, because warfarin has a narrow therapeutic window of efficacy and a wide range of interindividual variability in response. Finding a correct dosage can be a delicate matter, involving the gradual upward titration of an initially low dose with regular monitoring of the coagulation rate using the international normalized ratio (which compares the blood's clotting ability at a given moment to a standardized measure) and adjustment of the dosage until the appropriate rate of coagulation is obtained. Too much warfarin places a patient at risk of a potentially fatal hemorrhage, while too little may increase a risk of blood clots and stroke.[32] The complexity of warfarin dosing is indicated by the fact that warfarin is the second most common drug (after insulin) implicated in emergency room visits—causing more than 43,000 emergency cases per year.[33]

A variety of factors can influence individual response to warfarin, including dietary intake of leafy green vegetables, alcohol consumption, age, weight, and liver function. In addition, the current label lists approximately 130 specific drugs reported to interact with warfarin.[34] For many years, researchers have also observed population-based variation in response to warfarin associated with different races or ethnicities—particularly "Asian" or "east Asian." That is, studies have observed that on average, subjects identified as Asian may tend to have a different response to warfarin than subjects identified as belonging to different races, particularly "Caucasian."[35] Based on such observations, the FDA-approved label for Bristol Myers Squibb's brand-name warfarin, called Coumadin, states, "Asian patients may require lower initiation and maintenance doses of warfarin."[36] Race, then, has long been a part of the clinical conceptualization of warfarin response. It was widely assumed that a significant proportion of such variation was likely due to differing frequencies of certain alleles that affected drug response. In the absence specific information relating to such alleles, race was presumed to be a reasonable surrogate to finding the right dose of warfarin.[37] As one 2005 study concluded, "Warfarin dose requirements vary across ethnic groups even when adjusted for confounding factors, suggesting that genetic variation contributes to interpatient variability."[38] As in the article by Albain et al., "other factors" again created a space for geneticizing racial difference.

In the past decade, great strides have been made toward identifying specific genetic variations that have a significant impact on individual response to warfarin.[39] In particular, specific polymorphisms in the *CYP2C9* gene and *VKORC1* gene have been identified as accounting for 30 percent to 50 percent of variation in individual response to warfarin.[40] *CYP2C9* affects pharmacokinetics, or what a body does to a drug. People with certain *CYP2C9* alleles metabolize, or break down, warfarin more slowly than average—those people would need a lower dose of warfarin. *VKORC1*, in contrast, involves pharmacodynamics, or what a drug does to a body. It affects the production of vitamin K, which is vital to blood clotting. Warfarin works, in part, by suppressing the production of vitamin K. Individuals with certain *VKORC1* alleles might also need a lower dose of warfarin.[41] Each person has two copies of each gene. Carriers of two *CYP2C9*1* alleles, known as the *wild type* or standard type, are extensive metabolizers of warfarin. The two most common relevant *CYP2C9* variants are referred to as *CYP2C9*2* and *CYP2C9*3*.[42] The most common relevant *VKORC1* variant is referred to as *VKORC1 3673(1639G > A)*.[43] These variants have become particular targets for genetic testing.

With the proliferation of genetic data, one might think that race would cease to play a significant role in studies of warfarin response. Yet, as genetic studies grew in number, so did the use of race and related categories to assess variable frequencies of particular polymorphisms in specific population groups. Numerous studies observed that some relevant *CYP2C9* and *VKORC1* alleles vary in frequency across certain ethnic or racial groups.

Usually these studies employed such broad categories as Asian, Caucasian, Hispanic, or African American,[44] but some studies were more nation-specific, identifying allelic frequencies and response, for example, in Swedes, Koreans, Iranians, Japanese, and Israelis.[45]

Ironically, even as the significance of specific genetic variations has been more fully elaborated and characterized, there seems to have been an increase in such racial, ethnic, or nation-specific studies of allelic frequencies. In recent studies of the impact of genetics on warfarin response, it seems to have become an unstated norm to characterize gene frequency with reference to whatever racial, ethnic, or national group in which the study happened to be performed. For example, a report on warfarin and genetic testing issued in 2008 by the American Medical Association, the Critical Path Institute, and the Arizona Center for Education and Research on Therapeutics highlighted the significance *CYP2C1* and *VKORC1* but also emphasized for both that the "prevalence of gene variation differs depending on racial background," stating, for example, that "approximately 37% of Caucasians, 14% of African-Americans and 89% of Asians carry at least one variant copy of VKORC1."[46] The PharmGKB lists studies of this *VKORC1* variant, finding a range of frequencies in European populations from 39% in "Swedish" to 54% in "Spanish," with frequencies of 91% and 93% in "Chinese" and "Japanese," respectively.[47] This begs the question of why one would care about frequencies across racial or ethnic groups when it is possible to test directly for the gene itself, regardless of race. Yet genes, it seems, somehow take on an added interest when connected with race, or perhaps vice versa. Far from withering away, race is persisting and even proliferating as genetic information increases.

COMMERCIAL IMPERATIVES: LABELS, TESTS, AND MORE "ETHNIC" PRODUCT DIFFERENTIATION

By August 2007, enough data on the genetics of warfarin response had been published to convince the FDA to authorize a labeling change for

Coumadin explaining how specific genes might affect a person's response to the drug. In a conference call announcing the change, the FDA's Lawrence Lesko noted that "this marks the first time that such pharmacogenomic information has been included in a widely used drug. . . . This means that personalized medicine is no longer an abstract concept, but has moved into the mainstream, where it is recognized as a factor in a product used by millions of Americans."[48] An article in the journal *Medical Marketing & Media* enthused, "The FDA rang in the era of personalized medicine with a labeling change on blood thinner warfarin cautioning that patients with either of two genetic variations might respond differently to the drug."[49]

News reports of the FDA-mandated label change also noted some of its regulatory, legal, and commercial implications. Jane Woodcock, deputy commissioner and chief medical officer of the FDA, emphasized that the labeling update was "not a directive to doctors" to use genetic tests for warfarin therapy, since current clinical studies do not definitively support such a recommendation.[50] This caution was warranted, given the fact that no prospective clinical trials had yet been conducted comparing the outcomes of using genetic tests to guide warfarin dosing with existing practices. It reflected well-established understandings of the FDA's role in regulating drugs, not medical practice,[51] but also indicated a second concern involving potential legal claims of malpractice liability. A report in the *Wall Street Journal* noted that prior to the labeling change, a medical group called the Anticoagulation Forum wrote a letter to Lesko warning that doctors might rely too heavily on the genetic tests and fail to monitor patients closely enough. Some doctors might even delay starting a patient on warfarin until they had the results of a test in hand. The group asked that any new label "reflect the uncertainty" so doctors "wouldn't be held liable in court for failing to do the tests."[52] Even without a directive to test, large insurers like Aetna take account of such labeling changes when deciding whether to reimburse for a diagnostic genetic test. The labeling change therefore had significant implications for the growing industry of pharmacodiagnostics. Following the labeling change, a number of companies petitioned the FDA for approval of diagnostic kits that tested for a variety of *CYP2C9* and *VKORC1* polymorphisms related to warfarin response.[53]

A number of companies developed genetic tests related to warfarin response. These ranged from smaller, dedicated diagnostic companies, such as AutoGenomics, Nanosphere, and Osmetech, to new, large, full-service, direct-to-consumer genomics companies, such as 23andMe, DNA Direct, and deCODE Genetics. These latter companies offered so-called "home brew" tests that do not require specific FDA approval to be offered to the public.[54]

In this crowded market, one way for a company to differentiate its product was to obtain FDA approval for its particular test, thus certifying its clinical validity. A number of companies obtained such approval, including AutoGenomics, Nanosphere, ParagonDx, and Osmetech.[55] Beyond this, companies also highlighted their ability to provide distinctive services, such as fast turnaround time, additional consultation, or even help with processing insurance claims. Finally, because there are numerous alleles for both *CYP2C9* and *VKORC1* for which it is possible to test, some companies distinguished their tests by allele. The most commonly tested alleles are *CYP2C9*2* and *CYP2C9*3*, and *VKORC1* mutations at the -1639G > A position. Nanosphere, for example, distinguished its test in part by noting that it also tested for the *VKORC1(1173C > T)* allele.[56]

In the realm of allelic product differentiation, AutoGenomics came up with race, or "ethnicity," as a means to make its product stand out in a crowd. It did this by looking at some of the less common *CYP2C9* and *VKORC1* alleles and evaluating how their frequency varied across ethnic groups. As one news article on competition in the warfarin gene testing market put it:

> Among the 15 variants the INFINITI assay detects, several polymorphisms will be specific to particular ethnicities—such as the *4 variant identified exclusively among Japanese people and the 8773 SNPs in VKORC1 found in 21 percent of African Americans.
>
> Therefore, in marketing its test, *AutoGenomics will likely specifically target certain ethnic groups* [italics added], in addition to widely promoting it for the 200,000 to 500,000 patients who get initiated on warfarin each year.[57]

At the time of this story, AutoGenomics was a privately held company, based in Carlsbad, California. It described its mission as "to empower clinical laboratories with an automated cost effective solution to perform molecular testing that will significantly enhance work flow, cost efficiency, quicker turn-around time and result with enhanced patient care."[58] AutoGenomics offered an array of genetic tests on its website. Most were for research use only (RUO), meaning they had not obtained FDA approval and so could not be marketed to other test providers, such as hospitals or clinics, for direct use on patients. It also marketed four FDA-approved tests, including one warfarin assay. This particular assay, however, only covered the common $CYP2C9^*2$ and $CYP2C9^*3$ variations, and the $VKORC1\,3673(1639G>A)$ variant. It was not marketed with explicit reference to ethnicity. AutoGenomics also had an extended "Warfarin XP" assay that tested for six different $CYP2C9$ variants and eight $VKORC1$ variants, but it was not yet FDA approved and so was still only marketed for research use. Nonetheless, while its application for FDA approval of its basic warfarin gene test was still pending, AutoGenomics filled its website with information on differing allele frequencies across ethnic groups and argued for the Warfarin XP assay's distinctive abilities to test broadly across an array of ethnic groups.

One AutoGenomics web page, for example, ran with the title caption: "Warfarin XP: Enhanced Ethnic Characterization." The expanded panel test here explicitly linked genetics to ethnicity. In a section discussing the "clinical relevance" of the test, AutoGenomics discussed the frequency of certain less common variants directly in terms of frequency in "Japanese," "African-Americans," and "Caucasians." Here was a clear example of having specific alleles identified and testable, yet still using race to characterize the product. Why would AutoGenomics continue to use race if it had the gene identified? Certainly it was the gene variants, not the race, that made the difference in clinical response. When read against the above news report of marketing strategies, it becomes evident that AutoGenomics was layering ethnicity onto its more basic warfarin assay in order to differentiate its test and expand its market share.[59]

Most companies, including AutoGenomics, test for the three most common genetic variants affecting warfarin response. Ethnicity provided

AutoGenomics the basis for offering a second test that covered those three common variants plus an additional thirteen rarer variants. The ethnicities identified also conveniently corresponded to major racial groups—Asian (assuming Japanese comes to be taken as a stand-in for Asian), African (or African American), and European (Caucasian). It might seem at first blush that developing a test for less common alleles might narrow one's market, but when bundled with the test for common alleles and layered with racial identities the additional test becomes a potential means for capturing greater market share.

The salience of race in the marketing strategy employed by AutoGenomics was evident in a 2008 PowerPoint presentation (available as a download on its website) titled "Infiniti™ Warfarin XP: Because Ethnic Diversity Matters When Dosing with Warfarin."[60] The presentation begins with a slide noting the importance of the recent FDA relabeling of warfarin to include genetic data. It then discusses the variation across race of the particular *CYP2C9* and *VKORC1* alleles for which it tested, noting that its product was "THE ONLY TEST AVAILABLE THAT INCLUDES ALL RELEVANT VARIANTS!"[61] The inevitable conclusion was, "detecting 2C9 variants in addition to [the common] *2 and *3 is essential for broader identification of high risk metabolizers in several ethnic groups."[62] The presentation emphasized the need for an expanded panel testing for more variants. Ethnicity provided a rationale for offering an expanded test panel that differentiated the AutoGenomics test from others on the market.

One of the most explicit uses of race in relation to genetics to differentiate AutoGenomics' product occurs in a slide asserting that tests other than the AutoGenomics Infiniti platform would miss relevant genetic variants in "*virtually ALL* non-caucasian patents; Asian, African American, Chinese, Japanese, Hispanic, etc., would be missed using a panel limited to these variants."[63] The slide makes racial and ethnic identification appear to be essential to finding relevant genetic variants. In fact, the slide also refers to the common *2, *3, and 1173 variants that occur in *all* of these groups at differing frequencies. The only possible way to make sense of its claim about missing non-Caucasians is to assume it is referring to the patients with the rarer alleles, who would be missed by products that do not test for them. In developing its test, therefore, AutoGenomics was not just looking for genes; it was looking for racial and ethnic groups to whom it could market its product. In short, the slide attempts to translate racially identified gene frequencies into racially identified market share. Once again, finding specific genes did not cause race to wither away. To the contrary, it led to new ways to exploit race in the biomedical marketplace.

If AutoGenomics only tested for rare alleles—for example, *CYP2C9 *5*, *CYP2C9 *6*, or *CYP2C9 *11*—it might have difficulty gaining acceptance in the market against products that tested for the most common significant variants. Simply adding an array of rare alleles that only marginally increased the odds of finding a significant genetic variation could easily make the AutoGenomics test appear needlessly complex. Yet, by tying rare alleles to specific ethnic or racial groups, AutoGenomics provided a hook to draw in potential consumers. You might not know whether you have a rare allele, but you do know if you are black, white, or Asian. A product that says it tests for a rare allele found primarily in your racial or ethnic group is one you might choose.

AutoGenomics did not use race to identify relevant alleles but rather to 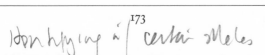 induce consumers to identify their own race or ethnicity (and hence themselves) with these alleles. AutoGenomics framed the test so that the African, Asian, or European race would become identified in the consumer's mind with an allele's frequency. Beyond this, for the product to actually succeed in the marketplace, biomedical professionals and insurance companies would have to similarly identify race with genetics in warfarin response. Through its product development and marketing strategies, then, AutoGenomics was not only selling a pharmacogenomics assay, it was producing and marketing a conception of race as genetic.

Ironically, following its 2008 approval of AutoGenomics' basic Warfarin Assay testing only for the three most common *CYP2C9* and *VKORC1* variants, the FDA required AutoGenomics to remove all "clinical relevance" material associated with its various RUO assays from its website.[64] The Warfarin XP expanded panel was not yet FDA approved; that is, it was permitted only for use in research. All references to race appeared under clinical relevance headings for Warfarin XP and were subsequently

Idon hpying in/ certai Meles

removed from the AutoGenomics website. Similarly, AutoGenomics also removed the "Because Ethnic Diversity Matters . . ." presentation from its website. Nonetheless, in 2009, Anand Vairavan, Marketing Manager and Personalized Medicine Specialist for AutoGenomics, insisted that "we still absolutely believe that Ethnic Diversity Matters when developing genetic tests to help with Warfarin dosing."[65] He noted that "we still do offer this assay and sell more of the Expanded Panel assay as opposed to the [FDA-approved] IVD assay."[66]

In this instance, regulatory approval extracted a trade-off among tactics for product differentiation. One the one hand, AutoGenomics gained the legitimacy and distinction conferred by the FDA approval. On the other hand, it was then forced to downplay the racial aspect of the Expanded Assay—at least until it gets FDA approval for that test as well. Nonetheless, the company's commitment to racialized marketing of its product remained clear and the Expanded Assay continued to be a more profitable test. AutoGenomics licensed the technology to several companies in Europe, one of which, the Swiss company Bühlmann Laboratories, continued to post AutoGenomics slides on its website describing the Expanded Assay with race-specific information. AutoGenomics thus worked to minimize the impact of this trade-off and maintain its commitment to producing and capturing a racialized market.[67]

Perhaps sensing the opportunity in the AutoGenomics approach, one of its chief competitors, the British molecular diagnostics firm Osmetech (which changed its name to GenMark Dx when it went public in 2010) filed a race-specific patent application in October 2009 titled "CYP2C9*8 alleles correlate with decreased warfarin metabolism and increased warfarin sensitivity."[68] The first claim of the patent involves "determining whether a subject possesses a CYP2C9*8 allele" to help guide warfarin dosing. The third claim specifies, "The method of claim 1 wherein said subject is African-American, black African, or of black African descent."[69] The patent has not yet been approved, and GenMark Dx has not yet issued any race-specific marketing claims, but the application lays the groundwork for such approaches in the future.

ALGORITHMS, INERTIA, AND RACE AS A RESIDUAL CATEGORY

FDA approval of a particular warfarin assay (from AutoGenomics or any other company) affirms the test's clinical *validity*. Such technical ability to test for a genetic variation is one thing, but establishing a genetic test's clinical *utility* (i.e., its effectiveness in real-life clinical settings) is another. For the tests to be worthwhile, a clinician needs to figure out how to use the information the tests produce—this is where algorithms come in. A dosing algorithm for warfarin (or any drug) compiles diverse data relating to factors influencing drug response, assigns values to different factors, and applies the values to compute an estimated optimal dosage for any given patient. Weight and age are common factors. For example, a dose of two 200-mg tablets of ibuprofen might be recommended for an average adult, whereas the recommendation for a two- to three-year-old child weighing between twenty-four and thirty-five pounds would be one 100-mg dose. In between, the recommendation for an eleven-year-old weighing between seventy-two and ninety-five pounds would be 300 mg.[70]

Warfarin dosing is far more complex due to the high interindividual variability of response and the severe consequences of overdosing or underdosing. Since the FDA announced its labeling change, much attention has been devoted to developing dosing algorithms that incorporate new genetic information regarding the *CYP2C9* and *VKORC1* polymorphisms. Such algorithms are designed to tell doctors what they should do with the data produced by diagnostic genetic tests, such as those marketed by AutoGenomics.

Prominent among recent genetic dosing algorithms is one constructed by the IWPC; the algorithm was published in February 2009 in the *New England Journal of Medicine*.[71] The IWPC is comprised of eminent biomedical researchers and institutions from around the world and is based in Stanford, California, under the auspices of the PharmGKB. To develop a genetic dosing algorithm, the IWPC analyzed warfarin dose-response information from over twenty-one sites in nine countries. The study was not the first to show the advantage of incorporating genetic information into prescribing patterns, but it was by far the largest and most inclusive to date, with information on more than five thousand patients.[72]

The study was based on the perceived need to develop a dosing algorithm using both genetic and clinical data gathered from a "diverse and large population."[73] In this context, "diverse" included the concepts of race or ethnicity. From the outset, the study's use of these concepts was problematic. As stated in the methods section, "Information on race or ethnic group was reported by the patient or determined by the local investigator."[74] On the one hand, this reflects the simple reality of using data collected from numerous sites across the globe. On the other hand, both self-report and external ascription of race raise significant issues in a biomedical context.

Such problems are only compounded in situations in which race is externally ascribed by a local investigator, because external ascriptions of race are often unreliable and also may change over time.[75] Despite these issues, the one sentence quoted above states the entirety of the study's consideration of how it used race. This contrasts starkly with the detailed elaboration of "genotype quality controls" and "statistical analysis" in the remaining two pages of the same methods section.[76]

To compose the algorithm, the IWPC researchers calculated warfarin dosing three ways: 1) based on standard clinical data; 2) based on clinical data and genetic variations; and 3) using fixed daily doses. In developing dosing algorithms for each patient, researchers genotyped three *VKORC1* alleles and six *CYP2C9* alleles. They also collected clinical data on such characteristics as age, height, weight, use of certain other drugs, and, of course, race. They then compared how closely their computational predictions matched the actual, clinically derived stable warfarin dosage for each patient. This was, therefore, a retrospective study and did not measure prospectively whether the use of a genetic dosing algorithm actually reduced adverse events.[77] The study demonstrated the possible utility of the genetic dosing algorithm, but also found that the greatest benefits accrued only to the roughly one-half of patients who were outliers (at the high and low ends of warfarin dosing).[78]

As for race, at one point the study presented a figure comparing "the predicted doses according to representative clinical or demographic characteristics, genotype combinations, race, and use or nonuse of amiodarone [an important interacting drug]."[79]

It concluded that the data "suggest that most of the racial differences in dose requirements are explained by genotype."[80] The text accompanying the figure itself states that "racial differences in the estimated dose become insignificant when genetic information is added to the model."[81] On page 15 of the supplemental materials, the study calculated the percentage of variance in dose explained by race (R^2). In the study's own terms, race accounted for 14.2 percent of variation when it was the *only* thing in the model. This would comport with the notion that race serves as a potentially useful surrogate when specific genetic variables are unknown. When pharmacogenetic data was added to the model, however, the contribution of race went from 14.2 percent down to 0.3 percent—that is, almost nothing.[82]

It would seem, then, that with this algorithm, warfarin dosing had reached the promised land of truly individualized pharmacogenomic practice. The study cast specific genetic information as rendering race "insignificant," just as advocates of using race as an interim proxy said it would. Yet when we turn to the supplemental material provided with the study and examine the actual dosing algorithm used (and recommended for further use), there we find race, still a prominent factor to be used by every doctor in every dosage calculation, apparently regardless of the fact that race was "insignificant" (see Table 6.1).

The accompanying "legend for the use of algorithm" further specifies: "Asian Race = 1 if self-reported race is Asian, otherwise zero; Black/African American = 1 if self-reported race is Black or African American, otherwise zero; Missing or Mixed race = 1 if self-reported race is unspecified or mixed, otherwise zero."[83]

Most immediately striking here is the straightforward use of whiteness as an unmarked norm in biomedical research. The IWPC algorithm is thus typical, and yet stunning, in that it is appearing at the end of a decade of heated discussion concerning the proper use of race in biomedical contexts, discussion that directly critiqued the use of "white" as the unmarked standard

TABLE 6.1 WARFARIN PHARMACOGENETIC DOSING ALGORITHM

	5.6044	
–	0.2614 ×	Age in decades
+	0.0087 ×	Height in centimeters
+	0.0128 ×	Weight in kilograms
–	0.8677 ×	$VKORC1\ A/G^{\dagger}$
–	1.6974 ×	$VKORC1\ A/A^{\dagger}$
–	0.4854 ×	$VKORC1$ genotype unknown[†]
–	0.5211 ×	$CYP2C9^{*}1/^{*}2$
–	0.9357 ×	$CYP2C9^{*}1/^{*}3$
–	1.0616 ×	$CYP2C9^{*}2/^{*}2$
–	1.9206 ×	$CYP2C9^{*}2/^{*}3$
–	2.3312 ×	$CYP2C9^{*}3/^{*}3$
–	0.2188 ×	$CYP2C9$ genotype unknown
–	0.1092 ×	Asian race
–	0.2760 ×	Black or African American
–	0.1032 ×	Missing or mixed race
+	1.1816 ×	Enzyme inducer status
–	0.5503 ×	Amiodarone status
=	Square root of weekly warfarin dose*	

*The output of this algorithm must be squared to complete weekly dose in milligrams.
†All references to $VKORC1$ refer to genotype for rs9923231.

from which all other races are cast as deviating.[84] The algorithm only makes a person present as a racialized subject if he or she is not white. Here, white people do not explicitly possess race; that is, their race is tacit and does not formally come into play in calculating dosage. They are the norm against which the race of other subjects is made to matter. Thus, "black" and "Asian" dosages are calculated as deviations from the unstated white norm.

It is also curious to note that the algorithm lumps together "mixed race" and "missing race." Here, having mixed race is made the equivalent of absent race. In both cases, a sort of statistical guess is being made to encompass the unknown. Through this association, the algorithm renders mixed race as mysterious and uncertain, a category without clear boundaries that is treated as the equivalent of absence in order to contain any challenge it might pose to the model. Yet how can this characterization of mixed race as a distinct category deal with estimates that anywhere between 30 percent to 70 percent of self-identified African Americans have some white relatives in their ancestral history or that a significant proportion of white-identified people have some multiracial background? Many of these people would likely register as either black or white. Thus, a self-identified black person and a self-identified white person, each with "mixed ancestry," would likely register respectively as black or white, even though both could also register under the same mixed race category. Moreover, once a value is assigned, the algorithm multiplies it by different amounts depending again on racial identification. Thus, a person of mixed African and European ancestry could be counted three different ways depending on whether they self-identified as "white," "black," or "mixed." This would be the case for everybody's mixed-race person of the moment, President Barack Obama. Alternatively, three siblings, each with the same proportion of "mixed" ancestry could be counted differently by this algorithm, again depending on how they self-identified. Perhaps more significantly, this model assumes some sort of "pure" notion of races as biologically bounded and distinct, perhaps capable of "mixture," but with such mixtures ultimately separable into preexisting, purportedly pure kinds, thus reinforcing genetically essentialist conceptions of races as biologically distinct entities.[85]

A similar dynamic is evident in a separate dosing algorithm published a year earlier by a team of researchers led by Brian Gage, of Vanderbilt University, a prominent warfarin researcher and member of the IWPC (as were several of the other researchers involved in the study). Declaring warfarin to be the "ideal drug to test the hypothesis that pharmacogenetics can reduce drug toxicity,"[86] this study contained a single race variable, specified as "African-American race" which ultimately accounted for 0.4

percent of variation in response to warfarin—almost the exact same (negligible) amount as in the IWPC algorithm.[87]

In both the Gage and the IWPC algorithm, race appears to be operating as a sort of residual category that has persisted through inertia. Race had long been a part of considering how individuals respond to warfarin. It was generally understood to be a surrogate for underlying genetic variation and therefore was included as a variable in numerous pregenomic studies. The use of race thus became a standardized norm in warfarin research. Once instantiated as normative practice, race simply appears to have persisted, almost reflexively, even in the face of data showing its minimal impact on dose-response variation. The inertial power of race was so strong that it persisted in the IWPC algorithm, even alongside explicit assertions of its insignificance. To the extent that race captured any substantive information (that is, to the extent that the 0.3 percent to 0.4 percent variation could be deemed significant), race must be understood as a sort of catchall category encompassing a residuum variation for which the researchers had no specific explanation. This brings us back to the observation by Yen-Revello, Aumen, and McLeod that race remains an appealing surrogate where "drug-genotype interactions remain unknown."[88] Apparently, however, race remains appealing even after drug-genotype interactions are discovered. This is because genotype generally will never explain *all* variation in drug response. There will always be some aspects of interindividual variation in drug response that remain "unknown." As long as the inertial force of race maintains it as a normative category in biomedical research, it may be possible for researchers to associate race with whatever residuum of unexplained variation they find in their studies.

The awkwardness of the use of race in the algorithm hearkens back to the discomfort noted by Duana Fullwiley in her study of California biomedical researchers. But with the IWPC dosing algorithm, we have a formal institutionalization of the imperative to render ambiguous racial identifiers as genetically bounded and fixed. In this particular promised land of genetically guided dosing, race did not wither away; on the contrary, it persisted—prominently and structurally.

RACE, COMMERCE, AND REGULATORY CLASH

There is also a commercial imperative driving the continued use of race in the face of genetic discovery. The Yen-Revollo, Aumen, and McLeod study alludes to it, noting that using race as a surrogate is also appealing "because personal genotyping is cost prohibitive." Simply stated, it is cheaper to identify a patient by race than by genotype. Beyond this, it turns out race can be economically relevant, not only as an alternative to genotyping but also as a complement to it. Thus, for example, a 2008 policy statement on gene testing for warfarin response issued by the American College of Medical Genetics (ACMG) states,

> CYP2C9*2 and *3 are found in the *major racial groups*, but with different allelic frequencies. *These alleles should be tested in all individuals.* There are also several rare alleles of CYP2C9 alleles that have different frequencies in different ethnic populations, and some alleles are preferentially found in only certain racial groups. Some CYP2C9 alleles, such as CYP2C9 *5, *6, and *11, are preferentially found in *African-descendent* populations at low allele frequencies, but are not found in *Asian-descendant* populations. On the other hand, the rare CYP2C9 *4 polymorphism has only been reported in individuals from Asia. The decision to test for polymorphisms other than CYP2C9 *2 and *3 *should be based on the populations being tested* by a laboratory and the capability to make patient management decisions informed by these less-frequently encountered alleles [italics added].[89]

Here race is front and center, right alongside specific genetic variation. Given the nature of genetic variation, it will always be possible to find certain genetic variations that occur at differing frequencies across racial groups. For example, one comprehensive review article found frequency variation ranging from 0.9 percent to 20 percent for at least one *CYP2C*2 allele in different "Caucasian" populations, and a range for "Africans" from

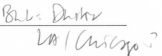

zero to 8.7 percent.[90] There certainly is a difference in frequency between Africans and Caucasians, but there is also significant overlap, and the overall variation within Caucasians seems to dwarf that between Africans and Caucasians. The question is which differences do the researchers *choose* to make matter and how?

A sense of how these choices are made is provided by an examination of the studies cited by the ACMG report to support its recommendation to take race into account. To support its assertion that "some CYP2C9 alleles, such as CYP2C9 *5, *6, and *11, are preferentially found in African-descendent populations at low allele frequencies, but are not found in Asian-descendant populations,"[91] the report cited the article "In-Vitro and In-Vivo Effects of the *CYP2C9*11* Polymorphism on Warfarin Metabolism and Dose" by Tai et al.[92] As is evident from the title, this study discusses only the *CYP2C9*11* polymorphism and says nothing about frequencies for the *5 and *6 alleles. Moreover, this was a study of 303 "Caucasians" and 101 "African-Americans"; it said nothing about allelic frequencies in Asian populations. Additionally, to support its assertion that "the rare CYP2C9*4 polymorphism has been found only in individuals from Asia,"[93] the ACMG report cited an article titled "A Case Report of a Patient Carrying *CYP2C9*3/4* Genotype with Extremely Low Warfarin Dose Requirement."[94] As is evident from this title, the study reported on a single patient—in this case, from Korea. The report itself noted, "This is the first report of a Korean patient with the *CYP2C9*3/*4* showing warfarin intolerance. The *CYP2C9*4* allele including 1076T>C (Ile359Thr) has been reported in only one Japanese subject."[95] The ACMG took a report of one Korean woman that also cited one additional Japanese subject and expanded it into a technically accurate but highly misleading assertion that this allele is only found in "individuals from Asia." There may well be studies out there providing better support for the ACMG assertions, but the ones it cited certainly are not sufficient. The ACMG report thus casually added to an accumulating sort of folk wisdom or common sense in the medical community promoting the continued relevance of race alongside the development of specific genetic information.

The basis for making the choice to frame allele frequency data in terms of race takes on a distinctly economic cast when considered in light of the statement's overall purpose of identifying which groups should get which tests. In the ACMG report, race becomes relevant at the margins, where allelic frequencies are low and variable across racially defined population groups. The ACMG in effect suggested using race as a screening mechanism to determine which individuals should get which genetic tests. Yet multiplex assays such as those offered by AutoGenomics (not to mention those now being offered by such genetic testing behemoths as 23andMe) are currently able to test efficiently for a range of alleles simultaneously. The only reason for preferentially assigning tests by race appears to be in the interest of economic gain rather than scientific efficiency. If testing for more alleles costs more, then race may be used to perform a sort of economic triage to focus on those for whom the test is most likely to produce a medically useful result.

Lawrence Lesko and other senior FDA officials have echoed the logic of the ACMG's report, stating, for example, that

the type of genomic data (e.g., which alleles, what genotypes) that needs to be evaluated, and when, is one of the critical issues in drug development and regulatory review. In some cases, consideration of racial/ethnic differences in the distributions of various alleles with no or reduced metabolic activity in the evaluation of dose-response relationships is important.[96]

The FDA officials went on to specify *CYP2C9* as one of the genes listed "for recommended polymorphic alleles to measure in specific population groups."[97] These groups, not surprisingly, are racialized as Caucasians, African Americans, and Asian Americans.[98] For the FDA, then, race remained not only a legitimate but an "important" factor in evaluating drug dose response—again, even as specific genes were being identified. In this conceptualization of the promise of pharmacogenomics, genes are not replacing race, they are complementing race.

All of this brings us back to AutoGenomics and its marketing campaign for its Warfarin XP Assay built around the proposition that "Ethnic Diversity Matters." The commercial value of this product was intimately tied to the statements of biomedical professionals, such as the ACMG, and federal regulators, such as Lesko at the FDA. Research, regulation, and commerce are thus mutually implicated in producing understandings of race as relevant to pharmacogenomics and in constructing consumers and clinicians who identify race with genetics when making medical decisions.

Research, regulation, and commerce, however, are not monolithic phenomena. Just as there has been ongoing debate among researchers concerning the utility of race in pharmacogenomics, there was also something of a regulatory clash between the FDA and the Centers for Medicaid and Medicare Services (CMS) concerning warfarin testing. The conflict grew out of the 2007 FDA labeling change for warfarin specifying the significance of specific alleles and the subsequent decision by the CMS that it was premature to offer Medicare reimbursement for pharmacodiagnostic warfarin-response tests. The labeling change gave urgency to efforts to develop viable genetic dosing algorithms and also provided a great impetus to companies to develop and market genetic tests.[99]

Most algorithms, such as those developed by the IWPC, are free. Gene tests are not. They average between three hundred and five hundred dollars per test. Payment for such tests obviously is central to their commercial success, and central to payment is insurance coverage. The problem for companies offering genetic tests is that the FDA recommendation was based on the clinical *validity* of the tests, while insurance coverage tends to be based on considerations of clinical *utility* and related concerns for cost-effectiveness.[100]

The clinical utility of genetic testing for warfarin dosing had not been established to the satisfaction of numerous insurers, including the CMS. One article in the *Wall Street Journal* noted that "major insurers such as Aetna Inc., WellPoint Inc. and Cigna Corp." did not cover the costs of such tests, in part because "some specialists say testing hasn't been proved to reduce the risks of the drug."[101] Even influential studies, such as the one conducted by the IWPC, were retrospective and did not measure whether

184

incorporating genetic data into dosing algorithms materially reduced adverse drug events (ADEs).[102] As University of Washington professor Ann Wittkowsky said of the FDA labeling decision, "It is fascinating science, but it is not yet ready for prime time."[103] Similarly, a 2008 report of the Secretary of Health and Human Services' Advisory Committee on Genetics, Health and Society (SACGHS) entitled "Realizing the Potential of Pharmacogenomics: Opportunities and Challenges," while referring to the use of *CYP2C9* and *VKORC1* testing to guide warfarin dosage as an early application of pharmacogenomics, nonetheless indicated that "much of the valuable evidence about pharmacogenomics is in the form of early scientific discoveries. Although this information has the potential to be useful, its clinical utility is not yet well understood."[104]

Additionally, Francis Collins, shortly after he stepped down as director of NHGRI, stated his belief that researchers still did not have the right type of evidence "to enable a clear statement to providers about whether this kind of genetic testing ought to be done prospectively before trying to prescribe this drug with all of its complications."[105] The FDA's own Deputy Commissioner and Chief Medical Officer, Janet Woodcock, noted that they would "have to wait for outcomes data" before actually changing the label to mandate genetic testing.[106]

So it was that in May 2009, the CMS announced its intention to deny Medicare coverage for pharmacogenomic testing to predict warfarin response, stating that "the available evidence does not demonstrate that [such testing] improves health outcomes in Medicare beneficiaries."[107] The CMS held out the possibility that coverage might be granted in the future, but only after a prospective, randomized trial found that using genetic testing to guide warfarin dosing lessens the frequency and severity of ADEs compared to standard methods.[108]

One news report of the CMS announcement also mentioned a study published in January 2009 in the *Annals of Internal Medicine* questioning the cost-effectiveness of using pharmacogenomics information in warfarin dosing.[109] Mark Eckman, the lead author on the study, pointedly criticized a previous study conducted jointly in 2006 by the American Enterprise Institute (AEI) and the Brookings Institution (estimating an annual savings of $100 million to $2 billion from integrating genetic testing into warfarin therapy) as "optimistic" in its assumptions.[110] The AEI-Brookings report was actually conducted by FDA staff and had been referenced by the FDA to support the drive toward incorporating pharmacogenomic data in drug submissions.[111] It was also cited by diagnostic companies, such as Iverson Genetic Diagnostics and Osmetech to support the marketing of their products. Such questioning of the tests' economic value further undermined the rationale for insurance coverage.[112]

As one might expect, the CMS announcement was not well received by companies offering genetic tests, especially given the fact that many private payors emulate CMS when determining whether to cover new technologies. Ramanath Vairavan, senior vice president of Sales and Marketing for AutoGenomics, opined,

> This illogical decision perhaps has been influenced by the lobbying of big pharma, that in spite of numerous prospective studies and publications that have clearly shown the benefit for genetic testing and the FDA relabeling of the drug, CMS has succumbed into making a contradictory decision that will certainly impact patient well being and the cost of healthcare. . . . As a manufacturer of the test we appeal to CMS to revisit this controversial decision at the earliest.[113]

Vairavan's concern regarding "big pharma" highlights the fact that the pharmacogenomics industry too is not monolithic. The marketing model for genetic tests ultimately depends on the ability to use genomics to identify which subjects should get which drugs—that is, to narrow the market for specific drugs. The more pharmacodiagnostics companies are able to identify genes that correspond with drug response, the greater will be the marker for their product. Each success for an AutoGenomics represents a potential threat to big pharmaceutical companies marketing blockbuster drugs to large undifferentiated populations. Yet, one review of the comments submitted to the CMS before it announced its intentions found that most of those opposing coverage (about 18 percent of the total) were "professional organizations, payors, and some healthcare providers." Those with the most immediate interest in the CMS decisions appear to have been those with an immediate stake in the payment for diagnostic tests.[114]

In the aftermath of the CMS decision, the Center for Medicine in the Public Interest (CMPI) announced plans to develop a proposal outlining areas in which the FDA and CMS "can harmonize the way they evaluate outcomes and guide treatment."[115] The CMPI is a conservative, free market–oriented group associated with the Pacific Research Institute, a think tank founded in 1979 whose stated vision is the promotion of "the principles of individual freedom and personal responsibility [which], the Institute believes . . . are best encouraged through policies that emphasize a free economy, private initiative, and limited government."[116] The CMPI announced its plans, in part, as a response to the CMS decision, thereby casting the CMS as an impediment to product development. Hence, the "harmonization" sought by the CMPI primarily involved getting the CMS to follow the more industry-friendly FDA in its attitude toward genetic testing for warfarin.

Hope was on the horizon for pharmacodiagnostic companies, however, as prospective studies of the clinical utility of pharmacogenomic dosing algorithms were designed and carried out. Prominent among these was the Clarification of Optimal Anticoagulation through Genetics, or COAG, trial, directed by the NHLBI. The study planned to enroll 1,200 patients and would cost nearly $10 million. In February 2009, Raynard Kingston, then acting director of the NIH asserted, "These efforts showcase NIH's firm commitment to building a future of personalized medicine—a future in which doctors will be able to prescribe the optimal dosage of medicine for each patient right from the start."[117]

In June 2010, Medco, a major PBM (not to be confused with the company of the same name that originally acquired the rights to BiDil in the early 1990s), published results in the *Journal of the American College of Cardiology* from a warfarin study using genetics to guide dosing that seemed to establish the clinical utility of genotyping patients. The study, however, was contested, and another major PBM, CVS Caremark's division, continued to deny warfarin genotyping coverage to its customers. Payors, in general, continued to be skeptical, citing the lack of data from large, randomized clinical trials proving that routine genetic testing to dose warfarin improves outcomes and lowers costs.[118]

Race does not seem to have played much of a role in the CMS decision or subsequent debates about the merits of insurance coverage for genetic tests. In the minutes of the February 2009 CMS meeting discussing genetic testing, there is barely a mention of race or ethnicity. Race, it seems, was much more important to FDA officials, such as Lawrence Lesko or Robert Temple, who saw it as a means to drive their agenda of pursuing pharmacogenomic drug development, than it was for CMS officials (and private insurers), who were focusing on the more contained and less easily racialized issues of cost-effectiveness. Warfarin was front and center as a poster child for the FDA's Critical Path Initiative as the first of a series of interviews posted on the FDA website to explore Critical Path projects focused on warfarin.[119] The FDA embraced race as a means to validate its institutional drive toward realizing the promise of "personalized medicine." The CMS, in contrast, did not have any particular use for race in making coverage determinations or in justifying its institutional position.

PATENTING RACE . . . AGAIN

The PTO provided an additional regulatory site for the racialization of warfarin response. Genetic testing companies, such as AutoGenomics, generally do not use race in their patents, which tend to cover the technical specifications of their assay platforms (the actual apparatus conducting the tests). Such companies reserve race for certain marketing efforts. Rather, it was particular warfarin researchers themselves who introduced race into the realm of intellectual property. On December 21, 2005, Yuan-Tsong Chen, Hsiang-Yu Yuan, and Jin-Jer Chen filed a patent application titled "Genetic Variants Predicting Warfarin Sensitivity."[120] The lead inventor, Yuan-Tsong Chen, was a Distinguished Research Fellow at the Genomics Center and director of the Institute of Biomedical Sciences at the Academia Sinica in Taipei, Taiwan.[121] He was also a professor in the Department of Genetics at

Duke University in Durham, North Carolina. The other inventors were also at the Academia Sinica, and the patent rights were assigned to that institution. The Academia Sinica was also a member of the IWPC and credited with supplying data to the dosing algorithm study published so prominently in the *New England Journal of Medicine* in February 2009.[122]

The abstract of the application states, "We discovered that a polymorphism in the promoter of the VKORC1 gene is associated with warfarin sensitivity. This polymorphism can explain both the inter-individual and *inter-ethnic* [italics added] differences in warfarin dose requirements."[123] The claims section includes the following:

1. A method of determining the dose range of a warfarin for a subject, comprising investigating the sequence of the promoter of the VKORC1 gene of the subject. . . .

9. The method of claim 1 wherein the subject is an *Asian* [italics added].

10. The method of claim 1 wherein the subject is a *Caucasian* [italics added].

11. The method of claim 1 wherein the subject is an *African*, *African American*, or *Hispanic* [italics added].[124]

Once again, the mention of race in the claims section is particularly significant, because the claims specify the legally operative scope of the patent, defining the formal legal metes and bounds of the territory covered by an invention. The force and authority of the U.S. government was thus conscripted into legitimating the use of race in relation to genetics in a manner that implies or infers that race itself is genetic. The basis for making such race-specific claims is to be found in studies of allelic frequencies that vary across population groups. The patent application reductively solidified such variation into a rigid racial difference that was then to be given the imprimatur of the state through the potential grant of patent protection.

A news report on Academia Sinica's role in the IWPC noted that it was carrying out a follow-up study of 600 patients in Taiwan to verify the predictive accuracy of the model. One of the Academia Sinica researchers asserted that "the result of the study on the island is significant in that it will serve as the dosing guideline for people of *ethnic Chinese origin* [italics added]. . . . This is the largest community in the world."[125] The report went on to note:

> The research efforts may turn out to be profitable as well. In 2005 Academia Sinica created a spin-off business called PharmiGene Inc., which focuses on the creation of personalized medicine products. The company has already used the scientific knowledge gained by Academia Sinica to manufacture several gene-detection kits, including a warfarin dosing prediction model developed in 2005.[126]

With PharmiGene and its race-specific patent, Academia Sinica was positioning itself to sell its warfarin tests to "people of ethnic Chinese origin," not only the largest "community" in the world, but also potentially the largest market. Race persisted as a viable basis for framing and capturing an emerging pharmacogenomic market.

As the Academia race-specific patent worked its way through the PTO, it encountered some problems. In January 2009, the patent examiner rejected certain claims in the application as obvious and anticipated by two patent applications filed by University of Washington researcher Mark Rieder (also a member of the IWPC), particularly the second, number 20080057500 (referred to as "Rieder II").[127] The Rieder application (a continuation of an earlier patent filed on October 18, 2004) was titled "Methods and compositions for predicting drug response."[128] The application directly referenced the *VKORC1* gene and warfarin response, stating in the abstract, "The present invention provides methods and compositions for determining individualized Warfarin dosages based on genotype of DNA polymorphisms and haplotypes derived from them in the VKORC1 gene."[129] Given the Academia Sinica application's explicit focus on *VKORC1*, this presented something of a problem.

In response, Yuan-Tsong Chen filed an "inventor's declaration" setting forth his reasons why the Rieder application did not negate his submission. He placed race at the center of his argument as he asserted,

Although only 4% [of] Caucasians carry the haplotypes [a group of linked genes] unrelated to warfarin response, i.e., H3-H6, these haplotypes constitute as high as 39% of the African-American population and as high as 19% in Hispanic Americans. . . . As another example, the total frequency of H3-H6 is 20% in ethnic groups other than Caucasians, African-Americans, Asians, and Hispanic-Americans. These teachings clearly indicate that haplotypes H3-H6, which according to Rieder II, are unrelated to warfarin response, CANNOT be ignored in the whole human population.[130]

Chen explicitly used race to show the relevance of haplotypes H3–H6 and thus differentiate his patent application from Rieder's. He added race to make his claims appear novel and non-obvious. The motivation here was not scientific, but legal and commercial. The connection of genes and race here primarily served the purpose of obtaining patent protection, not of furthering science.

Hearkening back to the role of patents in the case of BiDil, we can see how this situation is both similar and different. The story of BiDil involved using race to recapitalize the value of existing generic drugs. The need to create a patentable product and convince corporate backers of the drug's viability as a commercial product led Jay Cohn and NitroMed to use race as a frame for interpreting existing science, developing clinical trial protocols, compiling regulatory filings, and designing marketing campaigns. The Academia Sinica patent application process did not directly involve the reconfiguration of an existing product as racial in order to extend patent life, but it does show how race can be used to differentiate one product or process from another as a potential means to obtain patent protection. Both models exploited race in order to enhance the commercial value of scientific research. The use of race in warfarin patents is thus part of the larger and accelerating dynamic of using race in biotechnology research and product development.

CONCLUSION

The case of warfarin is emblematic of a larger dynamic coming to characterize the use of race beyond BiDil in biomedical research, development, and marketing. Not only is general use of racial and ethnic categories in biotechnology patents increasing, subsequent race-specific trials, marketing campaigns, and clinical education are also on the rise. Warfarin, however, is more than simply an additional case study. It brings to light a common dynamic underlying the general rise of racial patents and the persistence of racial profiling in biomedicine, even as specific genes are being identified. The experience of warfarin calls into question the entire rationale for using race in the "meantime" between current reality and the future promise of truly individual genomic medicine. It also illustrates the inertial power of race to remain prominent in a conceptual system of biomedical analysis once introduced, especially when buttressed by commercial imperatives. Finally, together with such examples as the study by Albain et al., it shows how race is being constructed as a residual category to explain any "unknown" aspects of drug response, creating a new space for the persistence of race in biomedicine.

7

FROM DISPARITY TO DIFFERENCE

The Politics of Racial Medicine

T HE STORY OF BIDIL and the related rise of race in biomedical practice
and patenting clearly raise concerns over the dangers of reifying race
in a manner that could lead to new forms of discrimination. BiDil,
however, is part of a much larger dynamic in which the purported "reality
of race" as genetic is used to obscure the social reality of racism. To the
extent that this dynamic succeeds in reductively reconfiguring health (and
other types of disparities) in terms of genetic difference, it casts personal
responsibility and the market as the appropriate arenas for addressing differential outcomes, and undermines rationales for deliberate state or insti-
tutional interventions to address discrimination.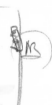

This is not to advocate "color-blind" medicine. On the contrary, there
are very real health disparities in this country that correlate with race. African Americans suffer a disproportionate burden of a number of diseases,
including hypertension and diabetes. Like heart failure, these are complex
conditions caused by an array of environmental, social, and economic, as
well as genetic, factors. Central among these is the fact that people of color
experience discrimination, both in society at large and in the health-care
system specifically. The question, once you identify these disparities in
health outcomes, is about how to address the underlying causes. Of course,
outcomes can have multiple causes, both social and genetic. But health

disparities are not caused by an absence of "black" drugs. As studies by the Institute of Medicine (IOM) among others make clear, they are caused by social discrimination and economic inequality.[1] The problem with marketing race-specific drugs is that it becomes easier to ignore the social realities and focus on the molecules.

TWENTY-NINE MEDICINES

Early on in the story of BiDil, the dynamic relation between markets and manipulated scientific data expanded to support larger claims about the legitimacy of developing race-specific drugs. In November 2004, in a special supplement on race and genetics, *Nature Genetics* published an article by Sarah Tate and David Goldstein titled "Will Tomorrow's Medicines Work for Everyone?"[2] Among other things, the article noted that "twenty-nine medicines (or combinations of medicines) have been claimed, in peer-reviewed scientific or medical journals, to have differences in either safety or, more commonly, efficacy among racial or ethnic groups."[3] This number was immediately taken up throughout the media and certain professional contexts as providing "further" evidence of supposedly "real" biological differences among races.

Reports of these striking results were almost invariably paired with a discussion of the near contemporaneous formal announcement of the A-HeFT results for BiDil. For example, after discussing BiDil, an article in the *Los Angeles Times* referred to "a report in the journal *Nature Genetics* last month [that] listed 29 drugs that are *known* [italics added] to have different efficacies in the two races."[4] Similarly, a *Times* (London) article asserted that "only last week, *Nature Genetics* revealed research from University College London *showing* [italics added] that 29 medicines have safety or efficacy profiles that vary between ethnic or racial groups."[5] Also, a *New York Times* editorial titled "Toward the First Racial Medicine" began with a discussion of BiDil and went on to note that "by one count, some 29 medicines show evidence of being safer or more effective in one racial group or another, suggesting that more targeted medicines may be coming."[6] Linking BiDil to the twenty-nine medicines was of course not accidental.[7] They were paired to give the impression that there was some "real" difference underlying racial response to these drugs.

One small problem with these stories: they totally misrepresented the findings and analysis of the Tate and Goldstein piece. Remember first that Tate and Goldstein asserted that these twenty-nine medicines have only been "claimed" to have racial differences in safety or efficacy. They went on in the next sentence to assert, "But these claims are universally controversial, and there is *no consensus* [italics added] on how important race or ethnicity is in determining drug response."[8] If one took the trouble to actually read the analysis of the claims, one would see that Tate and Goldstein considered only four of the twenty-nine medicines to provide "evidence of a genetic cause"[9] related to the differential drug response, and only an additional nine to provide evidence that "the association has a reasonable underlying physiological basis."[10] For the remaining sixteen medicines, Tate and Goldstein found either no demonstration of a physiological basis to any observed difference, nor any possible false-positive claims. Moreover, of the thirteen medicines with some supporting evidence of racial difference, three were ACE inhibitors—whose claims of racial difference have been thoroughly contested in professional literature— and one of these drugs was BiDil.[11] All of the thirteen drugs showing difference dealt with hypertension, and the ISHIB has issued guidelines arguing against race-specific treatment of hypertension on the grounds that any asserted population-based difference in response was not substantial enough to warrant denying effective therapy to the many blacks who would respond well to these drugs.[12]

One might dismiss the distortion of the Tate and Goldstein article as sloppy journalism. But the use, or rather misuse, of the twenty-nine medicines statistic was embraced in expert and often more conservative circles. I refer in particular to Jon Entine and Sally Satel, both fellows at the conservative AEI. Both have gained a good deal of notoriety for their popular

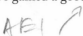

works of race and genetics: Entine, for his book *Taboo: Why Black Athletes Dominate Sports and Why We Are Afraid to Talk About It*,[13] and Satel for, among other writings, a prominent *New York Times Magazine* article titled "I Am a Racially Profiling Doctor."[14] Entine framed a 2004 AEI symposium on BiDil by noting that "only last month, the *prestigious* [italics added] journal *Nature Genetics* reported that at least 29 medicines have so far been identified that are either safer or more effective in certain *populations because of genetic* [italics added] differences between those population groups."[15] Satel echoed Entine's move in a more qualified manner later in the AEI symposium when she asserted, "Generally, when we're talking about BiDil and things like that, its skin color as a marker for genetic heritage."[16] Then, a month later, she repeated Entine's claim about the twenty-nine medicines and genetics almost word for word in an article for the conservative Manhattan Institute titled "Race and Medicine Can Mix without Prejudice: How the Story of BiDil Illuminates the Future of Medicine."[17] Not only did Entine and Satel elide any reference to Tate and Goldstein's qualifying analysis, they also extended the purported connection between race and drug response into the realm of genetics. BiDil provided the starting point for this move toward identifying race with genetic difference—a difference that the A-HeFT investigators themselves did *not* make.

Here then was another critical moment of reification. By connecting BiDil to the manipulated twenty-nine medicines statistic, Satel and Entine cast BiDil as the poster drug for the future of addressing racial difference—much as the corporate analysts cast it as the new paradigm for multicultural pharmaceutical marketing. Entine and Satel's message was that race and genetics correlated closely enough to provide a basis not only for general medical practice, but also for addressing specific health disparities. The related message was that the correlation also provides the basis for market-driven pharmaceutical development to produce new drugs, such as BiDil, to address these differences.

This is where reification in the context of medical practice intersects with broader strategies regarding commerce and the politics of difference. At work here is an appropriation of race as reified in the BiDil story to serve larger political agendas aimed at transmuting health disparities rooted in social and economic inequality into mere health "differences" rooted in biology and genetics. Attempts to address social "disparity" generally implicate the power of the state or other nonmarket institutions to intervene consciously both in the allocation of resources and the sanctioning of racist practices. In contrast, attempts to address genetic "difference" may be located at the molecular level and targeted by pharmaceuticals developed and dispensed through the purportedly impersonal forces of the market.

Implicit in the logic of conservatives such as Satel and Entine, who use BiDil to characterize disparate health outcomes in terms of genetics, is an argument that approaches to health disparities should be privatized. This argument goes far toward explaining why free market conservative organizations such as the AEI and the Manhattan Institute took such an interest in BiDil and the Tate and Goldstein article.

The next year Satel (with coauthor Jonathan Klick) and Richard Epstein, a law and economics professor at the University of Chicago, expanded upon these themes in a special issue of *Perspectives in Biology and Medicine*. Both pieces attacked the IOM's 2003 report *Unequal Treatment: Confronting Racial and Ethnic Disparities in Health Care*,[18] which chronicled an array of health disparities and connected them directly to social and economic issues of equity, access, and racism. Epstein posited that "the leap from disparity to discrimination is not, on balance, established,"[19] thereby rendering disparity to be the functional equivalent of mere difference and therefore without implications for issues of social justice. In addition, Satel and Klick complained that the IOM report was "too quick to diagnose bias," and objected that "many medical schools, health philanthropies, policymakers, and politicians are proceeding as if 'bias' were an established fact. In other words, they consider part of the solution to the disparity problem to be located in the arena of race politics."[20] As an alternative, Satel and Klick argued that

> understanding health disparities as an economic problem tied to issues of access to quality care and health literacy, rather than as a civil rights problem borne of overt or unconscious bias on the part of physicians, is

a more efficient and rational way to address the problem of differential health outcomes.[21]

In contrasting "race politics" with economics, Satel and Klick implied that the latter is somehow apolitical—a mere given reality that existed outside the history and social reality of institutionalized racial subordination in this country. Thus decontextualized, health disparities did not demand a coordinated political response, leaving the market as the appropriate arena for an individualized response to depoliticized health "differences."

In their articles, Satel and Epstein provided intellectual cover for reviving a previous and far more egregious attempt by U.S. Department of Health and Human Services (DHHS) secretary Tommy Thompson to transmute the IOM's focus on disparity into difference. In December 2003, the DHHS issued a report on health disparities, supposedly based on the IOM report. The DHHS report, however, dismissed the "implication" that racial differences in care "result in adverse health outcomes."[22] It turned out that top officials had directed DHHS researchers to drop their initial conclusion that racial disparities were "pervasive in our health care system," and to delete or recharacterize findings of "disparity" as mere evidence of health-care "differences."[23] For example, an earlier version of the report mentioned the term "disparity" thirty times in the "key findings" section, while the final report mentioned it only twice and left the term undefined.[24] DHHS officials accompanied this push to use the term "difference" to emphasize "the importance of . . . personal responsibility" for health outcomes.[25] Ultimately, Tommy Thompson backtracked when word of the report's manipulation was leaked by concerned DHHS staff. Nonetheless, Satel and Epstein effectively continued where Thompson stopped—emphasizing personal choice and market forces, rather than racism or inequality, as the basis of health "differences" among races. This approach exemplifies a dynamic identified by anthropologists George Ellison and Ian Rees Jones, whereby "the 'geneticization' of individual identity shifts responsibility for genetic conditions onto individuals," and the "collective geneticization of social identities shifts responsibility for social inequalities in health on shared values, beliefs and behaviours."[26]

Support for BiDil and the repudiation of the IOM report are related. Together they constitute a strategic move to locate the responsibility for individual health disparities in biology or "personal choice," rather than society. The implicit goals are to undermine calls for further state action to address the underlying racism that leads to disparities, and also to privatize the move to address health disparities by leaving it to market forces, exemplified by the drug development model of BiDil and the twenty-nine medicines. In the world of law, this is a way of saying that disparate impact is not due to discrimination, but due to natural forces, meaning that it is nobody's fault and therefore requires no conscious effort to redress.

This is not to say that genes play no role at all in disparities. To the contrary, disparities involve complex interplay of biological (including genetic), social, historical, political, economic, behavioral, and environmental factors. The danger comes from privileging reductive genetic and market-driven characterizations of disparities that come to command excessively disproportionate shares of scarce health-related resources. In 1995, Dorothy Nelkin and M. Susan Lindee observed that "images and narratives of the gene in popular culture reflect and convey . . . genetic essentialism." Genetic essentialism, they argued, represents a mode of biological reductionism resting on a fallacy that "reduces the self to a molecular entity, equating human beings, in their social, historical, and moral complexity, with their genes."[27] A similar dynamic may be at work in a genetic approach to disparities, which reduces not only the self but the entire social problem of disparities to genetics.[28]

FRAMES FOR DISPARITIES AND DIFFERENCE

Contemporary debates over the meaning and significance of racial disparities in health have deep roots. Tracing their development over the past century, particularly in relation to the legal construction of racial difference, elucidates a history of tension between two competing frames for characterizing social understandings and responses to disparities. I characterize these frames here as a distinct binary, but they really exist as a continuum with one side or another gaining different degrees of prominence in different eras or contexts. One the one side I place "markets," on the other "justice."

First, when identifying a race-based health disparity, one can locate its source in human bodies or in social conditions. The former tends to biologize race, marking racialized bodies as somehow defective, weak, or diseased, often at the molecular level; examples would include characterizations of heart failure as a "different disease" in African Americans. The latter tends to racialize social dynamics, marking society as somehow discriminatory or unjust; examples would include many of the findings of the IOM report concerning the social bases of disparities.

Second, having identified the source of the problem, the next step is to frame a locus of responsibility for addressing it. If the source has been located in racialized human bodies, then the tendency is to situate responsibility for addressing the problem in the individuals whose bodies are affected. This often takes the form of calls for "personal responsibility" in taking care of oneself. Examples would include the DHHS push to emphasize personal responsibility in the report to Congress on the IOM study of disparities. If the source of the problem is located in society, then the tendency is to situate responsibility for addressing the problem in the polity. Examples would include characterizations of health equality as a civil right.

Third, having identified the source or the problem and located responsibility for it, the final step is to formulate an approach to address it. Going down one track, if you have located the source of the problem in human bodies, perhaps at the genetic level, and situated responsibility in the individuals whose bodies are affected, then the tendency is to formulate privatized, market-based approaches to address the problem. Examples would include BiDil, a drug formulated to address purported disparities in heart failure at the molecular level, to be purchased from a pharmaceutical corporation by individual consumers taking responsibility for their condition. This approach was evident in a 2006 statement by Alan Levine, secretary of Florida's Agency for Health Care Administration, declaring that "in the case of BiDil, we have clearly identified a product targeted toward closing the racial disparity gap."[29] Going down the other track, if you have located the source of the problem in social conditions, and situated responsibility in the political community as a matter of justice, then the tendency is to formulate government-based policy initiatives to address the problem. Examples would include any of an array of civil rights–related laws that improve the social or economic conditions of minority populations, thereby improving their health.

Of course, many responses to disparities may reflect different mixes of these tracks or frames to health disparities. Thus, for example, a federal program may encourage market-based mechanisms to improve minority access to drugs in the marketplace. The disparities frame of "access" often emerges as an area around which Democrats and Republicans share a measure of agreement, as it implicates both government initiatives to reduce disparities and personal responsibility for individualized health-care choices in the market. The "access" approach involves the political community in formulating policy responses to a problem, but it also ultimately locates the problem of disparities in the individual bodies of the affected minorities. Calls for improved access to health care, then, may involve federal initiatives to help historically disadvantaged groups, but they are double-edged insofar as they are oriented around promoting market solutions to health disparities that characterize health care as a consumer good rather than a civil right. Moreover, diverse well-intentioned federal initiatives have both directly and indirectly promoted the framing of health disparities in terms that locate the problem in the bodies of individual members of geneticized racial groups.[30] In the context of using social identities such as race in public health research, Ellison and Jones have expressed the concern that recent "expansion in genetic technology will lead to a further focusing of the medical gaze onto individual risk factors and away from social, environmental and ecological factors."[31] The critical point, then, is to be sensitive to which particular frame is being deployed at any given point in a debate over the source, responsibility, or response to health disparities.

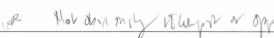

MARKETS AND JUSTICE: BACKGROUND

In 1896, Frederick Hoffman published *Race Traits and Tendencies of the American Negro* in the Publications of the American Economic Association.[32] Hoffman, a statistician at the Prudential Life Insurance Company, wrote the article for Prudential in response to a wave of state legislation banning discrimination against African Americans. Hoffman's aim was to establish the biological inferiority of the Negro as a basis for justifying Prudential's decision to exclude African Americans from access to insurance coverage. Prudential had begun cutting back on providing life insurance to African Americans as early as 1881 on the grounds that they suffered higher rates of mortality. Other insurance companies soon followed suit. State legislatures, particularly in the North, were wary of the growing power of the insurance industry and soon began enacting new statutes to regulate the industry; some of these included anti-discrimination provisions. Prudential decided to resist the new laws by asserting a "natural" biological basis for their discrimination. Leslie Ward, the vice president of Prudential, declared, "We are quite sure that mortality, even amongst the best of colored lives, would not compare favorably with the mortality amongst whites."[33]

Hoffman's task was to provide rigorous scientific analysis to undergird such claims. In his 330-page treatise, Hoffman compiled statistics, anecdotal observations, and eugenic theories to argue that "it is not in the conditions of life, but in the race traits and tendencies that we find the causes of excessive mortality."[34] Hoffman's work is replete with charts, measurements, and statistical observations, all purporting to establish the biological inferiority of the "American Negro" not only in basic mortality but in such physiological traits as "chest expansion," "physical strength," or resistance to disease.[35] Such observations built on Hoffman's conclusion in an article he had published four years earlier that "the time will come, if it has not already come, when the negro, like the Indian, will be a vanishing race."[36]

Of course, academics and expert commentators had been declaring the inferiority of the "negro race" for decades before Hoffman came on the scene.[37] What is distinctive about his work for Prudential is that it demonstrates the use of actuarial data to provide a gloss of objective scientific rigor to the construction of biological racial difference in a legal context in order to gain economic advantage in a competitive marketplace. This is the flip side of the BiDil story: where Jay Cohn used a purported race-based biological difference to *include* African Americans in a patent, Prudential was using biological difference to *exclude* African Americans from insurance coverage. Both involved using statistics to construct race as biological in a legal context to serve underlying commercial interests.

Hoffman's work did not go unchallenged. W.E.B. DuBois, in particular, presented a powerful critique, questioning Hoffman's methodology and noting that health outcomes of African Americans were comparable to those of immigrant groups with similar economic resources. Acknowledging "that in certain diseases the Negroes have a much higher rate than the whites," DuBois asked, "The question is: Is this racial? Mr. Hoffman would lead us to say yes, and to infer that it means that Negroes are inherently inferior in physique to whites." DuBois asserted, however, that such differences "can be explained on other grounds than upon race." Examining the data behind various differentials in morbidity and mortality, DuBois concluded "that the Negro death rate and sickness are largely matters of [social] condition and not due to racial traits and tendencies."[38]

Nonetheless, by and large, DuBois's critiques failed to gain traction in the broader scientific community and "Race Traits" remained the standard of excellence for statistical research into race and health for many years.[39] This dynamic, whereby assertions of race-based biological difference persist and eclipse rigorous criticisms, presages the experience, over a century later, of the Exner et al. article on racial differences in response to ACE inhibitors, which received far greater attention than subsequent critiques.

It was also in 1896 that the U.S. Supreme Court issued its infamous "separate but equal" decision in the case of *Plessy v. Ferguson*.[40] The Supreme Court rejected Homer Plessy's argument "that the enforced separation of the two races stamps the colored race with a badge of inferiority," finding "if this be so, it is not by reason of anything found in the act, but solely because the colored race chooses to put that construction upon it."[41]

Writing for the majority, Justice Henry Brown declared, "Legislation is powerless to eradicate racial instincts, or to abolish distinctions based upon physical differences, and the attempt to do so can only result in accentuating the difficulties of the present situation. . . . If one race be inferior to the other socially, the constitution of the United States cannot put them upon the same plane."[42]

Just as DuBois offered a trenchant critique of Hoffman's work that placed social forces front and center in analyzing mortality differentials, Justice John Marshall Harlan's eloquent dissent in *Plessy* argued that the social consequences of state action must be accorded constitutional recognition. "The arbitrary separation of citizens, on the basis of race," Harlan declared, "while they are on a public highway, is a badge of servitude wholly inconsistent with the civil freedom and the equality before the law established by the constitution. It cannot be justified upon any legal grounds."[43]

In its attempt to locate racial identity in the object of Plessy's body, Brown's brief opinion echoed Hoffman's massive compilation of statistics, which similarly grounded its defense of a "segregated" approach to life insurance underwriting by locating racial difference in the bodies of African Americans. Brown also located responsibility for stigma that might result from the law in the social realm, beyond the purview of the court. Brown argued that Louisiana could draw legal distinctions based upon "physical differences" without violating the Equal Protection clause of the Fourteenth Amendment, and if African Americans felt degraded by the law, that was their problem.[44] The state could act on biological difference but had no responsibility to redress harms related to social difference. The Supreme Court's opinion in *Plessy* thus legitimated the racial segregation of physical space by denying the legal significance of social differences that might be engendered by the law.[45] Hoffman similarly tried to justify a social (i.e., non-state-sponsored) segregation of insurance coverage by asserting the legal significance of purported biological differences among races.

Each of these foundational documents of twentieth-century race theory characterized the relative legal significance of social and biological differences in commercial contexts. In justifying racial subordination, they denied or obscured the significance of social or political forces, while elevating biological difference as a justification for state-sanctioned discrimination. This schema naturalizes racial difference and places any responsibility for addressing its implications beyond the purview of the state, more appropriately addressed by individual action or structured by commercial market considerations. For the past century, this characterization of racial difference has existed in tension (and often direct conflict) with the approach of those like DuBois and Harlan, who have sought to foreground the social basis of racial difference and assert a public, state responsibility for both creating and redressing inequalities embedded in such differences.

The 1954 case of *Brown v. Board of Education* repudiated Plessy's concept of "separate but equal" as "inherently unequal."[46] It did so by upending the logic that relegated the social beyond legal consideration, noting that "to separate [school children] from others of similar age and qualifications solely because of their race generates a feeling of inferiority as to their status in the community that may affect their hearts and minds in a way unlikely ever to be undone."[47] The opinion also marked a transition in the social sciences, away from Hoffman's biologization of racial difference toward DuBois's focus on the impact of social forces on the status and situation of racial groups. The Warren Court famously cited the work of social scientists such as Kenneth Clark and Gunnar Myrdal in supporting its legal recognition of the impact of segregation upon the hearts and minds of African American children.[48] Where Hoffman and Justice Brown foregrounded race as a biological concept in order to locate the responsibility for inequality in black bodies and minds, Clark, Myrdal, and the Warren Court foregrounded the social dynamics of race to locate responsibility for inequality in the state and the polity.

It is perhaps no coincidence that the early 1950s also saw the beginning of the end of the race-based insurance introduced by Prudential and others in the 1880s. For example, by the end of 1954, Metropolitan Life had eliminated most of its rules on race-based commissions and by 1958, almost all of its race-based practices with regard to differential commissions ceased. Still, reform did not come all at once, and certain other race-specific practices, including imposing different policy limits and medical examination requirements on black applicants, continued at least through the mid-1960s.[49]

From *Brown* to the passage of the Civil Rights Act in 1964 and the Voting Rights Act of 1965, the emergent civil rights revolution focused on securing government guarantees of fundamental citizenship rights for African Americans. Thomas and Mary Edsall, in their influential book *Chain Reaction*, have argued that the politics of this first era focused on equality of *opportunity* in a manner that galvanized a majority of the country and overcame conservative forces of racial resistance. After 1965, however, the civil rights agenda shifted its focus to "broader goals of emphasizing equal outcomes or results for blacks."[50] Statistics were essential to measuring such outcomes, and it is around this time that race-specific data from the Census Bureau started to become essential for gauging social, economic, and political discrimination in this country.[51] It is in this context, speaking before the Second National Convention of the Medical Committee for Human Rights in Chicago, Illinois, on March 25, 1966, that Dr. Martin Luther King Jr. declared, "Of all the forms of inequality, injustice in health care is the most shocking and inhumane."[52]

The civil rights shift in focus from *access* to fundamental rights of citizenship to *outcomes* secured through affirmative government action also gave rise to a conservative backlash, operationalized through Richard Nixon's "Southern strategy," which used race as a wedge issue, casting state action to enforce civil rights as an illegitimate grant of special privilege to minority groups. The new Republican strategy, carried to its acme by Ronald Reagan in the 1980s, focused on the concept of "equal opportunity" as opposed to "affirmative action."[53] The language of equal opportunity, often framed in terms of access, was clearly more acceptable than the language of affirmative action to what Kevin Philips termed the "emerging Republican majority."[54] The Edsalls argue that this was part of a broader shift from a "'liberal' paradigm centered on 'social responsibility,' in favor of a conservative paradigm centered around 'legitimate self interest.'"[55]

In the legal arena, this approach manifested in the Reagan Department of Justice (DOJ) position on school desegregation and affirmative action, which reoriented the government's role away from intervening to correct historical patterns of discrimination toward a focus on protecting individuals from specific acts of contemporary conscious discrimination.[56] Emblematic of this shift was the Reagan DOJ's assault on the 1971 Supreme Court decision in *Griggs v. Duke Power*.[57] In *Griggs*, the court found that employment policies that are facially neutral with regard to race (such as aptitude test scores) but nonetheless produce results that have a highly disparate impact on a minority racial group, might be found to violate Title VII of the Civil Rights Act. To justify such tests, an employer would have to show that there was a "business necessity for such test," which is a very high standard.[58] The critique was framed in terms of individual merit being subordinated to racial quotas. For example, Professor Linda Gottfredson of the University of Delaware argued that the logic of *Griggs* ignored "the whole issue of individual rights, and individual fairness . . . there is no provision for the constitutional rights, the civil rights of whites."[59]

Ultimately the Reagan DOJ's approach began to make headway with the Supreme Court as more conservative appointees shifted the court's ideological balance to the right. Later cases, beginning with *Richmond v. Croson*[60] (decided under Chief Justice William Rehnquist in 1989) and culminating in *Parents Involved in Community Schools v. Seattle School District No. 1*[61] (decided under Chief Justice John Roberts in 2007), effectively rolled back affirmative mandates in employment and school desegregation reaching back to *Brown*. A particular focus of these cases was on *individuals* as a locus for constitutional consideration. In a case such as *Croson*, this meant requiring institutions wishing to implement affirmative action programs to show particularized injury suffered by identifiable minority groups in the recent past. In her opinion for the majority, Justice Sandra Day O'Connor expressed the concern that

> to accept [a] claim that past societal discrimination alone can serve as the basis for rigid racial preferences would be to open the door to competing

claims for "remedial relief" for every disadvantaged group. . . . Those whose societal injury *is thought* to exceed some *arbitrary* level of tolerability then would be entitled to preferential classification. We think such a result would be contrary to both the letter and the spirit of a constitutional provision whose central command is equality.[62]

O'Connor's dismissal of the legal significance of the "societal injury . . . thought" to be experienced by minority groups echoes Justice Brown's similar dismissal, in *Plessy*, of claims about the stigma of segregation by asserting, "if this be so, it is not by reason of anything found in the act, but solely because the colored race chooses to put that construction upon it."[63] Brown might just as easily have said that African Americans' claims to societal injury resulting from enforced segregation were merely "*thought* to exceed some *arbitrary* level of tolerability" and hence did not deserve constitutional consideration. Both Brown and O'Connor characterized the social realities of racial discrimination as troublesome intrusions into legal analysis. Brown wants to ignore them; O'Connor to transcend them. Both saw race as obscuring a more proper focus on *individual* rights and identities.

Similarly, in *Parents Involved*, Chief Justice Roberts used a rhetoric of *individual* rights to strike down race-specific school assignments meant to achieve the ideal of desegregation called for in *Brown*. Roberts struck down the assignment plans because they did not "provide for a meaningful individualized review of applicants but instead rely on racial classifications in a 'nonindividualized, mechanical' way."[64] The state, here, was forbidden from considering race as a primary basis for assigning students to public schools. At first blush this might seem to be a logical culmination of *Brown*'s repudiation of *Plessy*'s state-mandated racial segregation. On closer examination, however, it is revealed to be quite the opposite. In mandating a "colorblind" approach to remedying past effects of racial discrimination, Roberts effectively located responsibility for addressing the consequences of racial discrimination in the private sphere of social life, beyond the purview of the state—exactly where Brown located it in his *Plessy* opinion. This "privatization" of discrimination is fully in line with the Reagan-era legacy of neoliberal (or neoconservative) valorization of private, market-based solutions as the appropriate means to address social problems.[65]

There is one additional echo of *Plessy* involving race-specific therapies such as BiDil. One of the central issues in *Plessy* was who was empowered to determine Homer Plessy's race. In Plessy's case, it was a railroad official who made the definitive determination that he was "colored." In upholding the Separate Accommodations Act, the Supreme Court not only endorsed the degrading legal principle of "separate but equal," but also implicitly validated the state's power to delegate to railroad officers the authority to make definitive determinations of racial identity. Thus, *Plessy* was not just about segregating people based upon their racial identity; it was also about establishing a legal framework for allocating power to determine racial identity.[66]

In the case of BiDil, in which insurance companies or the state (through Medicare or Medicaid) may only cover prescriptions that follow the label's race-specific indication, who is to determine the race of the patient? What happens if a person who hitherto self-identified as white, Asian, or Hispanic tells her doctor she is black in order to have a prescription for BiDil covered under her health insurance policy? More to the point, what if the health insurer disputes this claim? A similar situation could present itself in the case of Myriad's European patent on a genetic test for *BRCA2* in Ashkenazi Jewish women. What if a woman denied her Jewish identity in order to avoid paying Myriad's premium for a breast cancer test? Would the doctor, or Myriad itself, have standing to challenge that self-ascribed identity? In *Plessy*, the Supreme Court clearly decided that the state could empower its agents to override individual self-ascriptions of racial identity. When proprietary drugs or genetic tests are at stake, will corporations have similar powers?

To the extent that the Rehnquist or Roberts courts accord any legal recognition to the social conditions of racial discrimination, they have done so as an interim concept that is to be transcended. Thus, in *Richmond V. Croson*, Justice O'Connor juxtaposed group-based racial remedies against "the dream of a Nation of equal citizens in a society *where race is irrelevant* [italics added] to personal opportunity and achievement."[67] O'Connor reiterated her dream of a world where race was irrelevant in her 2003 opinion in *Grutter v. Bollinger*,[68] in which she anticipated that "25 years from now, the use of racial preferences will no longer be necessary to further the interest approved today."[69] O'Connor's dream of a country where race is irrelevant resonates with contemporary promises by biomedical researchers and clinicians yearning for a time when genetic information will similarly render race irrelevant. O'Connor was speaking of making race *socially and legally* irrelevant, whereas pharmacogenomic experts now speak of making race *biologically* irrelevant. The two sentiments are connected, though, by their common disdain for the social realities of group-based racial harms. Both view social concepts of race as impediments to progress, to be transcended and left to the dustbin of history. Both also valorize the individual as the ultimate target of intervention—legal or medical.

Neoconservative race theorists tolerate the use of race only when such schemes retain a primary focus on considering the individual attributes of persons being classified. As Justice Antonin Scalia wrote in his concurring opinion in the 1995 case of *Adarand v. Pena*, "Individuals who have been wronged by unlawful racial discrimination should be made whole; but under our Constitution there can be no such thing as either a creditor or a debtor race."[70] Similarly, biomedical researchers using race as an interim surrogate on the road to the promised land of personalized pharmacogenomic medicine focus on the *individual* bodies of patients to address what are often broad-based social determinants of health. Race-based pharmacogenomic practices ironically obscure or elide the social significance of group-based harms to health, much as Justice Scalia denied the significance of group-based harms to the civic standing of racial minorities. This approach aligns with a dynamic in law and politics identified by professor of law Dorothy Roberts, in which "race consciousness is decreasing in government social policy at the very moment it is increasing in biomedicine."[71]

All of this fits with the Edsalls' analysis of the ideology engendered by the Reagan revolution, which rejected "a 'liberal' paradigm centered on 'social responsibility,' in favor of a conservative paradigm centered on 'legitimate self interest.'" Applied to the framing of health disparities, this shift also marks the frames invoked to characterize health disparities in contemporary policy debates.[72]

RACE IN A BOTTLE:
THE POLITICS OF DISPARITIES TODAY

This brings us back to the significance of race-based pharmacogenomics for contemporary debates over the nature and proper response to health disparities in this country. The drive to geneticize race in the context of disparities implicates the idea of "racial formation," defined by sociologists Michael Omi and Howard Winant as "the sociohistorical process by which racial categories are created, inhabited, transformed, and destroyed."[73] From this perspective, the promotion of "race in a bottle"—of pharmaceutical solutions to disparities—can be understood as a "racial project" that, in Omi and Winant's terms, *is simultaneously an interpretation, representation, or explanation of racial dynamics, and an effort to reorganize and redistribute resources along particular racial lines.* Racial projects connect what race *means* in a particular discursive practice and the ways in which both social structures and everyday experiences are racially *organized*, based upon that meaning."[74] Racialized drugs and drug patents promulgate understandings of race as genetic in a manner that has the potential to recharacterize structural health disparities along lines of biology and individual behavior. They redistribute biomedical research and commercial resources away from political initiatives to redress social injustice and into the market. While framed in terms of addressing the health of minority populations, this redistribution does not involve the transfer of resources from privileged to subordinated groups. Rather, it involves leveraging the rhetoric of racial justice to engineer a transfer of resources from the public sphere to private markets. This privatization of race is fully in line with broader neoliberal dynamics of privatization.

Omi and Winant go on to argue that views of the state as "intervening" in racial conflicts obscure the fact that the state itself is racially structured. "The state," they assert, "*is* inherently racial. Far from *intervening* in racial conflicts, the state is itself increasingly the preeminent site of racial conflict."[75] One might well say the same thing about the realm of biomedicine. Current debates about using racial categories in medicine are not really about *intervening* in racial disparities; they are about how the broad structures of biomedical practice, from labs to clinics to product development and marketing, are themselves sites for producing and contesting meanings of race and difference. Biomedicine has long been racially structured. It does not exist outside of race relations—it actively constructs and shapes them.

The touchstone for current debates on disparities remains the 2003 IOM report *Unequal Treatment: Confronting Racial and Ethnic Disparities in Health Care.* This report was at the heart of the controversy involving Secretary Tommy Thompson's suppression of its findings and the subsequent conservative critiques from the likes of Sally Satel and Richard Epstein. The report itself defined disparities in health care as "racial or ethnic differences in the quality of healthcare that are not due to access-related factors or clinical needs, preferences [defined as patients' informed choices regarding health care], and appropriateness of intervention."[76] From the outset, then, the IOM report *excluded* issues of access and personal preferences from its consideration of disparities. This frame directed attention away from both market-driven issues, such as facilitating the provision of pharmaceutical products to minority consumers, and individualizing issues, such as changing personal preferences or behavior.

The report instead focused on 1) "the operation of healthcare systems and the legal and regulatory climate in which health systems function"; and 2) "discrimination at the individual, patient-provider level."[77] The frame for the first item clearly located disparities in social structures that were the responsibility of the political community to address. The frame for the second item was more individualizing, but focused on the behavior of health-care providers instead of patients, thereby implicating concerns for group-based prejudice—whether explicit or implicit—in the provision of health care.

As discussed earlier, much of the critique of the report attacked its focus on structural issues and argued for concentrating more on individual behavior and responsibility. The move from "disparities" to "difference" aimed to shift the frame of reference from social and political to individual and biological bases for the disparities chronicled by the IOM. This was accomplished, in part, through a blurring of the dual senses of the individual—social and biological—implicated by health disparities. Specifically, in terms of the initial frame of causation, the concept of "difference" (exemplified by Satel's geneticization of racial difference with respect to BiDil) locates the source of disparities in racialized individual biology. Second, in terms of the frame for responsibility in addressing the problem of disparities, the critique's focus on such issues as individual behavior and access to medical care (or medications) locates responsibility in racialized individual social conduct. The first frame constructs a pathology of racialized bodies and has roots going back to Hoffman's *Race Traits and Tendencies of the American Negro*. The second frame constructs a pathology of racialized social behavior that has similarly deep roots but is more directly traceable to the *Moynihan Report: The Negro Family*, issued by Senator Daniel Patrick Moynihan in 1965, suggesting that many poor black families were caught in a "tangle of pathology" contributing to their social and economic problems.[78] A focus on genes and personal responsibility combines concepts of biological and social pathology to locate responsibility for disparities firmly in the individual members of minority groups.

The blurring of the biological and the social to pathologize individual minorities relates more broadly to recent, more conservative approaches to health disparities that focus on altering individuals' behaviors and "empowering" individuals with increased access to products (including care and drugs) in the health marketplace. Thus, for example, in 2005, then Republican Senate Majority Leader (and medical doctor), Bill Frist, prominently called for approaches to disparities that "promote dignity and personal responsibility." While acknowledging historical and social forces that shape disparities, Frist nonetheless argued for a primary focus on programs that "will help decrease individuals' risky behavior." He noted that "the major causes of death among African Americans, for instance, are heart disease, cancer, stroke, accidents, and diabetes. Most of these are chronic diseases rather than acute illnesses, and all of these causes of death are at least arguably preventable."[79] By prevention, Frist meant action by individuals who take personal responsibility for their poor health outcomes. In this formulation, Frist acknowledged social determinants of health but then omitted them from his actual framing of the problem, which located responsibility primarily in the pathologies of "individuals' risky behavior."

Having individualized the problem of disparities, Frist called for fostering "competition" and "empower[ing] patents" by adopting

(1) market reforms to make the cost of health care more sensitive to consumer demand; (2) a more stable and consumer-friendly insurance market; (3) a variety of more affordable, consumer-directed health care products such as health savings accounts (HSAs); and (4) broader risk spreading and more effective risk adjustment throughout the individual and small-employer markets.[80]

Each of these remedies is firmly grounded in market-based approaches that promote individual "choice" and "access." It echoes an earlier request, in 2000, from Republicans in the National Governors Association for federal permission to "design [Medicaid] benefit packages to look more like commercial models," to "promote personal responsibility," and "to encourage choice through private health insurance."[81] In this model, health care is cast as a consumer good, not a civil right, and health itself becomes a matter of privatized risk-management.

Epidemiologist Philip Alcabes has identified a similar trend in epidemiology that reflects and reinforces the focus on personal responsibility instead of structural social determinants of health. He argues that contemporary discussions of race and health have been shaped by a misreading of the epidemiological concept of risk, which should be understood to apply to populations, not individual behavior. When combined with a focus on genetics in health disparities, this produces a mindset that "we do not deem it necessary, as part of a pursuit of better public welfare, to examine the structure of our social arrangements or . . . economic policies. . . . We do not have to fix the housing, provide health insurance or reopen the clinics. The problem is in the genes. There is nothing to be done." Describing individual members of minority populations as "at higher risk" for a disease allows us to make the individual the locus of the problem. "They carry risk in their genes," notes Alcabes. "They are socially suspect. They are implicated. And since we are innocent, we do not have to solve, or necessarily even examine, the vexing problems of modern society that truly make some people sick while others are well."[82]

The pharmaceutical industry has embraced the frame of health care as a consumer good in its approach to disparities. In 2007, the Pharmaceutical Research and Manufacturers of America (PhRMA) issued a report on "Medicines in Development for Major Diseases Affecting African Americans," enthusiastically titled "Nearly 700 Medicines in the Pipeline Offer Hope for Closing the Health Gap for African Americans."[83] Playing on the theme of addressing disparities, the report opens by declaring, "America's pharmaceutical research companies are developing 691 medicines for diseases that disproportionately afflict African Americans or diseases that are among the top 10 causes of death among African Americans. These medicines will help close the health disparity between African Americans and the rest of the population."[84] Of course, since most diseases in the United States disproportionately affect African Americans, this means that most pharmaceuticals on the market could be characterized as addressing disparities. Focusing on the market-oriented idea of access in the context of disparities, the report notes that "the reasons for the health disparity between African Americans and other Americans are complex and not completely understood." Instead of exploring some of those complex reasons, the report emphasized the market-oriented idea of access, noting that "lack of access to medical care is thought to play a role. African Americans, and all Americans, should have timely access to the medicines their physicians believe would work best for them."[85] Access to medicines in the U.S. context means adequate insurance coverage—either through commercial providers or through such federal programs as Medicare Part D, enacted in 2003 to provide prescription drug coverage to senior citizens.

In an earlier prominent statement on disparities, PhRMA lavished praise on a group called the Congressional Leadership Alliance to Eliminate Health Disparities.[86] Founded in February 2005 under the leadership of Gary Puckrein's NMHMF, the Alliance featured many prominent actors from the BiDil story, including Gary Puckrein himself; Michael Loberg, then CEO of NitroMed; and U.S. Representative Donna M. Christensen, who would go on later that year to testify forcefully for BiDil's approval before the FDA (after receiving substantial campaign contributions from NitroMed and its surrogates). Notably, the Alliance also prominently included former Speaker of the House, Newt Gingrich, who had made market-oriented approaches to health care a central focus of his political work after leaving Congress.[87]

The strange alliance of black Democrats, such as Christensen (and indeed the entire Congressional Black Caucus) with the likes of Newt Gingrich testifies to both the power and complexity of the politics behind BiDil and the drive to race-specific medicines. Bioethicists Yu, Goering, and Fullerton argue that support for BiDil from the African American community "can be viewed as strategically affirming the use of race in hopes of ultimately transforming the process of drug development and garnering more careful attention to the problem of health disparities."[88] Using Nancy Fraser's bivalent theory of justice (involving both recognition and redistribution) they argue that "the process of achieving recognition sometimes requires strategically affirming racial labels in the short term. As such, seeking recognition can allow for questionable, even potentially dangerous, partnerships in the name of promoting future justice."[89] Yu, Goering, and Fullerton recognize the dangers this approach poses for "reifying racial categories in medicine," but nonetheless offer the hope that such strategic partnerships may ultimately help to reduce disparities, "if done carefully, with clear and consistent qualifications about the meaning of race."[90]

There is much merit to this argument. But the weakest point in the strategy involves need to take great "care of the data." Even if the advocacy groups do take such care (which is questionable), they have no control over how their strategic allies will define and deploy racial categories. Moreover, Celeste Condit, professor of communications, has observed "a greater willingness among African Americans and other racialized groups to embrace rhetorics of difference," which she argues is part of a larger dynamic "that is articulating a new scientific legitimacy to biologically-based racial categories."[91] Where Yu, Goering, and Fullerton see the embrace of BiDil as a calculated risk to promote racial justice, Condit is concerned that African American embrace of a "difference perspective" had enabled support "for a medical approach that recognized different social groups as harboring different genes."[92]

Steven Epstein shares some of Condit's concerns about "the new focus on embodied difference" in approaching health disparities. He notes, on the one hand, that this approach "has coincided and cooperated with research on these disparities."[93] On the other hand, he cautions that "in other respects, this way of attending to difference—equating group identities with medically distinct bodily subtypes—has precluded direct attention to reducing inequalities in the domain of health, while encouraging the misleading notion that better health for all can best be pursued through study of the biology of race and sex."[94] Epstein explores in depth what he refers to as the "inclusion-and-difference paradigm," which reflects two goals: "the inclusion of members of various groups generally considered to have been underrepresented previously as subjects in clinical studies; and the measurement, within those studies, of differences across groups with regard to treatment effects, disease progression, or biological process."[95] Of particular note in relation to the curious confluence of diverse groups to support BiDil is Epstein's discussion of "categorical alignment," a tendency whereby "classification schemes that are already roughly similar become superimposed or aligned with one another."[96] He notes that racial categories had distinct meanings in the context of social movements, biomedical research, and state schemes of classification. Yet, Epstein argues, these distinct meanings could be blurred as "proponents of inclusion were able to act *as if* the social movement identity labels, the biomedical terms, and the state-sanctioned categories were all one and the same set of classifications—that is, that the politically salient categories were simultaneously the scientifically relevant categories."[97] Further reinforcing the drive toward categorical alignment are the powerful commercial incentives pharmaceutical corporations have to blur categorical distinctions in order to build ethnic niche markets for their products.

Epstein's attention to categorical alignment and the double edge of focusing on embodied difference in health disparities brings us back to a consideration of how symbols are effective in building community because of their imprecision.[98] BiDil was exactly such a symbol undergirding the Congressional Leadership Alliance and other similar coordinated efforts to cast drugs as an effective response to disparities. Money certainly played a role in building alliances, as NitroMed generously supported Christensen and other African American organizations, such as the ABC and the NAACP. But these and other groups concerned with health disparities understandably viewed BiDil as a long-overdue compensation for decades of blindness to the distinct needs and health concerns of the African American community. These groups, conceivably employing what Yu, Goering, and Fullerton would consider to be more nuanced and qualified understandings of race and the social bases of health disparities, could view BiDil as helping their community without accepting any implied messages of race as genetic. At the same time, conservatives such as Gingrich and industry groups such as PhRMA could embrace BiDil as a symbol of an approach to health "disparities" that transformed a thorny social issue of racial injustice into a market-oriented problem of increasing individual access to pharmaceutical products that address racial "difference" at the molecular level. The slippage between race as a social or genetic construct and between "disparities" or "difference" thus allows for political community-building among such odd bedfellows. Add to this the incentives pharmaceutical companies have to exploit such slippage for the purposes of ethnic niche marketing and you have a situation in which it is highly unlikely that any sort of care concerning the meaning of race will be consistently realized. As biologist Anne Fausto-Sterling notes, "Only rather slowly has the medical community realized that what appears at first to be an inclusive move—mandating participation by racially and sexually distinguishable groups in drug and other trials—might have a scorpion's sting, diverting attention from socioeconomic explanations of (and remedies for) health disparities."[99] How much more powerful might this dynamic prove when driven by commercial considerations of developing a market niche for a biomedical product?

Hailing the formation of the Congressional Leadership Alliance, PhRMA asserted that "one way to eliminate health care disparities is to ensure all patients have access to the health care they need. It is critical that patients and physicians have the freedom to choose the treatments that are right for each individual." PhRMA went on to praise "NMHMF's great work," declaring that the "medicines made by our member companies play an important role in helping to fight health care disparities."[100] Freedom of choice to purchase health and pharmaceuticals as consumer goods are at the heart of this corporate embrace of disparities.

In its report and praise for the Alliance, PhRMA was not geneticizing disparities so much as it was pharamaceuticalizing them in order to gain commercial advantage. The drugs it listed in the report (with the notable exception of BiDil) were recommended for use in all races. The report, then, did not directly racialize drugs so much as it racialized the diseases treated by the drugs, providing a basis for racially inflected marketing of the drugs to individuals with those diseases.

Yet, by racializing disease in the context of pharmaceuticals that operate at the molecular level, PhRMA's approach flows into the geneticization of race invoked by Satel in her embrace of BiDil and related critique of the IOM report. And so we come back to Linda Gottfredson, the critic of the holding in *Griggs v. Duke Power*, which allowed findings of racial discrimination based on the disparate impact of employer decisions. Speaking at an event sponsored by the conservative AEI to promote Jonathan Klick and Sally Satel's book, *The Health Disparities Myth: Diagnosing the Treatment Gap*, Gottfredson attributed race-based health disparities to "differences in an individual's cognitive abilities," arguing that "patients with lower general reasoning abilities are less likely to seek preventive care, know signs and symptoms of disease, and to adhere to treatment regimens."[101] Health literacy is certainly an important component for understanding health disparities, but by framing the issue in terms of "cognitive abilities," with the causes of disparities firmly located in the genetic constitution of racialized bodies, Gottfredson argued that the solution must entail efforts by health professionals to "improve their patients' understanding of the treatment procedures."[102] Gottfredson thus biologized the problem as a function of an individual's inherent nature, reviving dubious assertions from work such as Richard Hernstein and Charles Murray's *The Bell Curve*, that the ills of welfare, poverty, and an underclass are less matters of justice than biology.[103]

As for the *Health Disparities Myth* itself: Satel and Klick made the seemingly reasonable argument that socioeconomic factors explained health disparities better than race.[104] But this soon blurred into a critique that located responsibility for disparities in the individual. Echoing Gottfredson, Satel and Klick argued that "different racial groups have different behavioral profiles, and concentrating on the patient's side of decision-making" was "an essential element of improving minority health."[105] They argued that such behaviors "are less a characteristic of race, per se, than of class,"[106] but by focusing on *individual* behavior and economic circumstance, they totally ignored the fact that social and economic resources have been inequitably allocated for decades through systematic racially discriminatory application of government policies and private institutional racism.[107] Satel and Klick therefore ignored the IOM report's extensive analysis of structural, historical, and institutional causes of health disparities to argue simply that "the IOM panel . . . fail to make a persuasive case that physician bias is a significant cause of disparate care or health status."[108] This claim, in itself, was not necessarily unreasonable, but it obscured the IOM's extensive treatment of the issues contributing to health disparities that range far beyond physician bias. For example, the report's second of five major findings states, "Racial and ethnic disparities in health occur in the context of broader historic and contemporary social and economic inequality, and evidence of persistent racial and ethnic discrimination in many sectors of

American life." And its third finding states, "Many sources—including health system, healthcare providers, patients, and utilization managers— may contribute to racial and ethnic disparities in healthcare."[109] Moreover, insofar as the report did discuss bias, it did so in a measured and qualified manner, stating in its fourth finding, "Bias, stereotyping, prejudice, and clinical uncertainty on the part of healthcare providers may contribute to racial and ethnic disparities in healthcare. While indirect evidence from several lines of research supports this statement, a greater understanding of the prevalence and influence of these processes is needed and should be sought through research."[110] And yet, Satel and Klick titled the article that provided the basis for their book "Institute of Medicine Report: Too Quick to Diagnose Bias."[111] Given the measured tone of the actual IOM finding regarding bias, one might legitimately wonder whether it was Satel and Klick who were "too quick" in their diagnosis.

Focusing on individual provider bias, however, allowed Satel and Klick to situate their critique in the long line of racial backlash scholarship chronicled by the Edsalls in *Chain Reaction* with its focus on individual rather than structural racism and its concomitant emphasis on reverse discrimination.[112] Satel and Klick explicitly attacked "racial preferences in admission to medical school, racial sensitivity training for doctors, and legal action using Title VI of the Civil Rights Act," arguing that at best they are "trivial or irrelevant" and "potentially harmful at worst."[113] Satel and Klick thus implicitly cast health-care professionals, who are overwhelmingly white, as the aggrieved targets of unjust accusations of racism. Ironically, for a critique that emphasized the individual responsibility of people actually suffering from health disparities, Satel and Klick minimized the individual responsibility of those who provide the health care. Between Gottfredson and Satel and Klick (and their patrons at the AEI) we see a clear frame presented that locates the causes of disparities in individual bodies, not society; locates responsibility for dealing with disparities similarly in individuals, not the political community; and rejects government-sponsored policy interventions in favor of decentralized, market-oriented approaches to improving access.

In 2009, conservative blogger Jeffrey Temple favorably cited Satel in a commentary for the National Center for Public Policy Research (NCPPR) titled "Racism Is Not the Cause of Health Disparities." Echoing Tommy Thompson's approach to the original IOM report, Temple argued that those examining the issue "would be wise to seek the racial 'differences' in health issues rather than concentrating on finding 'disparity.'"[114] The NCPPR was established in 1982 "to provide the conservative movement with a versatile and energetic organization capable of responding quickly and decisively to fast-breaking issues." Temple's argument for shifting the frame from disparities to difference meshed seamlessly with the NCPPR's self-declared aim of "providing free market solutions to today's public policy problems."[115] Among other free market solutions advocated by the NCPPR is the privatization of Medicare.[116]

Genetics, of course, do play a role in health disparities, just as they play a role in all aspects of health. But as bioethicists Sankar et al. noted in a 2004 *Journal of the American Medical Association* article, its "direct contribution to the current pattern of health disparities in the United States is secondary to social and environmental influences."[117] Sankar and colleagues warn that "overemphasis on genetics as a major explanatory factor in health disparities could lead researchers to miss factors that contribute to disparities more substantially and may also tend to reinforce racial stereotyping, which may contribute to disparities in the first place."[118] They argue that "substantial evidence indicates that disparities in health status in the United States result largely from longstanding, pervasive racial and ethnic discrimination,"[119]pointing to such evidence as unhealthy housing and neighborhoods in areas with poor environmental quality, more dangerous jobs, and the effects of psychological stress caused by subjective experiences of racism.[120]

The contrast to Satel and Klick could not be more stark. Sankar and colleagues, however, are less concerned with such *negative* responses to the IOM report than with the problematic *positive* embrace of concerns for health disparities by powerful agencies of the federal government. They note that a "vision statement" issued by NHGRI after the release of the IOM report named as a "grand challenge" the need to develop "genome based tools" to disparities in health status. Such a focus may be understandable, given NHGRI's mission to promote genetics. Sankar and colleagues, however, go on to identity initiatives from several other institutes of the NIH that similarly placed genetics at the center of their health disparities initiatives. Among these were the National Institute of Arthritis and Musculoskeletal and Skin Diseases, the National Eye Institute, and the National Library of Medicine, whose "list of research priorities for health disparities put genetic research at the top, above research on environment and socioeconomic status, mechanisms of disease, and epidemiologic and risk factors."[121] With the best of intentions, federal mandates, once again, may be leading the way toward both the introduction of race into genetic research and the geneticization of health disparities research on race.

CONCLUSION

The politics of framing disparities reveals the double edge of using race in biomedical research and practice. Recognizing that race matters in health is not the same thing as agreeing upon *how* or *why* race matters. Racialized medicine has produced odd political bedfellows because of the ambiguity of race as a symbol. Nonetheless, behind that ambiguity lie distinct frames for conceptualizing racial difference and constructing its significance in the field of health. Contemporary scientific, legal, and commercial framings of race that locate its meaning in individual biology, beyond the concerns of the political community or the state, have deep roots going back at least to the era of Jim Crow. Resultant policies and legal doctrines are not inevitable, but have been and continue to be contested at many levels. Nonetheless, recent practice indicates a broad-based trend toward geneticizing health disparities in a manner that has powerful implications not only for our understandings of race but also for how we, as a society, choose to address the historical legacies of racial injustice in this country. Analysts of the ethical, legal, and social implications of the new genetics have devoted much time and attention to concerns that the genomics revolution might lead to new forms of distinctly genetic discrimination—hence the passage of the Genetic Information Nondiscrimination Act (GINA) of 2008 (P.L. 110–233, 122 Stat. 881). Despite such legitimate concerns, the drive to geneticize health disparities indicates that we must also be alert to the potential appropriation of genetics to obscure or justify existing racial inequalities.

CONCLUSIONS AND RECOMMENDATIONS

SOCIOLOGIST TROY DUSTER cautions that "it is . . . a mistake to uncritically accept old racial classifications when we study medical treatments. The task is to determine how the social meaning of race can affect biological outcomes."[1] The story of BiDil and the subsequent expanding embrace of race in biomedicine is a story of the failure of a wide variety of actors—from medical researchers to federal regulators to drug company executives—to heed Duster's admonition. Some doctors and scientists expressed similar concerns from the outset. One news report on BiDil quoted Craig Venter, who was CEO of Celera Genomics when it completed its rough draft of the human genome in 2001, as saying, "It is disturbing to see reputable scientists and physicians even categorizing things in terms of race. . . . There is no basis in the genetic code for race."[2] Joseph Graves, an evolutionary biologist then at Arizona State University, argued that "linking illness—or any other trait, like intelligence or athletic skill—to appearance is a fundamental scientific error."[3] He expressed the further concern that "scientists are often too quick to look for genetic explanations for disparities in health, when lifestyle may be the answer."[4]

BiDil does not address the social causes of heart failure, only the individualized biological ones. Such a therapy is administered based on understandings of biology. The patent submitted by Jay Cohn and Peter Carson was not for a method of treatment that merely correlated with a social group—it specified a chemical therapy for a black patient. It thereby characterized blacks as a biological group, and it received the approval of the federal government for this classification. NitroMed similarly obtained regulatory approval for BiDil as a drug to treat black people, conflating social with biological categories.

The drive to reduce disease to the level of the individual genome reflects a prototypically American emphasis on the autonomous, unencumbered individual as the primary subject of political and social concern.[5] This may appear to fly in the face of calls for "racial profiling" in medicine, but in fact there was an underlying and highly problematic logic at work here. In the context of the drive toward BiDil, those who argued for racial profiling in medicine asserted that it was permissible to use social categories of race as surrogates for biological characteristics that were understood to be "real" or "natural." Conversely, social, economic, and political differences that correlate with social categories of race were undervalued as important determinants of health. The implicit message here was that the purportedly biological differences identified by BiDil researchers deserved priority over the social differences identified by studies like the one conducted by the IOM.[6]

LEGAL AND POLICY IMPLICATIONS OF RACE AS BIOLOGY IN THE WAKE OF BIDIL

To the extent that such logic is extended into the realm of racial classifications in law, it has some additional troubling implications. First, in a general way, it may support certain efforts to further undermine already severely weakened commitments to affirmative action. Affirmative action programs use race as a social classification to redress past and present social, economic, and political injustice. As race becomes reimagined primarily in terms of biology (genetics in particular), such programs may increasingly come to be seen as based in ephemeral or insubstantial differences that are not the basis of legitimate classifications. In contrast, legal classifications based on so-called "real" differences based in biology may be put forth as sufficiently substantial to withstand the heightened or strict scrutiny required by equal protection doctrine under the Fourteenth Amendment to the U.S. Constitution.

Employers are already permitted under law to discriminate based on certain health conditions in which such discrimination is mandated as a "business necessity,"[7] or in other situations in which the health condition interferes with a "bona fide occupational qualification."[8] For example, it would be legal to discriminate against blind people when looking to hire a school bus driver. While the group "blind people" might be understood to constitute a "discrete and insular minority" that has historically experienced a measure of unjust discrimination, having sight would pass legal muster as a bona fide occupational qualification closely related to the compelling state interest of insuring the safety of both schoolchildren on the bus and pedestrians. The case for discrimination could become more complicated in the case of barring epileptics from being school bus drivers. Certainly, one would not want a school bus driver to have a seizure while on the road. But whereas the probability that a blind person cannot see the road is 100 percent, the probability that a person with epilepsy would have a seizure while driving is far lower. Nonetheless, the probability of such a seizure is also far higher than it would be for someone who did not have epilepsy. As a result, even though anyone can potentially have a seizure while driving, the greater probability that a person with epilepsy would have a seizure would probably justify discrimination in this context as sufficiently narrowly tailored to serve the compelling interest of protecting the lives of schoolchildren. However, what happens when we add to the equation the fact that many types of epilepsy can be effectively controlled through medication? For such cases, the probability of seizure goes down even further—at what point does the probability cease to justify discrimination?

To the extent that the federal government marks race as a "natural" biological category, it may open the door to new forms of race-based discrimination. In 2002, the Supreme Court held it permissible under the Americans with Disabilities Act (ADA) for Chevron to refuse to hire Mario Echazabal to work in a refinery because his hepatitis C would likely be aggravated by exposure to toxins at the refinery.[9] The ruling interpreted a section of the ADA that allowed employers to discriminate against workers whose condition posed a direct threat to others in the workplace.[10] At issue was whether the act also covered conditions that only posed a direct threat to the worker himself or herself. The court found that it did. Thus, it legitimized Chevron's discrimination against Echazabal on the basis of its assertion that his hepatitis C would likely pose a direct threat to him in the distinctive setting of a refinery. The ruling required an individualized medical assessment, yet it also recognized the legitimacy of discriminating against an individual based on a biological medical condition. Justice Souter's opinion reflected a general understanding that a work-related biological condition might provide a legal basis for discrimination.[11]

There is cause for concern, however, when one considers the implications of applying the logic of Souter's opinion to a situation in which racial categories have become biological. To the extent that legal institutions such as the PTO or the FDA come to mark certain biological conditions as "racial," race may become a surrogate not only for medical research but also for a wide array of legally sanctioned discrimination. Specifically, it deserves noting that while Echazabal was legally entitled to receive an individualized medical assessment of his health status—that is, having hepatitis C—the determination of whether that condition posed a direct threat to him under the ADA was still established by reference to probabilistic correlations between that condition and certain expected health outcomes in the presence of certain potentially aggravating factors in the environment. As race becomes correlated with various biological conditions, it takes only one further step to correlate race with a health threat.

In the not too distant past we have clear examples of discrimination based on a particular genetic condition being justified by only the most tenuous of probabilistic links to potential harm. Sickle cell trait has been the basis for differential genetic screening of populations and the outright exclusion from certain forms of employment. Is it coincidental that this sickle cell trait is among the most powerfully racially identified conditions in our culture? In the late 1960s, four black men died over an eleven-month period while going through basic combat training at a U.S. Army camp at the relatively high altitude of 4,060 feet. Autopsies revealed that all four had severe sickling of the red blood cells—although this could have been a consequence rather than a cause of their deaths. Nonetheless, a report of the deaths was published in the *New England Journal of Medicine* in 1970 and was followed up by a study conducted by the National Academy of Sciences (NAS). The NAS report found that the data were inadequate to support any specific conclusions but recommended that carriers of the sickle cell trait be excluded, inter alia, from copiloting an airplane. The U.S. Air Force Academy seized upon the NAS report to justify a new policy of excluding all blacks with the sickle cell trait—not the disease, just the trait. The policy continued until 1981, when a lawsuit finally prompted the academy to end its policy. Commercial air carriers adopted a similar policy that continued into the 1980s.

In this regard, it is instructive to reflect back upon the case of Echazabal. Just as the earlier Air Force Academy discrimination against blacks was done under the paternalistic guise of protecting them, so too was the decision upholding Chevron's discrimination against Echazabal ultimately justified in the name of protecting him from danger. The ADA's concern for health risks or "direct threats" introduces calculations of probabilistic correlation between biological condition and danger that draw upon claims put forth by biomedical researchers who assert correlations among race, genetics, and the risk of disease. This is not to say that these correlations are per se unreasonable, but it should alert us to be careful to prevent such correlations from becoming overly attenuated, especially when they are used in relation to race.[12]

In the 1998 case of *Norman-Bloodsaw v. Lawrence Berkeley Laboratory*, employees at Lawrence Berkeley Laboratory (LBL), a research institution jointly operated by the federal government and the University of California, brought suit when they discovered that LBL, without their knowledge or consent, had tested blood and urine from mandatory physical exams for syphilis, sickle cell trait, and pregnancy. This was the first class-action suit raising privacy and discrimination claims related to genetic testing in the workplace. The court ultimately found a cause of action to lie under Title VII of the Civil Rights Act of 1964 and under state and federal privacy claims. The screening, for sickle cell in particular, was differentially administered based on race: blacks were singled out for testing. While all the tests were offensive at a number of levels, of particular interest for our purposes is the fact that LBL, a major scientific research institution administered by one of the country's preeminent public universities, was, in practice, treating African Americans as a biological group to be screened for the sickle cell trait.[13]

LBL tried to justify its discriminatory practices by arguing that the aims of its testing program were to "protect employees from possible health hazards in their work environment."[14] The implicit claim here was that some defect in the employee's body justified the employer intrusion. In this case, the defective body was racialized as a condition of being rendered susceptible to external control in the form of genetic testing without informed consent. LBL's practices demonstrated no appreciation of either the fact that sickle cell trait is not limited to African Americans or the fact that merely having the trait does not necessarily predispose a carrier to any adverse health conditions. Rather, the social and cultural identification of sickle cell trait as "black" pervaded and warped the employment practices of a supposedly sophisticated scientific research institution in the 1990s.

More recently, in 2010, the NCAA adopted a new rule that requires sickle cell testing for Division I athletes.[15] One report on the proposed rule noted that "in the last decade, 21 football players have fallen ill during training and later died, and eight of those athletes was found to have sickle cell trait. The research so far is inconclusive."[16] This rule emerged as part of a settlement the previous year to a lawsuit filed by the family of a Rice University football player who had died due to complications resulting from sickle cell trait.[17] Clearly the intent was to protect the athletes, but it was also to protect the universities from lawsuits. Several questions remain: What happens after an athlete tests positive for the trait (not the disease, mind you, just the trait)? Is he or she barred from sports? The policy simply mandates "counseling" of the student. If a student's ability to attend college is dependent upon an athletic scholarship, how meaningful is this counseling, other than to provide legal cover for the institution, should the student decide to proceed in sports? Do students have to sign a waiver? The policy gives the student athlete the option of declining to take the test, but only upon condition of signing a written waiver releasing an institution from liability.[18] Will testing become a precondition of awarding athletic scholarships or perhaps grounds for rescinding them? The policy allows testing of prospective student athletes before they have enrolled.[19] Given the racialized nature of sickle cell in the United States, one can easily see the impending disproportionate impact of this policy upon black athletes. In other words, the test does not solve the problem; it merely racializes and displaces it.

Reviewing the NCAA policy, the Secretary of Health and Human Services' Advisory Committee on Heritable Disorders in Newborns and Children noted that "the history of sickle cell testing has been fraught with abuse of human rights."[20] The committee noted that the NCAA would not need to use genetic screening at all to protect student athletes if they adopted relatively straightforward guidelines used by the Department of Defense to prevent dehydration and exercise-related illness and further observed that "formal responses from the Sickle Cell Disease Association of America, Inc. and the American Academy of Pediatrics (AAP) to the NCAA rule do not support carrier screening as a means to reduce heat related illness or death."[21] There are many physical conditions that might affect student athletes for which tests are not done. Here, the distinctive interweaving of race, sports, and genetics in American culture must be understood as influencing the NCAA's actions.

One might think that the passage of GINA would largely alleviate such concerns. GINA was intended generally to prohibit discrimination in health coverage and employment on the basis of genetic information. But as legal scholar Mark Rothstein notes, "GINA was *not* enacted in response to a wave of genetic discrimination, defined as the adverse treatment of an individual based on genotype. . . . The real reason for enacting GINA was to assure people that they could undergo genetic testing without fear of genetic discrimination. As any clinical geneticist or genetic counselor will tell you, these fears are real."[22] Yet, the NCAA policy specifically involved mandatory genetic testing—though not in a health or employment context. Moreover, Rothstein argues that GINA's provision aimed at preventing workplace genetic discrimination "is infeasible and therefore is not being followed."[23] Of more direct relevance to the NCAA example, the Secretary's Advisory Committee noted that GINA "only applies to individuals who are asymptomatic (non-manifested condition). However, the current debate that sickle cell trait is associated with significant clinical indications during intense exercise can be argued as establishing a manifested genetic condition and excluded under GINA. This is only a legal theory for speculation today but may be the interpretation of the law tomorrow."[24]

Whether or not Rothstein's impressions or the committee's concerns about GINA prove out, as more biological conditions become racially identified, differential screening of individuals for those conditions and perhaps even outright group-based exclusions from employment, insurance, or other benefits may result. The mistreatment of African Americans with sickle cell trait is instructive here. It should be understood not as anomalous but as paradigmatic of problems that may develop as genetic knowledge and technologies continue to advance. In this regard, it is important to note that most efforts to address genetic discrimination focus on the production, circulation, and potential misuse of a particular individual's genetic information. Like GINA, statutes covering these problems tend to cover issues of privacy, information control, and the evaluation of individualized medical conditions.[25] Identifying certain biological conditions, especially genetic conditions, with racial groups presents challenges of a different order. Instead of implicating new forms of discrimination based on specific individualized genetic conditions, the re-biologization of race promises to entangle existing groups that have historically been subject to various forms of discriminatory treatment, such as African Americans, with new biological categories that are being produced through advances in the new genetics. The U.S. Air Force Academy, LBL, and the

NCAA did not single out blacks for screening based on access to private individual genetic information, but rather because of the identification of the social group "African American" with the biological group "sickle cell carrier."

Research that naturalizes racial boundaries has the potential to reinvigorate legally sanctioned race-based discrimination by recasting particular aspects of race in terms of biological difference.[26] Such discrimination is unlikely to appear in the familiar forms of the past. We should not expect to see direct segregation or exclusion of entire racial groups from rights and benefits based on their identification with genetic difference. Rather, subtler forms of differential treatment may arise based on tenuous correlations between genetic difference and racial groups; these correlations may lead to selective discrimination within those groups that is justified by reference to underlying "real" genetic distinctions. Harm may come not from deliberate animus toward a particular group but from which questions get asked, by whom, and to what ends.

A BIOMEDICAL ANALOGUE TO EQUAL PROTECTION

In many respects, the rise of ethnic biomedicine is a cautionary tale about what Martha Minow has called the "dilemma of difference": "When does treating people differently emphasize their differences and stigmatize or hinder them on that basis? And when does treating people the same become insensitive to their difference and likely to stigmatize or hinder them on *that* basis?"[27] In the case of biomedical research aimed at addressing race-based health disparities, however, this dilemma takes on a particular twist where treating people differently can simultaneously help and hinder them. Treating sickle cell anemia as a "black" disease has led to serious instances of stigma and unjust discrimination. It has also, however, enabled the political mobilization of elements of the African American community to campaign for increased funding for sickle cell research and other related health programs, which propelled the creation of the Office of Minority Health and the implementation of the Healthy People 2000 and 2010 initiatives.[28]

Race is a social category, but it has biological consequences. The two are not easily disentangled. Ignoring the relation between them can be as harmful as seeing them as essentially identical. The task becomes even harder when the imperatives of commerce and of the federal regulatory system combine to influence understandings of the nature and status of race as a category in biomedical research. In this country, biomedical progress has always been inextricably bound up with commerce. The issue, then, is not whether commerce should affect biomedical research or practice, but what the proper balance between commerce and science is. One of my concerns in this book has been to show how racialized medicine drives that balance out of whack. Certainly the choice of which drugs or diagnostics to develop has always been influenced by commercial considerations, but when commercial considerations affect not only the choice but the actual framing, interpretation, and presentation of scientific data, then something is wrong. Such has been the case, witting or not, with the distinctive rise of "ethnic" biomedicine in a postgenomic era. Moreover, the power of the state has become implicated in this dynamic as regulatory agencies, such as the PTO and the FDA, may be reinforcing and legitimizing ill-conceived understandings of racial difference as genetic. This has implications both for biomedical research and for broader social understandings of race.

To clarify our thinking, we must take to heart Troy Duster's admonition to use and understand racial categories as part of a "complex interaction of social forces and biological feedback loops."[29] We could begin by looking at the impact of federal mandates on biomedical practice. First, we must recognize the historical reality that there are already great troves of biomedical data that have been produced and classified with reference to the OMB-mandated racial categories. Additionally, there are some legitimate arenas for the continued use of such categories, especially for tracking social, economic, and legal phenomena involving racial discrimination or disparity. Nonetheless, at a minimum, any federal agency, institution, or individual conducting research with federal funds that reviews, approves, or uses race as a biological category or as a surrogate for a biological category should be required to offer a clarification of the terms of analysis and a justification for using them in such a manner. In this regard, it is instructive to consider that the PTO already has provisions directing patent examiners to reject applications for design patents that disclose subject matter "which could be deemed offensive to any race, religion, sex, ethnic group, or nationality."[30] The provisions also assert that "there is a further basis for objection in that the inclusion of such proscribed language in a Federal Government publication would not be in the public interest."[31] The PTO here seems to be acknowledging the significance of preventing the state from lending its imprimatur to improper uses of racial language. The basis is laid here for extending that concern from overtly offensive language to perhaps well-meaning but ill-conceived language that could promote a newly biologized understanding of racial difference.

In the years following the completion of the Human Genome Project, several prominent medical and scientific journals adopted editorial policies that reflected a similar concern. The statement from the editors of *Nature Genetics* might well serve as a model for a regulatory admonition to such agencies as the FDA or the PTO when they are asked to review applications such as those submitted by the developers of BiDil:

> The laudable objective to find means to improve the health conditions for all or for specific populations must not be compromised by the use of race or ethnicity as pseudo-biological variables. From now on *Nature Genetics* will therefore require that authors explain why they make use of particular ethnic groups or populations, and how classification was achieved. We will ask reviewers to consider these parameters when judging the merits of a manuscript—we hope that this will raise awareness and inspire more rigorous design of genetic and epidemiological studies.[32]

If the FDA or the PTO had been following such guidelines, the story of BiDil would likely have unfolded quite differently.

Requiring federal agencies to take a closer look at filings and applications that use race as a biological category could force applicants to provide more rigorous justification for their use of such terminology. The *Nature Genetics* guidelines for the use of racial categories thus serve a purpose in scientific review akin to what is known as *strict scrutiny* analysis in equal protection jurisprudence. Equal protection doctrine derives from the Fourteenth Amendment to the U.S. Constitution, which declares, "No State shall make or enforce any law which shall deny to any person within its jurisdiction the equal protection of the laws." Equal protection doctrine is used to evaluate state-mandated use of racial categories in such areas as school desegregation and affirmative action. While not necessarily directly applicable to the context of federal practice guidelines or regulatory approvals, courts and legal commentators have devoted considerable attention over the decades to developing guidelines and standards to assess and evaluate how racial and ethnic categories may be used appropriately to achieve specific goals.[33] Under equal protection doctrine, race is considered to be a "suspect classification," because of our history of racial oppression and the structural vulnerability of racial minority groups. Therefore, the state must justify the use of a racial classification by demonstrating that the classification is "narrowly tailored to serve a compelling state interest."[34] This is strict scrutiny. It requires a tight fit between the classification and the purpose or interest it serves in order to force out potentially invidious motivations behind the use of race in law. Where courts use strict scrutiny to expose invidious motives behind legal distinction based on suspect classifications, so too a harder administrative look at race when used as a biological category might reveal instances of its improper use.[35]

Professor of law Osagie Obasogie has urged federal agencies or advisory committees that new drug applications should be guided by a strict scrutiny framework similar to that employed in constitutional jurisprudence. He suggests that "once a general finding of safety and efficacy is made" a reviewing committee "questions whether there is a compelling state interest for a race-specific indication (an ongoing health disparity, the ineffectiveness of other treatments, etc.) and if the use of race is narrowly tailored such that race is not uncritically framed by government as a genetic variable while ensuring that other potential beneficiaries are not denied access."[36] Together with David Winickoff, Obasogie has also urged that in addition to traditional safety and efficacy thresholds, the FDA should adopt a null-hypothesis approach to race-specific drug approvals that would "at a bare minimum, require that clinical trials supporting race-specific indications show that a particular drug is not only better than existing treatments for the specified racial group but also no better than existing treatments for non-indicated groups."[37] They argue that this approach "would help ensure that these exclusions are as narrowly tailored as possible to 'the compelling state interest' of promoting public health."[38]

Similarly, I would suggest that whenever an applicant uses race in relation to biology before an agent of the state, a justification for the use should be required. This justification should involve, first, an assertion that the application serves a compelling interest and, second, a showing that the application uses race as biology in a way that is narrowly tailored to serving that interest. The second prong is necessary to force a distinction between observed correlations between certain biomedical conditions and certain socially identified racial groups, and racially specific genetic causation purported to underlie such correlations. Here that would mean providing compelling scientific evidence to support an assertion of race-specific genetic difference underlying any observed correlations. To date, no such differences have been identified by biomedical science. In cases such as that of BiDil, the first criterion would probably have been met. Providing an effective therapy for heart failure in African Americans would likely be a compelling interest, although the actual efficacy of BiDil in this regard is yet to be established. However, even if we assume that the first prong were met, the story of BiDil shows that this particular use of race in relation to biology was *not* narrowly tailored to serving that interest. In the language of equal protection analysis, BiDil's racial designation was both underinclusive and overinclusive: it would work in many people who were not black, and it would fail to work in certain people who were black.

Researchers can and should be able to decide how they choose to pursue their particular research agendas. But for years now, researchers and clinicians have been working under a variety of federal mandates that influence how, when, and whether they use racial and ethnic categories in their work. The time has come to examine those mandates and focus on them as targets for constructive intervention, rather than on the researchers and clinicians.

Many thoughtful attempts to articulate best practices for using racial and ethnic categories in biomedical research and clinical practice have involved discussions among social scientists, natural scientists, and medical professionals about how best to characterize and manage the social and/or scientific meaning of these categories. Largely absent from these considerations, however, has been an alternative approach with a long tradition of assessing how best to characterize and manage such classifications in a regulatory context: equal protection law.[39]

Concepts from equal protection analysis may be adapted to a biomedical context through comparison with existing biomedical analogues already in use in federal regulation of racial and ethnic classifications in research and clinical practice. Thus, for example, NIH guidelines for grant applicants and contract solicitations already require the inclusion of "a description of plans to conduct analyses to detect *significant differences* [italics added] in intervention effect by sex/gender, racial/ethnic groups, and relevant subpopulations, if applicable."[40] The guidelines go on to define "significant difference" as "a difference that is of clinical or public health *importance*, based on *substantial* [italics added] scientific data."[41] Similarly, the guidelines require such submissions to "include a description of plans to conduct *valid analysis* [italics added] by sex/gender, racial/ethnic groups, and relevant subpopulations, if applicable."[42] "Significant difference" and "valid analysis," like the equal protection standard of "narrow tailoring to serve a compelling state interest," involve terms of art that have been used constructively to manage racial and ethnic categories in diverse contexts. They have been defined over time and applied through an accretion of understanding, practice, and interpretation developed by the relevant professional communities. The model of equal protection analysis can be adapted to a biomedical context by using such analogous concepts as "significant difference" and "valid analysis" to evaluate the rigor and legiti-macy of uses of racial/ethnic classifications in relation to genetics.

Equal protection doctrine thus provides a useful model for developing guidelines to improve already existing and pervasive federal mandates governing the management of race and ethnicity in regulatory contexts. In addition to forcing out possible invidious motives, heightened scrutiny can also bring to light well-intentioned but careless or inconsistent use of racial and ethnic classifications.

To this end are proposed the following preliminary recommendations to consider in revising relevant federal mandates to address the use of race and ethnicity in biomedical research and clinical practice. They are orga-nized around a sequential scheme intended to parallel a general research plan of project conceptualization, design, and implementation. These rec-ommendations might be thought of as a regulatory analogue to the sort of guidelines on the use of racial and ethnic categories currently being con-sidered and adopted by some biomedical and scientific journals. They at-tempt to adapt or transpose the conceptual apparatus of equal protection law into the domain of biomedical research and clinical practice. It is hoped that they will provide the groundwork for further discussion of how federal mandates might be revised to help biomedical professionals keep genetic categories of population and social categories of race and ethnicity in a constructive relation to one another.

RECOMMENDATIONS

Federal regulations, mandates, guidelines, or other similar directives re-lating to federal funding, regulatory approval, or intellectual property protection for biomedical research and related products should be revised to require applications and related documents submitted to federal agen-cies that use or make claims based upon racial or ethnic categories to in-clude the following:

1. Definition

Population: Require a clear definition of the source of any population category being used and its scope and limits. Specify whether or to what extent shared biology and/or genetics is presumed to underlie the population classification chosen and the degree to which the classification also implicates nonbiological values (e.g., nationality, race/ethnicity, religion, geography, etc.).

Race/ethnicity: Require a clear recognition of the requirements of the OMB Revised Standards regarding the selection and use of racial/ethnic categories and an explicit statement of the social basis of those categories. This may take the form of including the OMB caveat: "The racial and ethnic categories set forth in the standards should not be interpreted as being primarily biological or genetic in reference."

Rationale: The OMB Revised Standards establish basic categories of race and ethnicity, but they do not dictate specifically how those categories are to be used or interpreted in different contexts. Thus, in practice, these categories are often merely starting points and are often elaborated upon and modified. The requirement of "definition" allows researchers and clinicians to adapt these categories to their own particular needs. It also ensures from the outset that such adaptation does not involve an inadvertent or inappropriate conflation of social categories of race and ethnicity with genetic population groupings.

2. Articulation

Population: Require articulation of the rationale for the particular population grouping(s) being used. Require articulation of the relation between the actual sample being used and the population category in which it is being placed. Specifically require articulation of the nature or degree of representativeness being asserted for the sample in relation to the population category chosen.

When genetically defined population categories are used, require clarification of the justification for any concurrent use of non-biological values, such as geopolitical nation-state boundaries or cultural groupings, to specify the location of descent populations. Nation-states may be used to describe geographic regions of the world from which certain populations recently descended—but such correlations must be justified and refined to clarify discontinuities between the nation-state boundaries and relevant geographic regions.

Race/ethnicity: Require articulation of and justification for any relationship asserted between any population-based genetic categories and any racial/ethnic categories. In particular, where appropriate, require articulation of whether race is being used as a *risk factor* (an attribute or exposure that, if present, directly increases the probability of a disease occurring and, if absent or removed, reduces the probability) or as a *risk marker* (an attribute or exposure that is associated with increased probability of disease, but is not necessarily a causal factor for a particular biomedical condition).

Rationale: The federal mandates create a powerful incentive for using racial and ethnic groupings to structure data and research or trial design. Once population groups and racial/ethnic groups are defined, it is important to require a clear articulation of how and why such categories are being used in the ongoing pursuit of the trial or research project.

Particular problems may arise when a relatively small sample size comes to stand as a proxy for successively larger groups. Thus, for example, the HapMap sample of forty-five Han Chinese in Beijing (a geographically situated ethnic group) may come to stand for all "Chinese" people (a historical geopolitical group) and then for all "Asians" (a continental group). As indeed, to a certain extent, they already have through the International HapMap Consortium referring to these samples as simply being from a part of "Asia."[43] This type of sequential expansion of correlation should be explicitly justified at each step.

3. Tight fit

Require a tight fit 1) between/among the population, racial/ethnic, and genetic categories being used; and 2) between the genetic category identified and the disease state/health issue or other biological activity being analyzed.

The tightness of the fit may be assessed by considering whether the relationship is based 1) on a "significant difference (or identity)" between/among the racial/ethnic and genetic categories used; and 2) on a "valid analysis" that connects both the relevant genetic category and its racial/ethnic correlate to the identified disease state or other biomedical condition.

Where race or ethnicity is being used as a risk factor, require a tight fit between the aspect of race or ethnicity identified as a risk factor and causal aspects of the condition.

Where race is being used as a risk marker, require an explicit articulation of the nature of the correlation asserted between the marker and the identified condition. Require the specification that such a correlation does not speak to underlying causal aspects of the condition.

Rationale: One of the most imposing challenges in using racial and ethnic categories in biomedical contexts is to prevent a sort of conceptual "slippage" that occurs through the elaboration of excessively attenuated relationships between racial and ethnic categories and purported biological and/or genetic correlates. Hearkening back to the example of the forty-five Han Chinese who come to stand for all of Asia, imagine further that this group of forty-five is identified as having a particular frequency of a specific genetic marker that *correlates* with a *higher likelihood* of having a particular genetic variation, which in turn *further correlates* with a *higher likelihood* of contracting a particular disease at some unspecified time in the future. This disease, in turn, may have multiple causes and be manifested in various forms with differing degrees of severity. This attenuated correlation becomes even more problematic when one realizes that the initial OMB-defined category of "race" itself is not tightly bounded in a social context but involves the use of proxy markers and historically contingent conceptions of racial identity that have changed substantially over time.[44]

It should also be noted that when differential health *outcomes* are being studied, the fit between racial/ethnic categories and biology will tend naturally to be very tight. For example, in health disparities research that studies the biomedical impact of differential access to medical care among specified black, Hispanic, Asian, and/or white populations, the fit between racial/ethnic categories and the biological health *outcomes* would be one of almost perfect identity.

Issues of "fit" will become more central in assessing projects using race and ethnicity as proxies to uncover purported underlying genetic *causes* of disease.

4. Purpose

Require a substantial health or scientific interest to be furthered by the use of racial or ethnic categorization in this context.

Rationale: The diverse federal mandates requiring the organization of data by race and ethnicity creates an incentive to use the data thereby produced—whether or not it is conceived of as directly relevant to the project at hand. Requiring the furtherance of a substantial health or scientific interest ensures that correlations between racial and ethnic categories and genetic categories will not be asserted post hoc with minimal justification. The standard of substantial interest is somewhat less rigorous than the compelling interest required under equal protection law. The rationale here is to recognize that biomedical research and clinical practice generally use racial and ethnic classifications for benign purposes.

5. Maintenance

The above-stated requirements must be met for each use of racial and/or ethnic categories throughout the relevant project or practice.

Rationale: This, again, is to prevent slippage. One common pitfall of existing approaches to using racial and ethnic categories in biomedical contexts is that researchers and clinicians may issue a sort of general disclaimer up front about race and ethnicity being social categories but then proceed through the rest of the project treating them as, in effect, primarily biological and/or genetic.

6. Caveat

If a researcher is unable to meet these requirements due to an inability to disentangle what he or she perceives to be complexly intertwined social/genetic/biological variables or categories, the application and/or related documents may still be submitted to the relevant federal agency *if* the researcher provides an explanation and prominently incorporates the OMB caveat that "the racial and ethnic categories set forth in the standards [or application, etc.] should not be interpreted as being primarily biological or genetic in reference."

Rationale: As a practical matter, individual researchers may find it difficult, given the design or nature of their projects, to break racial/ethnic and genetic population categories into their social, genetic, and nongenetic biological components. This is a major undertaking, but it is also necessary. The guidelines provide incentives to work out these issues, while the caveat allows researchers to proceed with their projects in a more deliberate manner while this difficult work progresses.

These recommendations are primarily *procedural* in nature. They preserve scientific autonomy and allow researchers and clinicians to define and act upon their own conceptions of the relevance of the OMB categories of race and ethnicity to their own work. They would apply only to applications and other related documents submitted to the federal government.

Race and ethnicity are powerful categories. They have important roles to play in understanding a wide array of health-related phenomena. They must, however, be used with care. There are significant differences between using such categories to identify disparities in health outcomes versus using them as proxies to try to identify underlying genetic causes of disease. It is hoped that these guidelines will promote more consistent and scientifically rigorous articulation, clarification, and application of these categories when submitting applications and related documents to relevant federal agencies.

The objective here is not to forbid the use of race as a category in federal policy, law, or regulation. Rather, it is to begin to articulate an institutional mechanism of guidelines whereby relevant administrative actors would be required to distinguish between uses of race as a sociopolitical category from uses of race as a biological and/or explicitly genetic category. The former can be used to track and/or redress historical inequities and current social prejudices. The latter, perhaps as a consequence of seeking relevant regulatory approvals for patents, products, and/or services, involves federal recognition of the use of race as a biological category.

In addition to these regulatory considerations of how and what the PTO and FDA should agree to sanction, there are myriad arenas in which the identification of particular racial groups with specific genetic conditions could have possible legal ramifications. For example, racially correlated disease information raises issues of employment or insurance discrimination already touched upon in the story of the sickle cell trait. In the realm of toxic torts, as gene–environment interactions become more fully understood, claims could be both organized and defended against by reference to racial categories.[45] It is also conceivable that a doctor might be sued for taking or failing to take race into account in making a diagnosis or prescribing treatment. How might this affect medical practice and the doctor–patient relationship—especially as drugs increasingly are being marketed directly to consumers? In the case of BiDil, what is a doctor to make of the fact that the FDA labeling specifies the drug for use only in black patients, whereas guidelines from the American Heart Association specify the same H/I combination as a generally legitimate therapy for anyone who is intolerant of ACE inhibitors?[46]

Just how law and policy may become implicated in such diverse areas over time is impossible to foresee. What is foreseeable, however, is that as new genomics information becomes available, a range of actors will continue to seek correlations between racial and biological groups. Such correlations will not and should not be ignored. However, it is imperative that they not be invoked casually or without sufficient consideration of the complex relations between race and biology. Demanding a clear and full articulation of the basis and justification for developing and employing such correlations should be considered an essential starting point for confronting the challenges to come.

NOTES

INTRODUCTION

1. White House Office of the Press Secretary, "Remarks by the President, Prime Minister Tony Blair of England (via satellite), Dr. Francis Collins, Director of the National Human Genome Research Institute, and Dr. Craig Venter, President and Chief Scientific Officer, Celera Genomics Corporation, on the completion of the first survey of the entire Human Genome Project," June 26, 2000, accessed December 28, 2010, http://www.ornl.gov/sci/techresources/Human_Genome/project/clinton2.shtml.

2. Samuel Levy, Granger Sutton, Pauline C. Ng, Lars Feuk, Aaron L. Halpern, Brian P. Walenz, Nelson Axelrod, et al., "The Diploid Genome Sequence of an Individual Human," *PLoS Biology* 5 (2007): e254, doi:10.1371/journal.pbio.0050254.

3. Examining the rise of biobanks, which store genetic samples for future study, Sandra Lee found that "the search for functional genetic variability is increasingly taken up in populations that are identified by conventional notions of 'race.'" Sandra Lee, "Biobanks of a 'Racial Kind': Mining for Difference in the New Genetics," *Patterns of Prejudice* 40 (2006): 448.

4. NitroMed, Inc., "NitroMed Receives FDA Letter on BiDil® NDA, a Treatment for Heart Failure in Black Patients," press release, March 8, 2001, accessed April 5, 2012, http://www.prnewswire.com/news-releases/nitromed-receives-fda-letter-on-bidil-r -nda-a-treatment-for-heart-failure-in-black-patients-71586147.html.

5. "FDA Approves BiDil Heart Failure Drug for Black Patients," *FDA News*, June 23, 2005, accessed July 5, 2005, http://www.fda.gov/bbs/topics/NEWS/2005/NEW01119.0 .html.

6. See, e.g., American Anthropological Association, "Response to OMB Directive 15: Race and Ethnic Standards for Federal Statistics and Administrative Reporting," September

1997, accessed March 28, 2012, http://www.aaanet.org/gvt/ombdraft.htm; American Anthropological Association, "Statement on Race," May 17, 1998, accessed March 28, 2012, http://www.aaanet.org/stmts/racepp.htm.

7. "Genes, Drugs and Race," Editorial, *Nature Genetics* 29 (2001): 239.

8. "Illuminating BiDil," Editorial, *Nature Biotechnology* 23 (2005): 903.

9. Paul E. Farmer, Bruce Nizeye, Sara Stulac, and Salmaan Keshavjee, "Structural Violence and Clinical Medicine," *PLoS Medicine* 3 (2006): e449, doi:10.1371/journal .pmed.0030449.

10. This is a paraphrase but, I believe, an accurate recollection of the exchange.

11. I generally agree with the approach of sociologists Michael Omi and Howard Winant to race as "an unstable and 'decentered' complex of social meanings constantly being transformed by political struggle." Michael Omi and Howard Winant, *Racial Formation in the United States: From the 1960s to the 1990s*, 2nd ed. (New York: Routledge, 1994), 55.

12. Omi and Winant, *Racial Formation*, 55.

13. Nancy Krieger, "If 'Race' Is the Answer, What Is the Question?—On 'Race,' Racism, and Health: A Social Epidemiologist's Perspective," *Is Race Real? A Web Forum Organized by the Social Science Research Council*, June 7, 2006, accessed December 22, 2010, http://raceandgenomics.ssrc.org/Krieger/#31.

14. Robert Service, "Going from Genome to Pill," *Science* 308 (2005): 1858.

15. Barbara J. Evans, David A. Flockhart, and Eric M. Meslin, "Creating Incentives for Genomic Research to Improve Targeting of Therapies," *Nature Medicine* 10 (2004): 1289.

16. See generally Mark Rothstein, ed., *Pharmacogenomics: Social, Ethical, and Clinical Dimensions* (Hoboken, N.J.: Wiley, 2003); Michelle Meadows, "Genomics and Personalized Medicine," *FDA Consumer Magazine* 39 (2005): 12, accessed March 28, 2012, http:// permanent.access.gpo.gov/lps1609/www.fda.gov/fdac/features/2005/605_genomics .html. The terms "pharmacogenetic" and "pharmacogenomic" are technically distinct but often used interchangeably. I will generally use the term "pharmacogenomic" throughout this book. As Adam Hedgecoe notes, "Recently there has been a move toward a consensus on the differences between the two terms, coming into line behind the idea that pharmacogenetics is about testing individuals for drug response, whereas pharmacogenomics is used more broadly to describe 'the concept of using whole genome information to predict drug action.'" Adam Hedgecoe, *The Politics of Personalised Medicine: Pharmacogenetics at the Clinic* (Cambridge: Cambridge University Press, 2004), 4; Francis S. Collins, Victor A. McKusick, and Karin Jegalian, "Implications of the Genome Project for Medical Science," accessed April 5, 2012 http://www.genome.gov/25019925; Sandra Lee, "Race, Distributive Justice and the Promise of Pharmacogenomics: Ethical Considerations," *American Journal of Pharmacogenomics* 3 (2003): 385.

17. C. Choi, "Prescriptions Go Personal," *The Scientist*, July 5, 2005, accessed July 6, 2005.

18. Ibid.

19. See Chapter 2 in this book.

20. National Human Genome Research Institute, "A Brief Guide to Genomics," accessed October 16, 2006, http://www.genome.gov/18016863.

21. Ibid.

22. Ibid.

23. National Human Genome Research Institute, "SNPs," accessed October 4, 2006, http://www.genome.gov/glossary.cfm [search for "SNPs"].

24. National Human Genome Research Institute, "Gene," accessed October 4, 2006, http://www.genome.gov/glossary.cfm [search for "gene"].

25. National Human Genome Research Institute, "Allele," accessed October 4, 2006, http://www.genome.gov/glossary.cfm [search for "allele"].

26. Levy et al., "Diploid Genome Sequence," e254; Francis Collins, "What We Do and Don't Know about 'Race,' 'Ethnicity,' Genetics and Health at the Dawn of the Genome Era," *Nature Genetics Supplement* 36 (2004): S13–15.

27. Troy Duster, "Buried Alive: The Concept of Race in Science," in *Genetic Nature/Culture: Anthropology beyond the Two-Culture Divide*, ed. A. Goodman, D. Heath, and M. S. Lindee (Berkeley: University of California Press, 2003), 265.

28. "Census, Race and Science," Editorial, *Nature Genetics* 24: 97–98.

29. Steven Epstein, *Inclusion: The Politics of Difference in Medical Research* (Chicago: University of Chicago Press, 2007), 28.

30. Prominent among these are Institute of Medicine's 2003 report: Brian D. Smedley, Adrienne Y. Stith, and Alan R. Nelson, eds., *Unequal Treatment: Confronting Racial and Ethnic Disparities in Health Care* (Washington, D.C.: National Academies Press, 2003).

31. Patricia Williams, *Seeing a Color-Blind Future: The Paradox of Race* (New York: Noonday Press, 1998), 52.

32. Duster, "Buried Alive," 45; Jonathan Marks, *Human Biodiversity: Genes, Race, and History* (Piscataway, N.J.: Transaction Publishers, 1995). For a powerful history of the politics of sickle cell anemia in the United States, see Keith Wailoo, *Dying in the City of the Blues* (Durham: University of North Carolina Press, 2001).

33. Richard Cooper, Katharina Wolf-Maier, Amy Luke, Adebowale Adeyemo, José R Banegas, Terrence Forrester, Simona Giampaoli, et al., "An International Comparative Study of Blood Pressure in Populations of European vs. African Descent," *BMC Medicine* 3 (2005): 2, doi:10.1186/1741-7015-3-2.

34. B. O. Tayo, M. Teil, L. Tong, H. Qin, G. Khitrov, Weijia Zhang, Quinbin Song, et al., "Genetic Background of Patients from a University Medical Center in Manhattan: Implications for Personalized Medicine," *PLoS ONE* 6 (2011): e19166, doi:10.1371/journal.pone.0019166.

35. M. J. Montoya, "Bioethnic Conscription: Genes, Race and Mexicana/o Ethnicity in Diabetes Research," *Cultural Anthropology* 22 (2007): 94–128.

1. ORGANIZING RACE

1. See, e.g., Esteban González Burchard, Elad Ziv, Natasha Coyle, Scarlett Lin Gomez, Hua Tang, Andrew J. Karter, Joanna L. Mountain, et al., "The Importance of Race and Ethnic Background in Biomedical Research and Clinical Practice," *New England Journal of Medicine* 348 (2003): 1170–1175; Richard S. Cooper, Jay S. Kaufman, and Ryk

Ward, "Race and Genomics," *New England Journal of Medicine* 348 (2003): 1166–1170; Elizabeth G. Phimister, "Medicine and the Racial Divide," *New England Journal of Medicine* 348 (2003): 1081–1082; Pamela Sankar and Mildred K. Cho, "Genetics: Toward a New Vocabulary of Human Genetic Variation," *Science* 28 (2002): 1337–1338.

2. NIH Revitalization Act of 1993, Pub. L. No. 103–43, 107 Stat. 122 (1993) (codified as amended in scattered sections of 42 U.S.C.).

3. Food and Drug Administration Modernization Act of 1997, Pub. L. No. 105–115, 111 Stat. 2296 § 115 (1997) (codified as amended in scattered sections of 21 U.S.C.).

4. Food and Drug Administration, "Guidance for Industry: Population Pharmacokinetics," 1999, accessed April 5, 2012, http://www.fda.gov/downloads/Drugs/Guidance ComplianceRegulatoryInformation/Guidances/UCM072137.pdf.

5. Ibid.

6. Food and Drug Administration, "Guidance for Industry: Collection of Race and Ethnicity Data in Clinical Trials," 2005, accessed April 5, 2012, http://www.fda.gov/down loads/RegulatoryInformation/Guidances/ucm126396.pdf.

7. Steven Epstein, *Inclusion: The Politics of Difference in Medical Research* (Chicago: University of Chicago Press, 2007), 76–82.

8. Ibid., 61–69.

9. Ibid., 72.

10. Ibid., 95–96.

11. Ibid., 83.

12. Ibid., 129.

13. United States Office of Management and Budget, "Revisions to the Standards for the Classification of Federal Data on Race and Ethnicity," October 30, 1997, accessed November 18, 2010, http://www.whitehouse.gov/omb/fedreg_1997standards/.

14. See, e.g., "Symposium on Race/Ethnicity and the 2000 Census," *American Journal of Public Health* 90 (2000): 1687–1781.

15. Melissa Nobles, *Shades of Citizenship: Race and the Census in Modern Politics* (Palo Alto, Calif.: Stanford University Press, 2000), 28, 44, 79–84. See also Margo J. Anderson, *The American Census: A Social History* (New Haven: Yale University Press, 1988); and Alice Robbin, "Classifying Racial and Ethnic Group Data in the United States: The Politics of Negotiation and Accommodation," *Journal of Government Information* 27 (2000): 133.

16. U.S. OMB, "Revisions to the Standards."

17. Nobles, *Shades*, 81–84; U.S. OMB, "Revisions to the Standards"; see also United States Census Bureau, "Racial and Ethnic Classifications Used in Census 2000 and Beyond," April 12, 2000, accessed April 5, 2012, http://www.pacificweb.org/DOCS/PopRaceAn cestry/Race/Racial%20and%20Ethnic%20Classifications%202000.pdf; see also Katherine K. Wallman, Suzann Evinger, and Susan Schechter, "Measuring Our Nation's Diversity: Developing a Common Language for Data on Race/Ethnicity," *American Journal of Public Health* 90 (2000): 1705.

18. Nobles, *Shades*, 75–79.

19. U.S. Census Bureau, "Racial and Ethnic Classifications."

20. Alice Robbin, "The Politics of Representation in the U.S. National Statistical System: Origins of Minority Population Interest Group Participation," *Journal of Government Information* 27 (2000): 435 ; see also Robbin, "Classifying," 149.

21. See Michael Omi, "Racial Identity and the State: The Dilemmas of Classification," *Law & Inequality* 15 (1997): 7, 10, 13; Robbin, "Classifying," 148–150.

22. Daniel J. Friedman, Bruce B. Cohen, Abigail R. Averbach, and Jennifer M. Norton, "Race/Ethnicity and OMB Directive 15: Implications for State Public Health Practice," *American Journal of Public Health* 90 (2000): 1714–1719; see also Nancy Krieger, "Counting Accountably: Implications of the New Approaches to Classifying Race/Ethnicity in the 2000 Census," *American Journal of Public Health* 90 (1990): 1687–1689; Edward Sondik, Jacqueline Wilson Lucas, Jennifer H. Madans, and Sandra Surber Smith, "Race/ Ethnicity and the 2000 Census: Implications for Public Health," *American Journal of Public Health* 90 (2000): 1687–1689.

23. Omi, "Racial Identity," 21.

24. National Institute of General Medical Sciences, "Human Variation Collections of the NIGMS Repository," accessed April 5, 2012, http://ccr.coriell.org/Sections/Collections /NIGMS/Populations.aspx?PgId=177&coll=GM; NIGMS, "DNA Polymorphism Discovery Resource," accessed April 5, 2012, http://www.genome.gov/10001552; National Center for Biotechnology Information, "Single Nucleotide Polymorphism," accessed April 5, 2012, http://www.ncbi.nlm.nih.gov/SNP/; NHGRI, "Developing a Haplotype Map of the Human Genome for Finding Genes Related to Health and Disease," accessed September 19, 2006, http://www.genome.gov/10001665; NCBI, "GenBank Overview," accessed April 5, 2012, http://www.ncbi.nlm.nih.gov/genbank/.

25. NIGMS, "NIGMS Human Genetic Cell Repository," accessed September 19, 2006, http://locus.umdnj.edu/nigms/ (accessed 9/19/06).

26. National Institute of General Medical Sciences, "Human Variation Collections of the NIGMS Repository," accessed April 5, 2012, http://ccr.coriell.org/Sections/Collections /NIGMS/Populations.aspx?PgId=177&coll=GM.

27. Coriell Institute for Medical Research, "Polymorphism Discovery Resource," accessed March 28, 2012, http://ccr.coriell.org/Sections/Search/Search.aspx?PgId=165&q=Poly morphism%20Discovery%20Resource.

28. Ibid.

29. An SNP is a DNA sequence variation that occurs when a single nucleotide (A, T, C, or G) in the genome sequence is altered. Each individual has many SNPs that together create a unique DNA pattern for that person.

30. NCBI, "GenBank Overview."

31. NHGRI, "Developing a Haplotype Map." On SNP analysis, see generally Noah A. Zaitlen, Hyun Min Kang, Michael L. Feolo, Stephen T. Sherry, Eran Halperin, and Eleazar Eskin, "Inference and Analysis of Haplotypes from Combined Genotyping Studies Deposited in dbSNP," *Genome Research* 15 (2005): 1594.

32. Mark J. Daly, John D. Rioux, Stephen F. Schaffner, Thomas J. Hudson, and Eric S. Lander, "High Resolution Haplotype Structure in the Human Genome," *Nature Genetics*

29 (2001): 229–232; Laura Helmuth, "Map of the Human Genome 3.0," *Science* 293 (2001): 583–585; NHGRI, "Developing a Haplotype Map."

33. International HapMap Consortium, "A Haplotype Map of the Human Genome," *Nature* 437 (2005): 1300.

34. Ibid.

35. Coriell Institute, "Human Variation."

36. International HapMap Consortium, "Integrating Ethics and Science in the International HapMap Project," *Nature Reviews Genetics* 5 (2004): 467–475.

37. "Gene Map Points to Personal Drugs," BBC News, October 26, 2005, http://news.bbc .co.uk/1/hi/health/4378624.stm.

38. Patricia Reaney, "Scientists Complete Map of Human Genetic Variation," *Boston Globe*, October 26, 2005, http://www.planetark.com/avantgo/dailynewsstory.cfm?newsid =33188.

39. Ronald Kotulak, "Genetic Map Offers Insight into Disease," *Baltimore Sun*, October 27, 2005, http://www.baltimoresun.com/news/health/balte.genes27oct27.1.5213070.story ?coll=bal-health-headlines.

40. J. C. Mueller, Elin Lõhmussaar, Reedik Mägi, Maido Remm, Thomas Bettecken, Peter Lichtner, Saskia Biskup, et al., "Linkage Disequilibrium Patterns and tagSNP Transferability among European Populations," *American Journal of Human Genetics* 76 (2005): 388.

41. International HapMap, "Integrating Ethics"; International HapMap, "A Haplotype Map."

42. L. Jorde, W. S. Watkins, M. J. Bamshad, M. E. Dixon, C. E. Ricker, M. T. Seielstad, and M. A. Batzer, "The Distribution of Human Genetic Diversity: A Comparison of Mitochondrial, Autosomal, and Y-Chromosome Data," *American Journal of Human Genetics* 66 (2000): 983.

43. Geoffrey C. Bowker and Susan Leigh Star, *Sorting Things Out: Classification and Its Consequences* (Cambridge: The MIT Press, 1999), 5–6.

44. See, e.g., Troy Duster, *Backdoor to Eugenics*, 2nd ed. (New York: Routledge, 1990); Morris W. Foster, "Ethical Issues in Developing a Haplotype Map with Socially-Defined Populations," National Human Genome Research Institute, accessed March 28, 2012, http://www.genome.gov/10001683.

45. Bowker and Leigh Star, *Sorting Things Out*, 4; Omi, "Racial Identity," 7.

46. Bowker and Leigh Star, *Sorting Things Out*, 196.

47. See, e.g., Stephen B. Thomas, "The Color Line: Race Matters in the Elimination of Health Disparities," *American Journal of Public Health* 91 (2001): 1046–1048; U.S. Department of Health and Human Services, Office of the Chief Information Officer, "HHS Policy for Improving Race and Ethnicity Data," October 24, 1997, accessed March 28, 2012, http://aspe.hhs.gov/datacncl/inclusn.htm.

48. Thomas, "Color Line," 1046–1047.

49. U.S. Department of Health and Human Services, Office of Disease Prevention and Health Promotion, "Healthy People: What Are Its Goals?" accessed September 19, 2006, http://www.health.gov/healthypeople/About/goals.htm.

50. Duster, *Backdoor*, 258–259, 272–273; Omi, "Racial Identity," 21.

51. Searches of articles in the PubMed database conducted November 18, 2010, using these terms yielded the following results: "African ethnicity": 42; "Asian ethnicity": 248; "European ethnicity": 65. In each case, the overwhelming majority of references occur after 2000.

52. See discussion of the rise of racial patents in Chapter 6.

53. Tony N. Frudakis and Mark D. Shriver, Compositions and methods for inferring ancestry, U.S. Patent Application 20040229231, filed August 19, 2003, and issued November 18, 2004.

54. See, e.g., http://www.ancestrybydna.com/. Useful analyses of the phenomenon of genetic ancestry tracing include: Duana Fullwiley, "The Biologistical Construction of Race: 'Admixture' Technology and the New Genetic Medicine," *Social Studies of Science* 38 (2008): 695–735; Alondra Nelson, "Bio Science: Genetic Ancestry Testing and the Pursuit of African Ancestry," *Social Studies of Science* 38 (2008): 759–783; and Kimberly TallBear, "Native-American-DNA.coms: In Search of Native American Race and Tribe," in *Revisiting Race in a Genomic Age*, Barbara Koenig, Sandra Soo-Jin Lee, and Sarah Richardson, eds. (Piscataway, N.J.: Rutgers University Press, 2008), 235–252.

55. Donna Haraway, *Modest_Witness@Second_Millennium.FemaleMan_Meets_OncoMouse: Feminism and Technoscience* (New York: Routledge, 1997), 291–320.

56. Anne Fausto-Sterling, "Refashioning Race: DNA and the Politics of Health Care," *Differences* 15 (2004): 1–37.

57. David Jones, "How Personalized Medicine Became Genetic, and Racial: Werner Kalow and the Formations of Pharmacogenetics," *Journal of the History of Medicine and Allied Sciences* (2011): 1, doi: 10.1093/jhmas/jrr046.

58. Ibid., 5.

59. Ibid., 33–34.

60. Urs Meyer, "Pharmacogenetics—Five Decades of Therapeutic Lessons from Genetic Diversity," *Nature Reviews Genetics* 5 (2004): 670.

61. Ibid.

62. The data presented in the text derives from searches conducted at the PubMed web portal, http://www.ncbi.nlm.nih.gov/pubmed, on September 30, 2010, using combinations of the terms "race," "ethnicity," "pharmacogenetics," and "pharmacogenomics." Searches were conducted in ten-year increments from 1960 to 2010. Thus, for example, the first search date—limited to 1/1/1960–1/1/1970—used the terms "race OR ethnicity," which manifested in the search engine as: "("continental population groups"[MeSH Terms] OR ("continental"[All Fields] AND "population"[All Fields] AND "groups"[All Fields]) OR "continental population groups"[All Fields] OR "race"[All Fields]) OR ("ethnology"[Subheading] OR "ethnology"[All Fields] OR "ethnicity"[All Fields] OR "ethnology"[MeSH Terms] OR "ethnicity"[All Fields] OR "ethnic groups"[MeSH Terms] OR ("ethnic"[All Fields] AND "groups"[All Fields]) OR ("ethnic groups"[All Fields]) AND ("1960/1/1"[PDAT] : "1970/1/1"[PDAT])."

63. Pamela Sankar, Mildred K. Cho, and Joanna Mountain, "Race and Ethnicity in Genetic Research," *American Journal of Medical Genetics* 143A (2007): 961–970, esp. 966.
64. Ibid.
65. Ibid., 967.
66. Cynthia Lee, "'Race' and 'Ethnicity' in Biomedical Research: How Do Scientists Construct and Explain Differences in Health?" *Social Science & Medicine* 68 (2009): 1187; H. Shanawani, L. Dame, D. A. Schwartz, and R. Cook-Deegan, "Non-Reporting and Inconsistent Reporting of Race and Ethnicity in Articles That Claim Associations among Genotype, Outcome, and Race or Ethnicity," *Journal of Medical Ethics* 32 (2006): 724–728. See also Timothy Caulfield, "Defining 'Race' as Defining the Problem," *Houston Law Review* 45 (2009): 1475–1482; Duana Fullwiley, "Race and Genetics; Attempts to Define the Relationship," *BioSocieties* 2 (2007): 221–237.
67. Anthony P. Cohen, *The Symbolic Construction of Community* (London: Ellis Harwood, 1985), 21.
68. See Richard Lewontin, *The Apportionment of Human Diversity*, Evolutionary Biology 6: 381–398 (1972). For an excellent overview of the history of scientific and cultural understandings of race, see generally Jonathan Marks, *Human Biodiversity: Genes, Race, and History* (Piscataway, N.J.: Transaction Publishers, 1995). For some influential statements on race by professional social science organizations, see, e.g., American Anthropological Association, "Response to OMB Directive 15: Race and Ethnic Standards for Federal Statistics and Administrative Reporting," September 1997, accessed March 28, 2012, http://www.aaanet.org/gvt/ombdraft.htm; AAA, "Statement on Race," May 17, 1998, accessed March 28, 2012, http://www.aaanet.org/stmts/racepp.htm; American Sociological Association, "The Importance of Collecting Data and Doing Social Scientific Research on Race," 2003, accessed March 28, 2012, http://www2.asanet.org/media/asa_race_statement.pdf.
69. AAA, "Statement on Race."
70. NHGRI, "Talking Glossary of Genetic Terms: Race," accessed September 30, 2010, http://www.genome.gov/Glossary/index.cfm?id=171.
71. For an elaboration of the concept of "care for the data," see Kim Fortun and Mike Fortun, "Scientific Imaginaries and Ethical Plateaus in Contemporary U.S. Toxicology," *American Anthropologist* 107 (2005): 49–50.
72. International Warfarin Pharmacogenetics Consortium, "Estimation of the Warfarin Dose with Clinical and Pharmacogenetic Data," *New England Journal of Medicine* 360 (2009): 753–764.
73. PharmGKB defines its mission as "to collect, encode, and disseminate knowledge about the impact of human genetic variations on drug response. We curate primary genotype and phenotype data, annotate gene variants and gene-drug-disease relationships via literature review, and summarize important PGx genes and drug pathways." PharmGKB, "Our Mission," accessed September 28, 2010, http://www.pharmgkb.org/.
74. Krista Conger, "Patients' Genetic Profiles Could Prevent Fatal Doses of Common Drug," *Stanford Report*, February 25, 2009, accessed March 29, 2010, http://news.stanford.edu/news/2009/february25/med-warfarin-022509.html.

75. International Consortium, "Estimation of the Warfarin," 753.

76. Ibid., 754.

77. International Consortium, "Estimation of the Warfarin," Supplementary Appendix S1a, accessed April 5, 2012, http://www.nejm.org/doi/suppl/10.1056/NEJMoa0809329 /suppl_file/nejm_intwarfpharmacons_753sa1.pdf.

78. International Consortium, "Estimation of the Warfarin," 754.

79. Bliss Broyard, *One Drop: My Father's Hidden Life—A Story of Race and Family Secrets* (New York: Little, Brown, 2007). See also Elaine K. Ginsberg, ed., *Passing and the Fictions of Identity* (Durham, N.C.: Duke University Press, 1996).

80. Mildred K. Cho and Pamela Sankar, "Forensic Genetics and Ethical, Legal and Social Implications beyond the Clinic," *Nature Genetics* 36 (2004): S9, citing K. A. Leech, *A Question in Dispute: The Debate about an 'Ethnic' Question in the Census* (London: Runnymede, 1989).

81. Celeste Condit, Alan Templeton, Benjamin R. Bates, Jennifer L. Bevan, and Tina M. Harris, "Attitudinal Barriers to Delivery of Race-Targeted Pharmacogenomics among Informed Lay Persons," *Genetics of Medicine* 5 (2003): 385.

82. Ariana Eunjung Cha, "Race Plays Role in New Drug Trials Treatment by Genetic Origin, Ethnicity Divides Medical Profession," *Washington Post*, July 28, 2003, A01, http:// www.washingtonpost.com/ac2/wp-dyn/A54171-2003Jul27?.html.

83. See, e.g., R. Hahn, "The State of Federal Health Statistics on Racial and Ethnic Groups," *Journal of the American Medical Association* 267 (1992): 268–271; R. Hahn, J. Mulinare, and S. Teutsch, "Inconsistencies in Coding of Race and Ethnicity between Birth and Death in U.S. Infants," *Journal of the American Medical Association*, 267 (1992): 259–263; R. Hahn, B. I. Truman, and N. Barker, "Identifying Ancestry: The Reliability of Ancestral Identification in the United States by Self, Proxy, Interviewer, and Funeral Director," *Epidemiology* 7 (1996): 75–80.

84. Cho and Sankar, "Forensic Genetics," S10.

85. Ibid., citing Alex L. Lowe, Andrew Urquhart, Lindsey A. Foreman, and Ian W. Evett, "Inferring Ethnic Origin by Means of an STR Profile," *Forensic Science International* 119 (2001): 17.

86. Ibid.

87. Fullwiley, "Race and Genetics," 225.

88. Duana Fullwiley, "The Molecularization of Race: Institutionalizing Human Difference in Pharmacogenetics Practice," *Science as Culture* 16 (2007): 12–15.

89. Ibid., 9–15.

90. Ibid., 14.

91. Ibid., 15.

2. THE BIRTH OF BIDIL

1. See, e.g., American College of Cardiology and American Heart Association, "ACC/ AHA Guidelines for the Evaluation and Management of Chronic Heart Failure in the

Adult," 2001, accessed April 5, 2012, http://circ.ahajournals.org/content/104/24/2996
.full; Milton Packer and Jay Cohn, "Consensus Recommendations for the Management
of Chronic Heart Failure," *American Journal of Cardiology* 83 (1999): 1A. Digitalis is the
traditional prototype of a class of drugs known as cardiac glycosides.

2. See, e.g., ACC/AHA, "Guidelines"; Packer and Cohn, "Consensus Recommendations."

3. See Joseph A. Franciosa, Anne L. Taylor, Jay N. Cohn, Clyde W. Yancy, Susan Ziesche, Adeoye Olukotun, Elizabeth Ofili, et al., "African-American Heart Failure Trial
(A-HeFT): Rationale, Design, and Methodology," *Journal Cardiac Failure* 8 (2002): 129.
See also NitroMed, Inc., "BiDil: Mechanism of Action," accessed April 5, 2012, http://
www.nitromed.com/hcp/mechanism.php; and NitroMed, Inc., "NitroMed and Merck
Form Strategic Collaboration," press release, January 7, 2003, accessed April 5, 2012,
http://www.evaluatepharma.com/Universal/View.aspx?type=Story&id=53082.

4. Keith Ferdinand, "Fixed-Dose Isosorbide Dinitrate-Hydralazine: Race-Based Cardiovascular Medicine Benefit or Mirage?" *Journal of Law, Medicine & Ethics* 36 (2008): 461.

5. See, e.g., Clyde W. Yancy, "The Role of Race in Heart Failure Therapy," Current Cardiology Reports 4 (2002): 218–225; Clyde W. Yancy, "Treatment of Heart Failure in African Americans: Clinical Update," *Ethnicity & Disease* 12 (2002): S25.

6. Yancy, "Role of Race," 218.

7. Ibid.

8. Ibid.

9. Ibid.

10. Ibid. Yancy does provide a caveat that "race is an arbitrary social/political designation,
and is pertinent as a crude marker of genetic variations only because of reproductive
isolation within any given race" (224). Yet this comes only after an extensive discussion
of what he characterizes as "an emerging database of potentially important genetic
variations that may explain" differences between black and white patients in heart failure (224).

11. Derek V. Exner, Daniel L. Dries, Michael J. Domanski, and Jay N. Cohn, "Lesser Response to Angiotensin-Converting-Enzyme Inhibitor Therapy in Black as Compared
with White Patients with Left Ventricular Dysfunction," *New England Journal of Medicine* 344 (2001): 1351, 1357.

12. Victoria Griffith, "FDA Paves the Way," *Financial Times* (March 8, 2001), 13; "This Heart
Drug Is Designed for African Americans," *Business Week* (March 26, 2001): 71; Geral-
dine Sealey, *Race and the Heart: 1st Drug Developed for Black Heart Failure Patients*,
ABCNews.com (March. 21, 2003), accessed April 6, 2012, http://abcnews.go.com
/Health/story?id=117554&page=1#.T38Azdl5Oro.

13. NitroMed, Inc., "BiDil® and the African American Heart Failure Trial (A-HeFT),"
http://www.nitromed.com/bildil/DOCS/background.html. This is a historical reference to the NitroMed website as it existed in December 2003. The url is no longer in use.

14. Jay N. Cohn, "Contemporary Treatment of Heart Failure: Is There Adequate Evidence
to Support a Unique Strategy for African-Americans? Pro Position," *Current Hypertensions Reporter* 4 (2002): 307. Cohn coauthored the study by Exner et al., "Lesser Re-

sponse." See also Peter Carson, Susan Ziesche, Gary Johnson, and Jay N. Cohn, "Racial Differences in Response to Therapy for Heart Failure: Analysis of the Vasodilator-Heart Failure Trials," *Journal of Cardiac Failure* 5 (1999): 178.

15. This logic is made quite clear in NitroMed's own statement on BiDil. See NitroMed Inc., "BiDil."

16. Jay N. Cohn, Donald G. Archibald, Susan Ziesche, Joseph A. Franciosa, W. Eugene Harston, Felix E. Tristani, W. Bruce Dunkman, et al., "Effect of Vasodilator Therapy on Mortality in Chronic Congestive Heart Failure: Results of a Veterans Administration Cooperative Study," *New England Journal of Medicine* 314 (1986): 1547. At the time, it was believed that this beneficial impact was due to a distinctive hemodynamic effect produced by the H/I combination. However, since no other vasodilator regimen has had a similar effect, it is now believed that the combination may have a distinctive effect on levels of nitric oxide (NO) in the blood. NO is believed to help protect against damage to the heart that may result in heart failure. See, e.g., ACC/AHA, "Guidelines"; Packer and Cohn, "Consensus Recommendations"; W. J. Paulus, Stefan Frantz, and Ralph A. Kelly, "Nitric Oxide and Cardiac Contractility in Human Heart Failure: Time for Reappraisal," *Circulation* 104 (2001): 2260.

17. Jay N. Cohn, Gary Johnson, Susan Ziesche, Frederick Cobb, Gary Francis, Felix Tristani, Raphael Smith, et al., "A Comparison of Enalapril with Hydralazine-Isosorbide Dinitrate in the Treatment of Chronic Congestive Heart Failure," *New England Journal of Medicine* 325 (1991): 303.

18. "Boehringer Mannheim Pharmaceuticals Corporation to Market New Medco Heart Drug," *PR Newswire*, Nov. 9, 1993.

19. Jay Cohn et al., "Comparison of Enalapril," 303; J. F. Williams Jr., et al., "ACC/AHA Guidelines for the Evaluation and Management of Heart Failure: Report of the American College of Cardiology/American Heart Association Task Force on Practice Guidelines (Committee on Evaluation and Management of Heart Failure)," *Journal of American College of Cardiology* 26 (1995): 1387.

20. The reports were numerous, bearing on a variety of characteristics measured in the trials. It appears that none of these reports disaggregated the data by race until the 1999 publication of Carson et al., "Racial Differences in Response to Therapy for Heart Failure," 178.

21. Jay N. Cohn, Method of reducing mortality associated with congestive heart failure using hydralazine and isosorbide dinitrate, U.S. Patent 4,868,179, filed April 22, 1987, and issued Sept. 19, 1989.

22. Ibid.

23. U.S. Trademark Registration 1896747, registered May 30, 1995, accessed April 7, 2012, http://trademarks.justia.com/743/17/bidil-74317284.html.

24. "Should've Asked for a Second Opinion (Medco Research Inc.'s Research on Drug BiDil Rejected by FDA)," *Business North Carolina*, July 1997, 14; see also "FDA Panel Rejects Medco's CHF Drug on Mortality Stats," *Medical Industry Today*, February 28, 1997 (noting an estimated total "cardiovascular market" at four billion dollars and a total market for BiDil at between $25 and $60 million).

25. "Medco's New BiDil Heart Failure Drug Formulation Begins Human Bioequivalence Testing," *PR Newswire*, November 7, 1994.

26. "Medco Research Finds BiDil® Bioequivalent and Re-Acquires Rights from Boehringer-Mannheim Pharmaceuticals Plans to Submit NDA," The Free Library (April 2, 1996), accessed April 6, 2012, http://www.thefreelibrary.com/MEDCO RESEARCH FINDS BIDIL(R) BIOEQUIVALENT AND RE-ACQUIRES RIGHTS . . . -a018149821.

27. "Medco Research Files NDA for BiDil®," The Free Library (July 3, 1996), accessed April 6, 2012, http://www.thefreelibrary.com/MEDCO RESEARCH FILES NDA FOR BIDIL(R)-a018449474.

28. Center for Drug Evaluation and Research, Cardiovascular and Renal Drugs Advisory Committee, Transcript from the 80th Meeting of the Food and Drug Administration, February 27–28, 1997, p. 14, accessed April 6, 2012, http://www.fda.gov/ohrms/dockets /ac/97/transcpt/3264T1.PDF.

29. Ibid., 212–214. Among other findings against BiDil, the Advisory Committee recommended unanimously that "there was no statistically significant effect on mortality for V-HeFT I" (193).

30. "Medco Drug Hits FDA Wall," *Triangle Business Journal*, February 27, 1997, accessed December 18, 2003, http://triangle.bizjournals.com/triangle/stories/1997/02/24/daily12 .html.

31. Cohn, Method of reducing.

32. Center for Drug Evaluation, "Transcript," 53.

33. "Minutes of Meeting between FDA and Dr. Jay Cohn and Wyeth-Ayerst," January 11, 1991, BiDil Administrative Correspondence, 210, http://www.accessdata.fda.gov/drug satfda_docs/nda/2005/020727_S000_Bidil_AdminCorres.pdf.

34. FDA and Medco, "Meeting Minutes," December 19, 1996. BiDil Administrative Correspondence, 173, http://www.accessdata.fda.gov/drugsatfda_docs/nda/2005/020727 _S000_Bidil_AdminCorres.pdf.

35. Center for Drug Evaluation, "Transcript," 53.

36. Center for Drug Evaluation, "Transcript," Center for Drug Evaluation & Research, Cardiovascular & Renal Drugs Advisory Comm., Minutes from the 80th Meeting of the Food and Drug Admin. 2 (Feb. 27–28, 1997), http://www.fda.gov/cder/foi/adcomm /97/cardac_022797_summin_agen_quest.pdf (last visited Oct. 11, 2003), at 2.

37. Ibid.

38. Center for Drug Evaluation, "Transcript," 21.

39. Center for Drug Evaluation, "Transcript," 20–21.

40. Of course, the investigators could have broken down the data into any one of a large number of other possible subgroups: the V-HeFT I and II reports listed at least twenty-two baseline characteristics that could each have provided an alternative basis for retrospective analysis of efficacy, independent of race. See, e.g., Susan Ziesche, Frederick R. Cobb, Jay N. Cohn, Gary Johnson, and Felix Tristani, "Hydralazine and Isosorbide Dinitrate Combination Improves Exercise Tolerance in Heart Failure: Results from V-HeFT I and V-HeFT II," *Circulation* Supplement 87 (1993): 6:V1-56. In fact, a 1993

article by Cohn suggested a number of variables that might impact therapeutic responses, but did not include race. He identified such issues as: "Do women respond the same as men? Do individuals with coronary disease respond differently than those with cardiomyopathy? Does ventricular geometry influence response to therapy? Are there biochemical or hormonal markers that will affect the response to specific intervention?" Jay N. Cohn, "The Vasodilator-Heart Failure Trials (V-HeFT). Mechanistic data from the VA Cooperative Studies. Introduction," *Circulation* Supplement 87 (1993): 6:VI-1, VI-2. Each of Cohn's questions marked a potential subgroup for analysis, but interestingly none of his questions concerned race.

41. Food and Drug Administration Modernization Act of 1997, Pub. L. 105–115, § 115, 111 Stat. 2296, 2313.

42. President William J. Clinton, "Remarks in Apology for Study Done in Tuskegee," White House Office of the Press Secretary, May 16, 1997, accessed March 28, 2012, http://clinton4.nara.gov/New/Remarks/Fri/19970516-898.html. In the Tuskegee Syphilis Study, conducted under the auspices of the U.S. Public Health Service from the 1930s to the 1970s, black men with syphilis were allowed to go untreated for years, even decades, after effective treatments were discovered in the 1940s, in order to provide researchers with information on the progression of the disease. See, e.g., A. M. Brandt, "Racism and Research: The Case of the Tuskegee Syphilis Study," in *Sickness and Health in America*, J. W. Leavitt and R. Numbers, ed. (Madison: University of Wisconsin Press, 1985), 331–346; Susan Reverby, *Examining Tuskegee: The Infamous Syphilis Study and Its Legacy* (Chapel Hill: University of North Carolina Press, 2009); James Jones, *Bad Blood: The Tuskegee Syphilis Experiment* (New York: Simon and Schuster, 1992).

43. Carson et al., "Racial Differences," 178.

44. Ibid., 182.

45. Ibid., 186.

46. Ibid., 183, 186; "NitroMed to Seek Heart Failure Indication for BiDil," *Medical Industry Today*, September 13, 1999, 71; NitroMed, Inc., "NitroMed Acquires BiDil™ New Drug Application for Treatment of Congestive Heart Failure," press release, September 10, 1999, accessed April 6, 2012, http://www2.prnewswire.com/cgi-bin/stories.pl?ACCT=104&STORY=/www/story/09-10-1999/0001018907&EDATE=.

47. Jay N. Cohn and Peter Carson, Methods of treating and preventing congestive heart failure with hydralazine compounds and isosorbide dinitrate or isosorbide mononitrate, U.S. Patent 6,465,463, filed September 8, 2000, and issued October 15, 2002.

48. Jay Cohn, interview by Joe Palca, National Public Radio, June 16, 2005, accessed June 29, 2010, http://www.npr.org/templates/story/story.php?storyId=4705662.

49. This finding is based on a search of the PubMed database using the terms "author: Cohn JN and (race or African or ethnic) And date bef: 1/1/2000," conducted March 5, 2010. The search did yield one passing mention of race, but only as one of several variables in a study for which no difference was found.

50. The filing stated: "Dr. Jay N. Cohn. In January 1999, as amended in January 2001, we entered into a collaboration and license agreement with Dr. Jay N. Cohn. Under the

agreement, Dr. Cohn licensed to us exclusive worldwide royalty-bearing rights to technology and inventions owned or controlled by Dr. Cohn and that relate to BiDil for the treatment of cardiovascular disease. . . . Pursuant to the agreement, Dr. Cohn was appointed to our scientific advisory board, entered into a consulting agreement with us and was granted an option to purchase 10,000 shares of our common stock." SEC Filing 03858247, NitroMed, Inc., S-1, Registration, August 20, 2003, 46, accessed March 1, 2010, http://ipoalerts.edgar-online.com/EFX_dll/EDGARpro.dll?FetchFilingHTML1?ID=in_2416828&SessionID=up9UHJMREAzXUIo.

51. Ibid., 41.

52. Ibid., 38–39.

53. Peter Carson, Gary Johnson, Peter Singh, Ross Fletcher, and Jay Cohn, "Differences in Vasodilator Response by Race and Heart Failure: V-HeFT," *Journal of the American College of Cardiology* 23 (1994): 382A.

54. See, e.g., Sheldon Krimsky, "The Profit of Scientific Discovery and Its Normative Implications," *Chicago-Kent Law Review* 75 (1999): 15. Krimsky notes, "The new federal initiatives on technology transfer and academic-industry-government collaborations were responsible for a marked rise in university patents. In 1980, American university patents represented one percent of all U.S. origin patents. By 1990, the figure rose to 2.4%. Within that decade, the number of applications for patents on NIH-sponsored inventions increased by nearly 300%" (22).

55. Jay N. Cohn, "Lessons from V-HeFT: Questions for V-HeFT II and the Future Therapy of Heart Failure," *Hertz* 16 (1991): 270. Reviewing the course of the V-HeFT trials, Cohn noted: "The natural evolution of V-HeFT would have mandated that the vasodilator regimen [to be combined with enalapril in V-HeFT III] would be the combination of the hydralazine and isosorbide dinitrate, which has been so effective in V-HeFT I and V-HeFT II. Unfortunately, the need for financial support has made it necessary that the vasodilator be an agent with potential commercial interest. Thus, a calcium antagonist has been substituted in V-HeFT III for the hydralazine nitrate combination, and it will be felodipine—a calcium antagonist with considerable vasoselectivity." Cohn, "Vasodilator-Heart Failure," VI-2-VI-3; see also Jay N. Cohn, "Treatment of Infarct Related Heart Failure: Vasodilators Other Than ACE Inhibitors," Invited Editorial, *Cardiovascular Drugs & Therapy* 8 (1994): 120.

56. Cohn, "Vasodilator-Heart Failure," VI-2-VI-3.

57. Ibid.

58. U.S. Patent No. 4,868,179; interview with Anne Taylor, Principal Investigator and Chairperson: A-HeFT, in Minneapolis, MN, November 11, 2002. Of course, six pills a day is still considered a lot. Indeed, doctors generally do not expect to see a great improvement in patient compliance with a drug regimen until the dosage is down to two times per day.

59. Center for Drug Evaluation, "Transcript," 210.

60. Cohn and Carson filed the first provisional application on September 8, 1999. U.S. Patent Provisional Application 60/152,616. The patent was ultimately issued in 2002 as U.S. Patent No. 6,465,463 (issued Oct. 15, 2002).

61. Roger E. Schechter and John R. Thomas, *Intellectual Property: The Law of Copyrights, Patents and Trademarks* (West Group, 2003), 291–292, 404, 421–430.

62. Correspondence, "Non-Final Rejection: Application No. 09/658,261," Raymond J. Henley III (Examiner) to Edward D. Greiff (Hale & Dorr, LLP), December 5, 2001.

63. Correspondence, "Response and Amendment under 37 C.F.R. s. 1.111: Application No. 09/658,261," Edward D. Greiff (Hale & Dorr, LLP) to Raymond J. Henley III (Examiner), May 6, 2002.

64. Correspondence, "Final Rejection: Application No. 09/658,261," Raymond J. Henley III (Examiner) to Edward D. Greiff (Hale & Dorr, LLP), May 6, 2002.

65. SEC Filing, Form S-1/A, Registration No. 333–108104, NitroMed, Inc., 11, October 2, 2003, accessed December 7, 2003, http://www.sec.gov/Archives/edgar/data/927829 /000104746903032333/a2119126zs-1a.htm.

66. Joseph Loscalzo, Joseph A. Vita, Michael D. Loberg, and Manuel Worcel, "Compositions for Treating Vascular Diseases Characterized by Nitric Oxide Insufficiency," U.S. Patent Application 20100068267, filed September 22, 2009, issued March 18, 2010.

67. Ibid.

68. See, e.g., Cheryl I. Harris, "Whiteness as Property," *Harvard Law Review* 106 (1993): 1746, 1768–1791.

69. See NitroMed, Inc., "The A-Heft Coalition," http://www.nitromed.com/BiDil.asp. This is a historical reference to the NitroMed website as it existed in March 2005. The url is no longer in use.

70. See, e.g., Gary Peller, "Race Consciousness," *Duke Law Journal* (1990): 758–834. Critical race theory is a large and diverse area of scholarship. For several useful anthologies, see also K. Anthony Appiah and Amy Gutmann, *Color Conscious* (Princeton, N.J.: Princeton University Press, 1996); Kimberle Crenshaw, Neil Gotanda, Garry Peller, and Kendall Thomas, eds., *Critical Race Theory* (New York: The New Press, 1995).

71. Melissa Nobles, *Shades of Citizenship: Race and the Census in Modern Politics* (Palo Alto, Calif.: Stanford University Press, 2000), 14–22; Minority Health and Health Disparities Research and Education Act of 2000, 42 U.S.C. § 202 (2000). U.S. Office of Minority Health, "About OMH" (2005), accessed March 28, 2012, http://minorityhealth.hhs.gov /templates/browse.aspx?lvl=1&lvlID=7; Center for Research on Genomics and Global Health, "About," accessed December 6, 2010, http://crggh.nih.gov/about.cfm.

72. Food and Drug Modernization Act of 1997, Pub.L. No. 105–115, 111 Stat. 2296. National Institutes of Health Revitalization Act of 1993, 42 U.S.C. § 201 (1993). Food and Drug Modernization Act of 1997, Pub.L. No. 105–115, 111 Stat. 2296. U.S. National Institutes of Health, "NIH Guidelines on the Inclusion of Women and Minorities as Subjects in Clinical Research," 2000, accessed February 9, 2006, http://grants.nih.gov/grants /funding/women_min/guidelines_update.htm; U.S. Food and Drug Administration, "Guidance for Industry: Collection of Race and Ethnicity Data in Clinical Trials," 2005, accessed April 6, 2012, http://www.fda.gov/downloads/RegulatoryInformation /Guidances/ucm126396.pdf. For studies of social causes of disparities, see, e.g., Institute of Medicine of the National Academies, *Unequal Treatment: Confronting Racial and Ethnic Disparities in Health Care*, 2003; National Institutes of Health Revitalization

Act of 1993, 42 U.S.C. § 201 (1993). On the criteria for FDA drug review, see, e.g., Michelle Meadows, "The FDA's Drug Approval Process: Ensuring Drugs Are Safe and Effective," U.S. Food and Drug Administration, 2000, accessed April 6, 2012, http://www.questia.com/googleScholar.qst?docId=5002484206.

73. NitroMed, Inc., "NitroMed Receives FDA Letter on BiDil® NDA, a Treatment for Heart Failure in Black Patients (Mar. 8, 2001)," accessed April 6, 2012, http://www.prnewswire.com/news-releases/nitromed-receives-fda-letter-on-bidil-r-nda-a-treatment-for-heart-failure-in-black-patients-71586147.html; Cohn and Carson, "Methods of Treating and Preventing."

74. National Minority Health Month Foundation, "Organizations Unite to Support BiDil's Approval for Heart Failure, Rebuff Designation as 'Race-Only Drug,'" June 15, 2005, accessed April 6, 2012, http://www.drugs.com/nda/bidil_050615.html.

75. Stephanie Saul, "U.S. to Review Heart Drug Intended for One Race," *New York Times*, June 13, 2005, A1.

76. Doris Gellene, "Heart Pill Intended Only for Blacks Sparks Debate," *Los Angeles Times*, June 16, 2005, accessed May 24, 2011, http://articles.latimes.com/2005/jun/16/business/fi-bidil16.

77. L. Boyce, "BiDil Controversy Raises Specter of Racial Profiling in Medicine," *Minnesota Spokesman Recorder*, November 24, 2004, accessed May 12, 2005, http://spokesman-recorder.com/news/Article/Article.asp?NewsID=50810&sID=4.

3. STATISTICAL MISCHIEF AND RACIAL FRAMES FOR DRUG DEVELOPMENT AND MARKETING

1. NitroMed, Inc., "NitroMed Receives FDA Letter on BiDil® NDA, a Treatment for Heart Failure in Black Patients (Mar. 8, 2001)," accessed April 6, 2012, http://www.prnewswire.com/news-releases/nitromed-receives-fda-letter-on-bidil-r-nda-a-treatment-for-heart-failure-in-black-patients-71586147.html; Jay N. Cohn and Peter Carson, Methods of treating and preventing congestive heart failure with hydralazine compounds and isosorbide dinitrate or isosorbide mononitrate, U.S. Patent 6,465,463, filed September 8, 2000, and issued October 15, 2002.

2. Ibid.

3. Ibid.

4. NitroMed, Inc., "NitroMed Initiates Confirmatory BiDil® Trial in African American Heart Failure Patients," press release, March 17, 2001, accessed April 6, 2012, http://www2.prnewswire.com/cgi-bin/stories.pl?ACCT=104&STORY=/www/story/03-17-2001/0001449774&EDATE=. The 2:1 ratio was reiterated by A-HeFT's principal investigator.

5. Daniel L. Dries, Derek V. Exner, Bernard J. Gersh, Howard A. Cooper, Peter E. Carson, and Michael J. Domanski, "Racial Differences in the Outcome of Left Ventricular Dysfunction," *New England Journal of Medicine* 340 (1999): 609. This was the

study Clyde Yancy used to make the case that heart failure was a "different disease" in blacks.

6. Ibid., 616.

7. Ibid., 612.

8. Ibid., 609.

9. Samantha Saha, letter to the editor, *New England Journal of Medicine* 341 (1999): 81, citing N. Krieger, D. R. Williams, and N. E. Moss, "Measuring Social Class in US Public Health Research: Concepts, Methodologies, and Guidelines," *Annual Review of Public Health* 18 (1997): 341.

10. See, e.g., William W. Dressler, "Lifestyle, Stress and Blood Pressure in a Southern Black Community," *Psychosomatic Medicine* 52 (1990): 182; Michael J. Klag, Lewis Kuller, Josef Coresh, and Paul K. Whelton, "The Association of Skin Color with Blood Pressure in US Blacks with Low Socioeconomic Status," *Journal of the American Medical Association* 265 (1991): 599; D. R. Williams, "Black-White Differences in Blood Pressure: The Role of Social Factors," *Ethnicity & Disease* 2 (1992): 126; Nancy Krieger and Stephen Sidney, "Racial Discrimination and Blood Pressure: The CARDIA Study of Young Black and White Adults," *American Journal of Public Health* 86 (1996): 1370; see also E. Harburg, John C. Erfurt, Louise S. Hauenstein, Catherine Chape, William J. Schull, and M. A. Schork, "Socio-Ecological Stress, Suppressed Hostility, Skin Color, and Black-White Male Blood Pressure: Detroit," *Psychosomatic Medicine* 35 (1973): 276; Clyde W. Yancy, "Heart Failure in African Americans: A Cardiovascular Enigma," *Journal of Cardiac Failure* 6 (2000): 183.

11. I am not a statistician. I have never even taken a course in statistics. I am a qualitative historian who runs screaming out of the room at the mere mention of "cliometrics." I am a nonpracticing lawyer who blows a gasket when confronted with the tidier-than-thou formulations of the law and economics crowd. One of the most disconcerting aspects of this whole story is that someone like me could so readily demolish such a powerful statistic with only a modicum of skepticism, intellectual curiosity, and persistence. To obtain the current statistic of 1.1:1, I went to the CDC Wonder mortality tables (http://wonder.cdc.gov), typed in an information request for the most recent year available (1999) for the category of Heart Failure (ICD 10 I50.0), and asked for age-adjusted compressed mortality rates by race measured by the closest fiscal year standard population (FY2000). The results were an age-adjusted death rate for all blacks of 20.5 per million and all whites of 18.9. The black-to-white ratio is approximately 1.08:1. The source of the Wonder mortality data set is the CDC's Office of Analysis and Epidemiology at the National Center for Health Statistics. Seeking longer-term numbers, the compressed mortality from the years 1979 to 1998 using a FY2000 standard population leads to a ratio of roughly 1.14:1. If you use a FY1970 standard population the ratio rises to 1.27:1. This higher number over the longer term fits with data released in the CDC's *Morbidity and Mortality Weekly Report* (*MMWR*) noting that between 1980 and 1995 there was a steady narrowing in the gap between blacks and whites for mortality from heart failure. Indeed, looking at mortality rates for individuals age 65 and older (among

whom approximately 94% of heart failure deaths occurred in 1994) the *MMWR* observed, "Because of greater declines in death rates from heart failure among black adults, from 1980 to 1995 the black:white ratio for men narrowed from 1.3:1 to 1.1:1 and for women from 1.4:1 to 1.1:1." CDC, Changes in Mortality from Heart Failure—United States, 1980–1995," *Morbidity and Morality Weekly Report* 47(30), August 7, 1998, 633–637, accessed November 20, 2002, http://www.cdc.gov/mmwr/preview/mmwrhtml /00054249.htm.

12. On racial disparities in health, see, e.g., Institute of Medicine (IOM), *Unequal Treatment: Confronting Racial and Ethnic Disparities in Health Care* (Washington, D.C.: National Academies Press, 2002); and U.S. Department of Health and Human Services (DHHS), *Healthy People 2010: Understanding and Improving Health*, 2nd ed. (Washington, D.C.: U.S. Government Printing Office, 2000); and Secretary's Advisory Committee on National Health Promotion and Disease Prevention Objectives for 2020. *Phase I Report: Recommendations for the Framework and Format of Healthy People 2020*, 2010, accessed January 8, 2011, http://www.healthypeople.gov/hp2020/advisory/PhaseI/PhaseI .pdf.

13. See, e.g., M. J. Montoya, "Bioethnic Conscription: Genes, Race and Mexicana/o Ethnicity in Diabetes Research," *Cultural Anthropology* 22 (2007): 94–128; and Sandra Soo-Jin Lee, Joanna Mountain, and Barbara A. Koenig, "The Meanings of 'Race' in the New Genomics: Implications for Health Disparities Research," *Yale Journal of Health Policy, Law, & Ethics* 1 (2001): 33–75, esp. 64.

14. G. Kienzlen, "BRCA2 Patent Upheld," *The Scientist*, July 1, 2005, http://www.the-scientist .com/news/20050701/01.

15. M. Gessen, "Jewish Guinea Pigs," *Slate*, July 26, 2005, http://slate.msn.com/id/2123397; On eugenics, see generally, e.g., Daniel Kevles, *In the Name of Eugenics* (Cambridge, Mass.: Harvard University Press, 1998); Paul Lombardo, *Three Generations, No Imbeciles: Eugenics, The Supreme Court, and* Buck v. Bell (Baltimore, Md.: Johns Hopkins University Press, 2008).

16. NitroMed, Inc., "NitroMed Receives FDA Letter on BiDil® NDA, a Treatment for Heart Failure in Black Patients (Mar. 8, 2001)," accessed April 6, 2012, http://www .prnewswire.com/news-releases/nitromed-receives-fda-letter-on-bidil-r-nda-a-treatment -for-heart-failure-in-black-patients-71586147.html; http://www.nitromed.com; Nitro-Med, Inc., "NitroMed Initiates Confirmatory BiDil® Trial in African American Heart Failure Patients," press release, accessed April 6, 2012, http://www2.prnewswire.com/cgi -bin/stories.pl?ACCT=104&STORY=/www/story/03-17-2001/0001449774&EDATE=.

17. G. Guterman, "Shades of Doubt and Fears of Bias in the Doctor's Office," *The Chronicle of Higher Education*, May 25, 2001, accessed December 16, 2002, http://chronicle.com /free/v47/i37/37a01601.htm#race.

18. "Trials for 'Ethnic' Drug," Editorial, *Science* 291 (2001): 2547; E. Marshall, "Trial for 'Ethnic' Therapy," *Science Now*, March 26, 2001, accessed December 12, 2002, http:// sciencenow.sciencemag.org/cgi/content/full/2001/326/2; "HF Drug Trial Planned for

Black Patients," *Today in Cardiology*, July 2001, accessed August 20, 2002, http://www
.cardiologytoday.com/200107/frameset.asp?article=AHeFT.asp; V. S. Elliot, "FDA May
Approve New Heart Drug for Blacks," *Amednews.com*, March 26, 2001, accessed May
24, 2002, http://www.ama-assn.org/amednews/2001/03/26/hlsc0326.htm; Association
of Black Cardiologists, press release, "Association of Black Cardiologists Supports Enrollment in the First Heart Failure Study Specifically for African Americans," July 21,
2002, accessed April 6, 2012, http://www.thefreelibrary.com/Association+of+Black+
Cardiologists+Supports+Enrollment+in+the+First . . . -a089209762.

19. K. M. Small, Reagan J. Kelly, Mehdi A. Keddache, Bruce J. Aronow, Gregory A.
Grabowski, Harvey S. Hahn, Karen L. Case, et al., "Synergistic Polymorphisms of Beta
1 and Alpha 2C Adrenergic Receptors and the Risk of Congestive Heart Failure," *New
England Journal of Medicine* 347 (2002): 1135–1142; R. Zimmerman, "Pair of Genes Is Said
to Increase Risk of Heart Failure in Blacks," *Wall Street Journal*, October 10, 2002.

20. National Heart, Lung, and Blood Institute (NHLBI), "Facts about Heart Failure," accessed December 3, 2002, http://www.nhlbi.nih.gov/health/public/heart/other/hrtfail
.htm. This is a historical reference to the NHLBI website as it existed in December
2003. The url is no longer in use.

21. NHLBI, "Data Fact Sheet: Congestive Heart Failure in the United States: A New Epidemic," accessed December 3, 2003, http://www.nhlbi.nih.gov/health/public/heart/other
/CHF.htm. This is a historical reference to the NHLBI website as it existed in December 2003. The url is no longer in use. "Congestive heart failure" (CHF) and "heart failure" (HF) are often used interchangeably, although technically the former is a subset of
the latter. Nonetheless, CHF mortality comprises the vast majority of all HF mortality.
BiDil is specified for treatment of CHF.

22. NHLBI, "Morbidity and Mortality: 2002 Chartbook on Cardiovascular, Lung, and
Blood Diseases," accessed December 3, 2002, http://www.nhlbi.nih.gov/resources/docs
/02_chtbk.pdf, 39. This is a historical reference to the NHLBI website as it existed in
December 2003. The url is no longer in use.

23. Dries et al., "Racial Differences," 609–616.

24. Ibid.

25. Ibid.

26. Ibid.

27. Ibid.

28. R. F. Gillum, "Heart Failure in the United States, 1970–1985," *American Heart Journal*
113 (1987): 1043–1045.

29. R. F. Gillum, "The Epidemiology of Cardiovascular Disease in Black Americans," *New
England Journal of Medicine* 335 (1996): 1597–1599.

30. R. F. Gillum, "Heart Failure," 1043.

31. Ibid.

32. Ibid.

33. Ibid.

34. Centers for Disease Control, "Changes in Mortality from Heart Failure—United States, 1980–1995."

35. Ibid.

36. Peter Carson, Susan Ziesche, Gary Johnson, and Jay N. Cohn, "Racial Differences in Response to Therapy for Heart Failure: Analysis of the Vasodilator-Heart Failure Trials," *Journal of Cardiac Failure* 5 (1999): 178–187, 186.

37. Clyde W. Yancy, "Editorial: Heart Failure in African Americans: A Cardiovascular Enigma," *Journal of Cardiac Failure* 6 (2000): 183–186; Clyde W. Yancy, "Heart Failure in Blacks: Etiological and Epidemiological Differences," *Current Cardiology Reports* 3 (2001): 191–197; Clyde W. Yancy, "The Role of Race in Heart Failure Therapy," *Current Cardiology Reports* 34 (2002): 218–225, 224.

38. Yancy, "Role of Race," 224.

39. University of Texas Southwest Medical Center at Dallas (UTSMCD), "New Release: Disparities in Black Americans' Response to Heart Failure Therapies May Signal Different Disease," May 15, 2002, accessed December 4, 2002, http://www.newswise.com /articles/2002/5/BLACKHRT.SWM.html.

40. Center for Science in the Public Interest (CSPI), "Integrity in Science," accessed July 2, 2010, http://www.cspinet.org/cgi-bin/integrity.cgi.

41. L. Braun, "Race, Ethnicity, and Health: Can Genetics Explain Disparities?" *Perspectives on Biology and Medicine* 45 (2002): 159–174. In a later study of the use of racial and ethnic categories in biomedical research, Sankar, Cho, and Mountain examined 330 randomly selected articles published between 2001 and 2004 that reported on genetic research and used one or more words from a defined list of race, ethnicity, or population terms. They found that no article actually defined or discussed the concepts of race or ethnicity being used. Pamela Sankar, Mildred K. Cho, and Joanna Mountain, "Race and Ethnicity in Genetic Research," *American Journal of Medical Genetics, Part A* 143A (2007): 961–970, esp. 961.

42. See, e.g., William W. Dressler, "Lifestyle, Stress and Blood Pressure," 182–198; Harburg et al., "Socio-Ecological Stress," 276; Michael J. Klag et al., "Association of Skin Color," 599–602; Nancy Krieger and Stephen Sidney, "Racial Discrimination and Blood Pressure," 1370; D. Raphael, *Social Justice Is Good for Our Hearts: Why Societal Factors—Not Lifestyles—Are Major Causes of Heart Disease in Canada and Elsewhere* (Toronto: CSJ Foundation for Research and Education, 2002); D. R. Williams, "Black-White Differences in Blood Pressure: the Role of Social Factors," *Ethnicity and Disease* 2 (1992): 126–141.

43. See, e.g., Klag et al., "Association of Skin Color," 599–602; Krieger and Sidney, "Racial Discrimination and Blood Pressure," 1370.

44. R. S. Cooper, Katharina Wolf-Maier, Amy Luke, Adebowale Adeyemo, José R. Banegas, Terrence Forrester, Simona Giampaoli, et al., "An International Comparative Study of Blood Pressure in Populations of European vs. African descent," *BMC Medicine* 3 (2005): 2, http://www.biomedcentral.com/1741-7015/3/2.

45. R. F. Gillum, "The Epidemiology of Cardiovascular," 1598.

46. Dries et al., "Racial Differences," 612.

47. Saha, letter to the editor, 287.

48. Jonathan Kahn, "Getting the Numbers Right: Statistical Mischief and Racial Profiling in Heart Failure Research," *Perspectives in Biology and Medicine* 46 (2003): 473–483.

49. See, e.g., NitroMed, Inc., press release, "NitroMed Stops Heart Failure Study—A-HeFT—in African Americans Due to Significant Survival Benefit of BiDil-R; Company Makes BiDil Available to All Patients in Study," July 19, 2004, accessed April 6, 2012, http://www.stockjunction.com/index.php?option=com_content&view=article &id=3292&catid=14:uncategorized&Itemid=14.

50. NitroMed, Inc., "BiDil® Named to American Heart Association's 2004 'Top 10 Advances,'" press release, January 11, 2005, http://www.mi3.com/pressreleases/2005.01.11 .NitroMed.pdf.

51. NitroMed, Inc., "FDA Accepts NitroMed's New Drug Application Resubmission for BiDil; Submission Granted a June 23, 2005 PDUFA Date," press release, February 3, 2005, accessed December 6, 2010, http://www.drugs.com/nda/bidil_050203.html.

52. To obtain this information, I visited the CDC's Wonder website (see note 11). The percentages are derived from queries for information concerning compressed mortality by race, age-adjusted for ages 45 to 64 and ages 65 and above. In the over-65 age group, the crude death rate for blacks is 142.9 per 100,000; for whites it is 153.3 per 100,000.

53. Derek V. Exner, Daniel L. Dries, Michael J. Domanski, and Jay N. Cohn, "Lesser Response to Angiotensin-Converting-Enzyme Inhibitor Therapy in Black as Compared with White Patients with Left Ventricular Dysfunction," *New England Journal of Medicine* 344 (2001): 1351–1357; "Vasotec I.V. Injection," *Physicians' Desk Reference* 2105 Thomson PDR, 57th edition (November 2002).

54. U.S. Food and Drug Administration, "Guidance for Industry: Collection of Race and Ethnicity Data in Clinical Trials," 2005, accessed April 6, 2012, http://www.fda.gov /downloads/RegulatoryInformation/Guidances/ucm126396.pdf.

55. Daniel L. Dries, Mark H. Strong, Richard S. Cooper, and Mark H. Drazner, "Efficacy of Angiotensin-Converting Enzyme Inhibition in Reducing Progression from Asymptomatic Left Ventricular Dysfunction to Symptomatic Heart Failure in Black and White Patients," *Journal of the American College of Cardiology* 40 (2002): 311.

56. J. S. Kalus and J. M. Nappi, "Role of Race in Pharmacotherapy of Heart Failure," *The Annals of Pharmacotherapy* 36 (2002): 471.

57. K. C. Ferdinand, Claudia C. Serrano, and Daphne P. Ferdinand, "Contemporary Treatment of Heart Failure: Is There Adequate Evidence to Support a Unique Strategy for African-Americans? Con Position," *Current Hypertensions Reports* 4 (2002): 311; Paul G. Shekelle, Michael W. Rich, Sally C. Morton, Col. Sid W. Atkinson, Wenli Tu, Margaret Maglione, Shannon Rhodes, et al., "Efficacy of Angiotensin-Converting Enzyme Inhibitors and Beta-Blockers in the Management of Left Ventricular Systolic Dysfunction According to Race, Gender, and Diabetic Status," *Journal of the American College of Cardiology* 41 (2003): 1529.

58. J. S. Kaufman, T. T. Nguyen, and R. S. Cooper, "Race, Medicine, and the Science behind BiDil: How ACE-Inhibition Took the Fall for the First Ethnic Drug," *Review of Black Political Economy* 37 (2010): 115–130, esp. 121.

59. Ibid., 118.
60. Ashwini R. Sehgal, "Overlap between Whites and Blacks in Response to Antihypertensive Drugs," *Hypertension* 43 (2004): 569–570.
61. Steven Epstein, *Inclusion: The Politics of Difference in Medical Research* (Chicago: University of Chicago Press, 2007), 219.
62. Kaufman et al., "Race, Medicine, and the Science," 126.
63. NitroMed, Inc., "NitroMed Initiates Confirmatory BiDil® Trial in African American Heart Failure Patients," press release, accessed April 6, 2012, http://www2.prnewswire.com/cgi-bin/stories.pl?ACCT=104&STORY=/www/story/03-17-2001/0001449774&EDATE=.
64. Sheryl Gay Stolberg, "Skin Deep: Shouldn't a Pill Be Colorblind?" *New York Times*, May 13, 2001, 4.

4. CAPITALIZING [ON] RACE IN DRUG DEVELOPMENT

1. Food and Drug Administration, "Drug Approval Package, BiDil, Medical Review, NDA 20–727," May 12, 2005, 12, http://www.accessdata.fda.gov/drugsatfda_docs/nda/2005/020727_S000_Bidil_MedR.pdf.
2. Food and Drug Administration, "Drug Approval Package, BiDil," 43; Derek V. Exner, Daniel L. Dries, Michael J. Domanski, and Jay N. Cohn, "Lesser Response to Angiotensin-Converting-Enzyme Inhibitor Therapy in Black as Compared with White Patients with Left Ventricular Dysfunction," *New England Journal of Medicine* 344 (2001): 1351–1357.
3. "FDA Approves BiDil Heart Failure Drug for Black Patients," *FDA News*, June 23, 2005, accessed July 5, 2005, http://www.fda.gov/bbs/topics/NEWS/2005/NEW0119.0.html.
4. "FDA May OK Advisory Panel Call for African American Heart Drug," *FDA Weekly*, June 17, 2005.
5. See, e.g., Marcia Angell, *The Truth about Drug Companies* (New York: Random House, 2004); Jerry Avorn, *Powerful Medicines: The Benefits, Risks, and Costs of Prescription Drugs* (New York: Vintage, 2004); Boston Consulting Group, "A Revolution in R&D: How Genomics and Genetics Are Transforming the Biopharmaceutical Industry," 2001, accessed July 5, 2005, http://www.bcg.com/publications/files/eng_genomicsgenetics_rep_11_01.pdf; Merrill Goozner, *The $800 Million Pill: The Truth behind the Cost of New Drugs* (Berkeley: University of California Press, 2004).
6. Alexandria Pešić, "Drugmakers Will Make 'Aggressive Changes' to R&D This Year, Say Researchers," *In-Pharma Technologist.com*, January 10, 2011, accessed January 13, 2011, http://www.in-pharmatechnologist.com/Industry-Drivers/Drugmakers-will-make-aggressive-changes-to-R-D-this-year-say-researchers/?c=kzr4kgmw%2FivrOjg1Oxas%2Bw%3D%3D&utm_source=newsletter_daily&utm_medium=email&utm

_campaign=Newsletter%2BDaily. The year the FDA approved BiDil, pharmaceutical giant Eli Lilly estimated that that cost could rise to $2 billion by 2010. A. Berensen, "Blockbuster Drugs Are So Last Century," *New York Times*, July 3, 2005, D1; C. Choi, "Prescriptions Go Personal," *The Scientist*, July 5, 2005, accessed July 6, 2005, http://www.the-scientist.com/2005/6/20/S12/1.

7. See, e.g., "A Revolution in R&D," Boston Consulting Group.

8. Adam Hedgecoe and Paul Martin, "The Drugs Don't Work: Expectations and the Shaping of Pharmacogenetics," *Social Studies of Science* 33 (2003): 327–364.

9. Penelope Manasco and Theresa Arledge, "Drug Development Strategies," in *Pharmacogenomics: Social, Ethical, and Clinical Dimensions*, ed. Mark Rothstein (Hoboken, NJ: John Wiley & Sons, 2003): 83–97.

10. Colin Campbell, Personal communication with author in 2003.

11. A. Berensen, "Blockbuster Drugs"; C. Choi, "Prescriptions Go Personal."

12. "FDA Label for BiDil Approved on 6/23/05," BiDil label, accessed July 7, 2005, http://www.fda.gov/cder/foi/label/2005/020727lbl.pdf.

13. "FDA May OK," *FDA Weekly*.

14. Ricardo Alonso-Zaldiva, "Panel Urges Heart Drug for African Americans," *Los Angeles Times*, June 17, 2005, accessed July 7, 2005, http://news.yahoo.com/s/latimests/20050617/ts_latimes/panelurgesheartdrugforafricanamericans.

15. Gregory Petsko, "Color Blind," *Genome Biology* 5 (2004): 119; Taslin Rahemtulla and Raj Bhopal, "Pharmacogenetics and Ethnically Targeted Therapies," *British Medical Journal* 330 (2005): 1036–1037.

16. C. E. Reeder and W. Michael Dickson, "Economic Implications of Pharmacogenomics," in *Pharmacogenomics: Social, Ethical, and Clinical Dimensions*, M. Rothstein, ed., (Hoboken, N.J.: Wiley, 2003), 243.

17. NitroMed, Inc., "BiDil® Tablets, NDA 20–727: FDA Advisory Committee Briefing Document," June 16, 2005, 10, 16, accessed July 8, 2005, http://www.fda.gov/ohrms/dockets/ac/05/briefing/2005–4145B2_02_01-NitroMed-Background.htm.

18. Andrew Moran and Richard Cooper, "Isosorbide Dinitrate and Hydralazine in Blacks with Heart Failure," *New England Journal of Medicine* 352 (2005): 1041.

19. NitroMed, Inc., "BiDil® Tablets," 23.

20. James Kingsland, "Colour-Coded Cures," *New Scientist* 186 (2005): 42–47.

21. See Andrew Pollack and Lawrence K. Altman, "Large Trial Finds AIDS Vaccine Fails to Stop Infection," *New York Times*, February 24, 2003, accessed February 25, 2003, http://www.nytimes.com/2003/02/24/scinece/24VACC.html.

22. See ibid.; Jon Cohen, "VaxGen's Sketchy Statistics," *Science Now*, February 27, 2003, accessed February 27, 2003, http://sciencenow.sciencemag.org/cgi/content/full/2003/227/1.

23. Jay N. Cohn, "The Vasodilator-Heart Failure Trials (V-HeFT). Mechanistic Data from the VA Cooperative Studies. Introduction," *Circulation* Supplement 87 (1993): VI-1, VI-2.

24. Victoria Stagg Elliott, "Color-Blind? The Value of Racial Data in Medical Research," *Amednews.com*, January 5, 2004, http://www.ama-assn.org/amednews/2004/01/05/hlsa0105.html, quoting Mark Feinberg, M.D., Ph.D., Professor of Medicine and HIV Specialist at Emory University School of Medicine.

25. NitroMed, Inc., "Annual Report," SEC Form 10-K, March 10, 2005, 38, accessed July 11, 2005, http://investors.nitromed.com/phoenix.zhtml?c=130535&p=irol-secToc&TOC=aHRocDovL2NjYm4uMTBrBrd2l6YXJkLmNvbS94bWwvY29udGVudHMuP2lwYWdlPTMzMjU1MzcmcmVwbz10ZW5r5r.

26. Food and Drug Administration, "Transcript of Meeting," Center for Drug Evaluation and Research, Cardiovascular and Renal Drug Advisory Committee, June 16, 2005, 180, accessed July 8, 2005, http://www.fda.gov/ohrms/dockets/ac/05/transcripts/2005-4145T2.pdf.

27. Ibid., 301–302.

28. Ibid., 388.

29. Robert Temple and Norman Stockbridge, "BiDil for Heart Failure in Black Patients: The U.S. Food and Drug Administration Perspective," *Annals of Internal Medicine* 146 (2007): 1, 57–62, 58.

30. Kirsten Bibbins-Domingo and Alicia Fernandez, letter to the editor, *Annals of Internal Medicine* 147 (2007): 3, 214–215, 214. This concern was echoed by John Flack, a professor of internal medicine at Wayne State University, who wrote of the BiDil data, "Subgroup analyses of clinical trials, although useful and hypothesis-generating, are very difficult to interpret with confidence as they are not protected by the randomization (potential confounders, known and unknown, are not equally distributed between contrasted groups). Furthermore, results reported in subgroup analyses are not always replicated in prospective trials testing the same hypotheses." John M. Flack, "Editorial Commentary on Fixed Combination Isosorbide Dinitrate/Hydralazine for Nitric-Oxide-Enhancing Therapy in Heart Failure," *Expert Opinion Pharmacotherapy* 8 (2007): 276.

31. Temple and Stockbridge, "BiDil for Heart Failure," 58.

32. G. T. Ellison, Jay S. Kaufman, Rosemary F. Head, Paul A. Martin, and Jonathan D. Kahn, "Flaws in the U.S. Food and Drug Administration's Rationale for Supporting the Development and Approval of BiDil as a Treatment for Heart Failure Only in Black Patients," *Journal of Law and Medical Ethics* 36 (2008): 457. I was a coauthor of this article, but the others really did the heavy lifting.

33. FDA, "Transcript of Meeting," 396.

34. Ibid., 308.

35. "Memorandum of Teleconference between NitroMed and FDA Division of Cardio-Renal Drug Products," April 7, 2005, BiDil Administrative Correspondence, 111, http://www.accessdata.fda.gov/drugsatfda_docs/nda/2005/020727_S000_Bidil_AdminCorres.pdf.

36. Ibid.

37. Ibid., 104.

38. Ibid., 104.

39. That would be me.

40. FDA, "Transcript of Meeting," 394.

41. Ibid., 307–308, 355.

42. Center for Drug Evaluation and Research, Cardiovascular and Renal Drugs Advisory Committee, Transcript from the 80th Meeting of the Food and Drug Administration, February 27–28, 1997, 156.

43. Ibid.

44. Ibid., 164.

45. Ibid., 168.

46. Ibid., 171.

47. FDA, "Transcript of Meeting," 304.

48. Ibid., 305–306.

49. John Henkel, "Orphan Drug Law Matures into Medical Mainstay," *FDA Consumer* 33 (1999): 29–32, accessed November 3, 2010, http://permanent.access.gpo.gov/lps1609/www .fda.gov/fdac/features/1999/399_orph.htm.

50. "FDA Approves BiDil Heart Failure Drug for Black Patients," *FDA News*, June 23, 2005, accessed July 5, 2005, http://www.fda.gov/bbs/topics/NEWS/2005/NEW0119.0.html.

51. Andrew Webster, Paul Martin, Graham Lewis, and Andrew Smart, "Integrating Pharmacogenetics into Society: In Search of a Model," *Nature Reviews Genetics* 5 (2004): 663–669; FDA, "Guidance for Industry: Pharmacogenomic Data Submissions," Food and Drug Administration, 2005, accessed December 12, 2005, http://www.fda.gov/cder /guidance/6400fnl.htm.

52. Temple and Stockbridge, "BiDil for Heart Failure," 58.

53. Robert Temple and Norman Stockbridge, "In Response," *Annals of Internal Medicine* 147 (2007): 3, 215–216.

54. Committee on Evaluation and Management of Heart Failure "ACC/AHA Guidelines for the Evaluation and Management of Heart Failure: Report of the American College of Cardiology/American Heart Association Task Force on Practice Guidelines," *Journal of the American College of Cardiology* 26 (1995): 1387.

55. See, e.g., Marcia Angell, *The Truth*, 157–171; Carl Elliott, "Pharma Goes to the Laundry: Public Relations and the Business of Medical Education," *Hastings Center Report* 34 (2004): 18–23; Katherine Greider, *The Big Fix: How the Pharmaceutical Industry Rips Off American Consumers* (New York: Public Affairs, 2003), 63–86.

56. "Examining the Evidence: Optimizing Heart Failure Management in African American Patients," Annual Meeting of the International Society on Hypertension in Blacks, July 17, 2005, accessed July 13, 2006, http://www.ishib.org/ishib2005/program.htm. "Pitt School of Pharmacy's 'Helpful Hands for Healthy Hearts' Program to Educate Minority Community about Cardiovascular Disease," press release, University of Pittsburgh Medical Center, July 11, 2005, accessed May 14, 2006, http://newsbureau.upmc. com/Medsurg3/PharmHelpingHands05.htm; FDA, "Transcript of Meeting," 210–211; Federal Elections Commission, "Campaign Finance Reports and Data," accessed May 28, 2005, http://www.fec.gov/disclosure.shtml; Association of Black Cardiologists, "2004

Annual Report," accessed May 4, 2010, http://www.abcardio.org/graphics04/ABC
_Annual_Report04.pdf.

57. National Minority Health Month Foundation, "Organizations Unite to Support BiDil's Approval for Heart Failure, Rebuff Designation as "Race-Only Drug," press release, June 15, 2005, accessed July 11, 2005, http://www.nmhmf.org/newsroom06142005.htm.

58. "Health Alert: New Heart Medication for African Americans," WISTV, June 16, 2005, accessed May 12, 2006, http://www.wistv.com/Global/story.asp?S=3485957& nav=0RaSb8bM.

59. HCD Research, "Physicians Believe Drugs Targeted for Ethnic and Racial Groups May Provide Therapeutic Advantages," press release, June 23, 2005, accessed May 12, 2006, http://biz.yahoo.com/bw/050623/235492.html.

60. L. Boyce, "BiDil Controversy Raises Specter of Racial Profiling in Medicine," *Minnesota Spokesman Recorder* (November 24, 2004): 1.

61. "Analysts Estimates: SG Cowen," CBS Marketwatch.com, October 27, 2004, accessed May 1, 2005, http://netscape5.marketwatch.com/tools/quotes/snapshot.asp?symb=NTMD &sid=1566926&siteid=mktw.

62. Michael Loberg, "Remarks on Behalf of NitroMed, Inc. at the Pacific Growth Equities 2005 Life Sciences Growth Conference," June 6, 2005, accessed May 12, 2006, http://phx .corporate-ir.net/phoenix.zhtml?p=irol-eventDetails&c=130535&eventID=1070377. This url provided access to a live web stream of the event and is no longer active.

63. Ibid.

64. Stephanie Saul, "Maker of Heart Drug Intended for Blacks Bases Price on Patients' Wealth," *New York Times*, July 8, 2005, accessed May 1, 2006, http://www.nytimes.com /2005/07/08/business/08hdrug.html?pagewanted=print.

65. Michael Loberg, "Webcast–NitroMed Presentation at UBS Global Life Sciences Conference," September 26, 2005, accessed September 27, 2005, http://event.streamx.us/event /default.asp?event=ubs20050926. This url provided access to a live web stream of the event and is no longer active.

66. Ibid.; Michael Loberg, "NTMD Web Cast at 23rd Annual JP Morgan Healthcare Conference," January 10, 2005, http://www.mapdigital.com/jpmorgan/healthcare05 /ondemand.html#n. This url provided access to a live web stream of the event and is no longer active.

67. "Nitromed Opportunity Is 'Substantially Improved'" *Forbes Magazine*, July 5, 2005, accessed May 5, 2006, http://www.forbes.com/markets/2005/07/05/0705automarketscan18 .html.

68. Diedtra Henderson, "NitroMed Heart Drug for Blacks Approved," *Boston Globe*, June 24, 2005, accessed December 12, 2006, http://www.boston.com/yourlife/health/diseases /articles/2005/06/24/nitromed_heart_drug_for_blacks_approved/.

69. Ibid.

70. NitroMed, Inc., "NitroMed Completes $31.4 Million Private Financing," press release, June 14, 2001, accessed April 7, 2012, http://www2.prnewswire.com/cgi-bin/stories.pl ?ACCT=104&STORY=/www/story/06-14-2001/0001514000&EDATE=.

71. Vince Parry, "The Art of Branding a Condition," *Medical Marketing & Media* 38 (2003): 43. See also Kalman Applbaum, "Pharmaceutical Marketing and the Invention of the Medical Consumer," *PLoS Medicine* 3 (2006): e189.

72. See, e.g., "NitroMed to Sell 6 Mln IPO Shares for $11–$13 Each," *Reuters*, October 2, 2003, accessed December 7, 2003, http://biz.yahoo.com/rf/031002/health_nitromed _ipo_2.html; NitroMed, Inc., "NitroMed, Inc., Announces Its Initial Public Offering," press release, November 5, 2003, accessed April 7, 2012, http://www.rhoventures.com /e0dd6344-3daa-474f-b9de-a00e888c83db/archived-news-2003-details.htm.

73. Strategic Research Institute, 5th Annual Multicultural Pharmaceutical Marketing & PR Conference, March 25–26, 2004, Princeton, New Jersey, accessed April 7, 2012, http://www.minorityprofessionalnetwork.com/caldata.asp?id=13086.

74. Victoria Griffith, "FDA Paves the Way for First 'Ethnic' Drug," *Financial Times*, March 8, 2001, 13, quoting Jay Cohn.

75. Derek V. Exner, Daniel L. Dries, Michael J. Domanski, and Jay N. Cohn, "Lesser Response to Angiotensin-Converting-Enzyme Inhibitor Therapy in Black as Compared with White Patients with Left Ventricular Dysfunction," *New England Journal of Medicine* 344 (2001): 1357.

76. Sally Satel, "I Am a Racially Profiling Doctor," *New York Times Magazine*, May 5, 2002, 56.

77. Sally Satel, "Medicine's Race Problem," *Policy Review* 110 (2001): 55, accessed December 17, 2003, http://www.policyreview.org/DEC01/satel.html.

78. Jon Entine, "The Straw Man of Race," *World & I* 16 (2001): 294, accessed December 27, 2004, http://www.jonentine.com/reviews/straw_man_of_race.htm, quoting Dr. Cohn.

79. Clyde W. Yancy, "Does Race Matter in Heart Failure?" *American Heart Journal* 146 (2) (2003): 205.

80. See, e.g., Michael Omi and Howard Winant, *Racial Formation in the United States: From the 1960s to the 1990s* (New York: Routledge, 1994), 54–55.

81. "FDA Approves BiDil Heart Failure Drug for Black Patients," *FDA News*, June 23, 2005, accessed July 5, 2005, http://www.fda.gov/bbs/topics/NEWS/2005/NEW0119.0.html.

82. See, e.g., "Multicultural Pharmaceutical Market Development Forum to Feature Expert Panel on Chain Pharmacy and OTC Marketing," *PR Newswire*, March 15, 2005, accessed April 7, 2012, http://www.aol.hispanicbusiness.com/news/newsbyid.asp ?id=21640.

83. See http://www.srinstitute.com/ApplicationFiles/web/WebFrame.cfm?web_id=324.

84. Ibid.

85. See Kevin Davies, "Coming Attractions: Advances in Genomic Medicine," *Bio IT-World*, accessed March 28, 2012, http://www.bio-itworld.com/archive/030805/firstbase .html.

86. "Cardiovascular Marketing: Budgets, Staffing and Strategy," http://www.researchand markets.com/reportinfo.asp?report_id=53547&t=0&cat_id=16.

87. "Clinical Trials Target Specific Ethnic Groups," accessed April 7, 2012, http://www .prnewswire.com/news-releases/clinical-trials-target-specific-ethnic-groups-72437617 .html.

88. Michael Loberg, "NitroMed Webcast at 23rd Annual JP Morgan Healthcare Conference"; see also Michael Loberg, "NitroMed Webcast Presentation at UBS Global Life Sciences Conference."

89. Tamara E. Holmes, "Vigilante Awarded BiDil Ad Campaign," December 27, 2004, accessed January 26, 2005, http://www.blackenterprise.com/ExclusivesEKOpen.asp ?id=981.

90. Ibid.

91. On product differentiation in marketing, see Theodore Levitt, *The Marketing Imagination* (New York: The Free Press, 1986), 128.

92. Anna Helgadottir, Hakon Hakonarson, Jeffrey Gulcher, and Mark Gurney, "Susceptibility gene for myocardial infarction, stroke, and PAOD; methods of treatment," U.S. Patent Application 20070280917, filed November 9, 2005, and issued December 6, 2007.

93. Anna Helgadottir, Hakon Hakonarson, Jeffrey Gulcher, and Mark Gurney, "Susceptibility gene for myocardial infarction, stroke, and PAOD; methods of treatment," U.S. Patent Application 20060019269, filed March 30, 2005, and issued January 26, 2006.

94. Anna Helgadottir, Andrei Manolescu, Agnar Helgason, Gudmar Thorleifsson, Unnur Thorsteinsdottir, Daniel F Gudbjartsson, Solveig Gretarsdottir, et al., "A Variant of the Gene Encoding Leukotriene A4 Hydrolase Confers Ethnicity-Specific Risk of Myocardial Infarction," *Nature Genetics* 38 (2006): 68–74.

95. "DeCode IDs Tablet Problem, Suspends Pivotal Trial," *FierceBiotech*, October 6, 2006, accessed December 4, 2010, http://www.fiercebiotech.com/story/decode-ids-tablet -problem-suspends-pivotal-trial/2006-10-06; Maureen Martino, "DeCode feels the sting of financial crisis," *FierceBiotech*, October 15, 2008, accessed December 4, 2010, http://www.fiercebiotech.com/story/decode-feels-sting-financial-crisis/2008-10-15.

96. Helgadottir et al., "Susceptibility gene," U.S. Patent Application 20070280917.

97. Ibid.

98. See generally Michael B. Fowler, "Hypertension, Heart Failure, and Beta-Andrenergic Blocking Drugs," *Journal of the American College of Cardiology* 52 (2008): 1078, commenting on the use of beta-blockers for hypertension and heart failure.

99. IMS World Health, "Top Therapeutic Classes by U.S. Dispensed Prescriptions," 2010, accessed October 4, 2010, http://www.imshealth.com/deployedfiles/imshealth/Global /Content/StaticFile/Top_Line_Data/Top%20Therapy%20Classes%20by%20U.S.RXs .pdf.

100. Brian Orelli, "New Beta Blocker on the Crowded Street," *Motley Fool*, December 17, 2007, http://www.fool.com/investing/dividends-income/2007/12/19/new-beta-blocker-in -a-crowded-forest.aspx.

101. Forest Laboratories, Inc., "Bystolic™, a Novel Beta Blocker, Is Now Approved by the FDA for the Treatment of Hypertension," press release, December 18, 2007, http:// www.frx.com/news/PressRelease.aspx?ID=1088188; Forest Laboratories, Inc., "Nebivolol Lowers Blood Pressure in Mild-to-Moderate Hypertensive Patients as Demonstrated in a Study Published in the *Journal of Clinical Hypertension*," press release, September 4, 2007, http://www.frx.com/news/PressRelease.aspx?ID=1047743; Forest

Laboratories, Inc., "UPDATE: Nebivolol Lowers Blood Pressure in African Americans with Stage I-II Hypertension as Demonstrated in a Study Published in the *Journal of Clinical Hypertension*," press release, November 1, 2007, http://www.frx.com/news/Press Release.aspx?ID=1071168.

102. See, e.g., Sidney Goldstein, "Beta Blocker Therapy in African American Patients with Heart Failure," *Heart Failure Reviews* 9 (2004): 161; see also Paul G. Shekelle, Michael W. Rich, Sally C. Morton, Col. Sid W. Atkinson, Wenli Tu, Margaret Maglione, Shannon Rhodes, et al., "Efficacy of Angiotensin-Converting Enzyme Inhibitors and Beta-Blockers in the Management of Left Ventricular Systolic Dysfunction According to Race, Gender, and Diabetic Status: A Meta-Analysis of Major Clinical Trials," *Journal of the American College of Cardiology* 41 (2003): 1529; Clyde W. Yancy, "Race-Based Therapeutics," *Current Hypertension Reports* 10 (2008): 276.

103. Elijah Saunders, William B. Smith, Karen B. DeSalvo, and Will A. Sullivan, "The Efficacy and Tolerability of Nebivolol in Hypertensive African American Patients," *Journal of Clinical Hypertension* 9 (2007): 867.

104. International Society for Hypertension in Blacks, "Drug for Hypertension Shows Promise as Future Treatment for Hypertensive African Americans," press release, July 17, 2005, http://www.ishib.org/ishib2005/resource/PDF/rel_saunders_ishib05_fin.pdf.

105. "New Data Reported as Nebivolol Moves Toward Launch in the United States," *MedScape Today*, January 17, 2008, http://www.medscape.com/viewarticle/568786_4.

106. "Beta Blocker Controls High Blood Pressure in Blacks," *Daily News Central*, July 18, 2005, http://health.dailynewscentral.com/content/view/1308/63.

107. "New Data Reported," *MedScape Today*.

108. Ibid.

109. FDA, "Bystolic Label and Approval History," http://www.accessdata.fda.gov/scripts/cder/drugsatfda/index.cfm?fuseaction=Search.Label_ApprovalHistory.

110. Frank Perier, "Forest Laboratories, Inc. at UBS Global Specialty Pharmaceuticals Conference—Final," *Fair Disclosure*, June 2, 2009.

111. "Bystolic," *Medical Media & Marketing*, January 9, 2009, accessed October 4, 2010, http://www.mmm-online.com/bystolic/article/100587/#.

112. "Invitation to Program on Bystolic," PA Pharmacists Association, February 14, 2008, http://www.papharmacists.com/2-14-08_%20a%20program%20on%20Bystolic.doc. This url provided access to a lecture announcement for the event and is no longer active.

113. Ibid.

114. American Pharmacists Association, "New Product Bulletin: Bystolic," 2008, 13, accessed October 4, 2010, http://www.pharmacist.com/AM/TemplateRedirect.cfm?template=/CM/ContentDisplay.cfm&contentID=18317.

115. "The monthly drug cost per patient for nebivolol is currently flat-priced at $30.90. In comparison, the monthly drug costs per patient for traditional beta-blockers used in the management of HTN are as follows: $0.15–$0.60 for atenolol, $0.60–$2.40 for metoprolol tartrate, $2.40–$6.00 for carvedilol, and $7.20–$21.60 for labetalol. Likewise, the

monthly drug costs per patient for traditional beta-blockers used in the management of HF are as follows: $2.40–$6.00 carvedilol, $3.60–$12.90 for metoprolol succinate, and $8.70–$13.20 for bisoprolol." "National PBM Drug Monograph Nebivolol (Bystolic®)," VHA Pharmacy Benefits Management Services and the Medical Advisory Panel, June 2008; Frank Perier, "Forest Laboratories, Inc."

116. Forest Laboratories, Inc., "Chairman's Letter," 2011, http://investor.frx.com/investor _center/chairmans_letter.

117. "The Hits Keep on Coming," *Medical Marketing & Media*, October 2008, MMM online.com, 57–58.

118. B. Séguin, B. Hardy, P. A. Singer, and A. S. Daar, "Bidil: Recontextualizing the Race Debate," *Pharmacogenomics Journal* 8 (2008): 171.

119. S.-M. Huang and Robert Temple, "Is This Drug or Dose for You?: The Impact of Consideration of Ethnic Factors in Global Drug Development, Regulatory Review, and Clinical Practice," *Clinical Pharmacology & Therapeutics* 84 (2008): 291.

120. One study of twenty-eight major American newspapers found 167 articles on BiDil published between May 3, 2001, and May 23, 2007. Simrat Harry and Timothy Caulfield, "BiDil, Clinical Trials and the Popular Press: An Exploration of Newspaper Coverage," *Health Law Review* 17 (2008): 1, 46–50.

121. David Armstrong, "NitroMed Halts Marketing of Drug," *Wall Street Journal,* January 16, 2008, accessed March 2, 2010, http://online.wsj.com/article/SB120044147052292697.html.

122. "Nitromed Shares Tumble as Personalized Drug Fails to Catch On," *USA Today*, August 3, 2006, accessed November 4, 2010, http://www.usatoday.com/money/industries /health/2006–08–03-nitromed_x.htm; Mass High Tech Staff, "NitroMed's Low Stock Price Prompts Nasdaq Warning," September 15, 2008, accessed November 4, 2010, http://www.masshightech.com/stories/2008/09/15/daily32-NitroMeds-low-stock-price -prompts-Nasdaq-warning.html?action=emailfriendform.

123. Craig M. Douglas, "NitroMed agrees to Be Sold for $36M," *Boston Business Journal*, January 30, 2009, accessed March 15, 2010, http://boston.bizjournals.com/boston/stories /2009/01/26/daily68.html.

124. Bradley Huggett, "BiDil Flops," *Nature Biotechnology* 26 (2008): 252.

125. Ed Silverman, "For BiDil, the Future Isn't Black and White," *Pharmalot*, August 2, 2007, accessed March 5, 2010, http://www.pharmalot.com/2007/08/for-bidil-the-future -isnt-black-and-white/.

126. Kenneth Bate, Pacific Growth Equities, Life Sciences Growth Conference, June 13, 2006, San Francisco, California, http://www.corporate-ir.net/ireye/confLobby.zhtml?ticker =NTMD&item_id=1315808.

127. For a discussion of formulary tiers, see, e.g., RegenceRx, "Pharmaceutical Benefits Management, Therapeutic Class Review, Cardiovascular Agents, Isosorbide Dinitrate/ Hydralazine (BiDil®)," November 2005, http://www.regencerx.com/docs/physicianRx /cardiovascular-bidil-1105.pdf.

128. Ibid.

129. "Combination Isosorbide Dinitrate/Hydralazine (BiDil®) VHA [Veterans Health Administration] Pharmacy Benefits Management Strategic Health Care Group and the

Medical Advisory Panel," *National Formulary Review*, 2006, accessed March 6, 2010, http://www.pbm.va.gov/Clinical%20Guidance/Drug%20Monographs/Isosorbide %20Dinitrate%20-%20Hydralazine%20Fixed-Dose%20Combination.pdf.

130. William Holtz, FoxKiser, counsel to Nitromed, "Petition FDA on Bioequivalence: Citizen Petition to FDA Division of Dockets Management," April 26, 2008, accessed April 7, 2012, http://www.fda.gov/ohrms/dockets/dockets/06p0174/06p-0174-cp00001 -01-vol1.pdf.

131. Christine Bechtel, Director, Executive Operations Staff, Center for Drug Evaluation and Review, FDA, correspondence, May 3, 2006, accessed November 5, 2010, http://www.bidil.com/hcp/files/BiDil_vs_generics.pdf.

132. NitroMed, Inc., "There Are No Generic Equivalents for BiDil—The Evidence, Slide Show for Health Care Providers," NitroMed, Inc., accessed February 10, 2010, http://www.bidil.com/hcp/files/BiDil_vs_generics.pdf.

133. NitroMed, Inc., "Study: Identical Doses of BiDil Components Are Not Bioequivalent to the Fixed Dose Combination—BiDil—Used in A-HeFT," press release, March 26, 2007, accessed November 4, 2010, http://www.drugs.com/clinical_trials/ study-identical-doses-bidil-components-not-bioequivalent-fixed-combination-bidil -heft-391.html.

134. FDA, "Questions: BiDil for Heart Failure," Cardio-Renal Advisory Committee, February 27, 1997, BiDil Administrative Correspondence, 165, http://www.accessdata.fda.gov /drugsatfda_docs/nda/2005/020727_S000_Bidil_AdminCorres.pdf.

135. Jonathan Denne, "'Substantial Evidence' from a Replicated Secondary Analysis, Followed by a Single Prospective Confirmatory Study," *Drug Information Journal* 42 (2008): 131–138. See also, generally, Stefan Timmermans and Marc Berg, *The Gold Standard: The Challenge of Evidence-Based Medicine and Standardization in Health Care* (Philadelphia, Pa.: Temple University Press, 2003).

136. "Response of FDA's Robert Temple to *Scientific American* Article," *FDAWebview*, August 8, 2007.

137. "BiDil's Clinical Story," PowerPoint slide packet offered to health care professionals, accessed April 7, 2012, http://www.bidil.com/hcp/files/BiDilClinicalStory.pdf.

138. Danielle Frank, Thomas H. Gallagher, Sherrill L. Sellers, Lisa A. Cooper, Eboni G. Price, Adebola O. Odunlami, and Vence L. Bonham, "Primary Care Physicians' Attitudes Regarding Race-Based Therapies," *Journal of General Internal Medicine* 25 (2010): 384–389.

139. NitroMed Analyst Day BiDil launch overview presentation and webcast, July 15, 2005, http://phx.corporate-ir.net/phoenix.zhtml?p=irol-eventDetails&c=130535& eventID=1093384. This url provided access to a live web stream of the event and is no longer active.

140. Mark Jewel, "Drug Maker Breaking New Ground with Grassroots Marketing of BiDil," *Associated Press*, April 11, 2006, accessed March 6, 2010, http://www.targetmarketnews .com/storyid04170602.htm.

141. Malorye Allison, "NitroMed Is Feeling the Pressure but Still Betting on Marketing to Save BiDil," *XConomy*, November 28, 2007, accessed November 4, 2010, http://www

.xconomy.com/boston/2007/11/28/nitromed-is-feeling-the-pressure-but-still-betting-on-marketing-to-save-bidil/.

142. ICFAI Centre for Management Research, "RACE Specific Drug 'BiDil': NitroMed's Marketing Challenge," case study, ICMR, Hyderabad, India, 2006, 5.

143. Ibid.

144. M. Witten, "Humpty Dumpty," *House, M.D.*, Fox Television, aired September 27, 2005.

145. E. R. Shipp, "Commentary: When Meds Target Blacks," *NY Daily News*, July 24, 2004, accessed February 1, 2005, http://www.nydailynews.com/news/ideas_opinions/story/215390p-185450c.html.

146. Ibid.

147. Ibid.

148. S. M. Reverby, "Special Treatment: BiDil, Tuskegee, and the Logic of Race," *Journal of Law and Medical Ethics* 36 (2008): 478.

149. Ibid., 479.

150. Ibid., 480.

151. Steve Stiles, "Conventional Wisdom on Race-Based Disparities in Heart-Failure Care Challenged," *Heartwire*, June 17, 2008, http://www.theheart.org/article/875963.do.

152. Kaiser Family Foundation, "Today's Topics in Health Disparities—Race and Genetics: The Future of Personalized Medicine," transcript of live webcast, August 20, 2008, 33, accessed March 13, 2010, http://www.kaisernetwork.org/health_cast/uploaded_files/082008_tthd_transcript.pdf.

153. Emily Singer, "Beyond Race-Based Medicine. 'Let's Move Beyond Race When Exploring Disease,' Says Clyde Yancy," *MIT Technology Review*, January 16, 2009, accessed February 26, 2010, http://www.technologyreview.com/biomedicine/21972/.

154. "NTMD Web Cast at 23d Annual JP Morgan Healthcare Conference," January 10, 2005, http://www.mapdigital.com/jpmorgan/healthcare05/ondemand.html#n.

5. RACE-ING PATENTS/PATENTING RACE

1. Donald Chisum, Craig Allen Nard, Herbert F. Schwartz, and Pauline Newman, *Principles of Patent Law 2* (New York: Foundation Press, 2001), 1–2.

2. Shubha Ghosh, "Race Specific Patents, Commercialization and Intellectual Property," *Buffalo Law Review* 56 (2008): 101, 103–108.

3. See, e.g., Nancy Kass, "The Implications of Genetic Testing for Health and Life Insurance," in *Genetic Secrets: Protecting Privacy and Confidentiality in the Genetic Era*, ed. Mark A. Rothstein (New Haven, Conn.: Yale University Press, 1999), 299–316; Mark A. Rothstein, "The Law of Medical and Genetic Privacy in the Workplace," in *Genetic Secrets*, 281. These concerns lay at the heart of the Genetic Information Non-Discrimination Act (GINA) (P.L. 110–233, 122 Stat. 881), enacted in 2008 to prevent the discriminatory use of genetic information in employment and insurance.

4. See, e.g., Michael J. Malinowski and Beth E. Arnold, *Biotechnology: Law, Business, Regulation* (New York: Aspen Publishers, 2002), §§ 2.01–07 (Supp. 2002). See generally E. Richard Gold, *Body Parts: Property Rights and the Ownership of Human Biological Materials* (Washington, D.C.: Georgetown University Press, 1996), 64–85; Rebecca S. Eisenberg and Robert P. Merges, "Opinion Letter as to the Patentability of Certain Inventions Associated with the Identification of Partial cDNA Sequences," *AIPLA Quarterly Journal* 23 (1995): 1; Michael A. Heller and Rebecca S. Eisenberg, "Can Patents Deter Innovation? The Anticommons in Biomedical Research," *Science* 280 (1998): 698; Arti K. Rai, "Fostering Cumulative Innovation in the Biopharmaceutical Industry: The Role of Patents and Antitrust," *Berkeley Technology Law Journal* 16 (2001): 813; Arti Rai, "Intellectual Property Rights in Biotechnology: Addressing New Technology," *Wake Forest Law Review* 34 (1999): 827; "Intellectual Property Rights and Research Tools in Molecular Biology," summary of a workshop held at the National Academy of Sciences, February 15–16, 1996, Washington, D.C., http://www.nap.edu/readingroom /books/property/; "Intellectual Property Rights: How Far Should They Be Extended," National Academy of Sciences, February 2–3, 2000, http://www7.nationalacademies .org/step/STEP_Projects_Feb_IPR_Conf_Agenda.html. This url provided access to the conference agenda for the event and is no longer active.

5. Richard Thompson Ford, "The Boundaries of Race: Political Geography in Legal Analysis," Harvard Law Review 107 (1994): 1841, 1847–1857, 1870–1878; Cheryl I. Harris, "Whiteness as Property," *Harvard Law Review* 106 (1993): 1707, 1713–1724.

6. George Lipsitz, *The Possessive Investment in Whiteness: How White People Profit from Identity Politics* (Philadelphia, Pa.: Temple University Press, 1998). See also Tom I. Romero II, "War of a Much Different Kind: Poverty and the Possessive Investment in Color in the Multicultural 1960 United States," *Chicano-Latino Law Review* 26 (2006): 69, discussing Lipsitz, *The Possessive Investment.*

7. Harris, "Whiteness," 1777–1791.

8. Romero, "War of a Much Different Kind."

9. Chisum et al., *Principles of Patent Law 2*, citing 35 U.S.C. § 154 (1994).

10. 35 U.S.C. § 101 (2000).

11. Ibid., § 102.

12. Ibid., § 103.

13. Ibid., § 112.

14. Ibid., § 103(a).

15. George Elliot, "A Brief Guide to Understanding Patentability and the Meaning of Patents," *Academic Medicine* 77 (2002): 1310. An oft-used negative example here would be the failure to meet the requirement by specifying the utility of a genetically engineered mouse to be "snake food."

16. 35 U.S.C. § 103(a).

17. Elliot, "Brief Guide," 1309–1314.

18. Ibid., 1310–1311.

19. 35 U.S.C. § 103(a).

20. Elliot, "Brief Guide," 1312.

21. My inquiry into this dynamic is animated by what Sheila Jasanoff has characterized as a concern "to understand how the legal process mediates among conflicting knowledge claims, divergent underlying values, and competing views of expertise in a democratic society." Sheila Jasanoff, *Science at the Bar: Law, Science, and Technology in America* (Cambridge, Mass.: Harvard University Press, 1995), xiv.

22. *Diamond v. Chakrabarty*, 447 U.S. 303, 305 (1980).

23. Ibid., at 309.

24. Utility Examination Guidelines, 66 Fed. Reg., at 1093.

25. See, e.g., Sheldon Krimsky, "The Profit of Scientific Discovery and Its Normative Implications," *Chicago-Kent Law Review* 75 (1999): 25–26. The following is a brief elaboration on this process. Deoxyribonucleic acid (DNA) is composed of ordered combinations of four nucleotides: adenine, guanine, thymine, and cytosine—generally abbreviated as A, G, T, and C. A given section of nucleotides along the double-helical strands of DNA may code for certain amino acids that, in turn, provide a particular protein. Protein synthesis occurs through a process in which the genetic information describing the protein is transcribed from the coding portion of the DNA molecule to a smaller "messenger" molecule of ribonucleic acid (RNA). This messenger RNA (mRNA) then combines with a ribosome and a third factor called transfer RNA (tRNA) to produce a protein. When scientists intervene in this process by adding the enzyme reverse transcriptase to the mRNA, they produce a new and discrete DNA "transcript" that codes for the particular protein. This transcript is known as a clone or complementary DNA (cDNA). See Michael Davis, "The Patenting of Products of Nature," *Rutgers Computer & Technology Law Journal* 21 (1995): 310–315.

26. Jasanoff, *Science at the Bar*, 895.

27. Issued patents have been formally approved by the PTO. Patent applications are currently pending before the PTO for review. Under new policies, applications are made available to the public while pending review. U.S. Patent and Trademark Office, "Frequently Asked Questions about Patents," accessed January 22, 2006, http://www.uspto.gov/web/offices/pac/doc/general/faq.htm.

28. Roger E. Schechter and John R. Thomas, *Intellectual Property: The Law of Copyrights, Patents and Trademarks* (St. Paul, Minn.: West Group, 2003), 404.

29. Ibid.

30. Ibid., 423–424.

31. The results are from searches of the U.S. PTO patent database conducted between August 25, 2005, and September 15, 2005, and between September 1, 2007, and September 7, 2007, using the web-based search engine available at http://www.uspto.gov. The search terms used included: Race, Racial, Ethnic, Ethnicity, Caucasian, Caucasoid, African, African-American, Negro, Negroid, Asian, Oriental, Mongoloid, Hispanic, Latino, Native American, Alaska Native, Pacific Islander. The terms "black" and "white" alone were too broad to be useful and so were qualified with the additional terms of "gene" or "genetic" or "nucleotide." Searches were also conducted using the

terms "Jewish" and "Jew," because of the distinctive history of the development of genetic screening technologies for diseases highly prevalent in Ashkenazi Jewish populations. The terms yielded an additional seven patents in each category. Yet because of this
chapter's focus on the OMB categories, these results have not been incorporated into
the present analysis. Selecting patents that imply or assert a genetic component to race
is an admittedly subjective basis for sorting the patents. The categorization of patents
that imply or assert a significant genetic component to race or ethnicity is meant to exclude those patents that use racial/ethnic categories as one of many general demographic characteristics, usually employed for organizing data, rather than identifying or
treating a particular physiological state. The categorization is meant to include those
patents that use racial/ethnic categories as a basis for asserting a distinctive prevalence
or etiology for a physiological condition, genetic variation, and/or drug response.

32. Schechter and Thomas, *Intellectual Property*, 409.
33. Ibid.
34. Teodorica L. Bugawan and Henry Erlich, Detection of susceptibility to autoimmune
    diseases, U.S. Patent Application No. 20040126794, filed September 25, 2003, and is-
    sued July 1, 2004.
35. Ibid.
36. Ibid.
37. Ibid.
38. Ibid.
39. Ibid.
40. Ibid.
41. Ibid.
42. During much of the nineteenth century, African Americans—both men and women,
    slave and free—served as the objects of much biomedical research. In the twentieth
    century, the Tuskegee experiments running from the 1930s to 1972, and the Department
    of Energy radiation experiments that disproportionately enrolled African Americans
    between 1944 and 1994, further demonstrated a medical interest in black bodies. None-
    theless, in the second half of the twentieth century, the importation of statistics into
    medical research and practice led a drive to create a standardized norm for research—a
    white male norm. This was particularly so in the case of pharmaceutical development, in
    which white males became the standard for research and the unstated, taken-for-
    granted norm against which other groups might be measured. See generally Harriet
    Washington, *Medical Apartheid: The Dark History of Medical Experimentation of Black
    Americans from Colonial Times to the Present* (New York: Random House, 2006); Susan
    Reverby, *Examining Tuskegee: The Infamous Syphilis Study and Its Legacy* (Chapel Hill:
    University of North Carolina Press, 2009); and see Steven Epstein, *Inclusion: The Politics
    of Difference in Medical Research* (Chicago: University of Chicago Press, 2007), 51.
43. Rene Bowser, "Racial Profiling in Health Care: An Institutional Analysis of Medical
    Treatment Disparities," *Michigan Journal Race and Law* 7 (2001): 111. For a recent discus-
    sion of the role of an unstated white norm in the context of equal protection, see Juan

Perea, "Buscando América: Why Integration and Equal Protection Fail to Protect Latinos," *Harvard Law Review* 117 (2004): 1446–1453.

44. Jay N. Cohn and Peter Carson, Methods of treating and preventing congestive heart failure with hydralazine compounds and isosorbide dinitrate or isosorbide mononitrate, U.S. Patent 6,465,463, filed September 8, 2000, and issued October 15, 2002.

45. Ibid.

46. Ibid.

47. Marco Guida, Linda Benson, and Penelope Hopkins, Method of identifying a polymorphism in CYP2D6, U.S. Patent Application 20030170651, filed June 5, 2002, and issued September 11, 2003. CYP2D6 is of particular interest to pharmaceutical corporations, because it is involved with drug metabolism.

48. Ibid.

49. Ibid.

50. Ibid.

51. Ibid.

52. Ibid.

53. Schechter and Thomas, *Intellectual Property*, 315–321.

54. See generally Jonathan Kahn, "What's the Use? Law and Authority in Patenting Human Genetic Material," *Stanford Law & Policy Review* 14 (2003): 417.

55. Schechter and Thomas, *Intellectual Property*, 363–364.

56. Bowser, "Racial," 111.

57. 35 U.S.C. § 103(a) (2000).

58. See, e.g., American Anthropological Association (AAA), "Response to OMB Directive 15: Race and Ethnic Standards for Federal Statistics and Administrative Reporting," September 1997, accessed March 28, 2012, http://www.aaanet.org/gvt/ombdraft.htm; American Sociological Association, "The Importance of Collecting Data and Doing Social Scientific Research on Race," 2003, accessed March 28, 2012, http://www2.asanet.org/media/asa_race_statement.pdf.

59. Schechter and Thomas, *Intellectual Property*, 393–394.

60. See, e.g., Nathaniel E. Gates, ed., *The Concept of "Race" in Natural and Social Science* (New York: Routledge, 1997); AAA, "Response to OMB Directive 15."

61. Schechter and Thomas, *Intellectual Property*, 397.

62. Ibid.

63. PTO, Patent Examination Policy—MPEP Staff—35 U.S.C. 112 1st para—Enablement of Chemical/Biotechnical Applications, Training Materials For Examining Patent Applications with Respect to 35 U.S.C. Section 112, First Paragraph-Enablement Of Chemical/Biotechnical Applications, accessed April 19, 2010, http://www.uspto.gov/patents/law/1pecba.jsp.

64. Ibid.

65. Amgen v. Chugai Pharmaceuticals, 927 F.2.d 1200, 1218 (Fed. Cir. 1991).

66. Regents of the University of California v. Eli Lilly and Co., 119 F.3.d 1559, 1567 (1997).

67. PTO, Biotechnology/Chemical/Pharmaceutical Customer Partnership meeting, December 3, 2008, http://www.cabic.com/bcp/.

68. J. Aquino, "PTO Personalized Medicine Session Illustrates Complex Issues Ahead," *Life Sciences Law & Industry Report* 3 (2009): 96.

69. Ibid.

70. Ibid.

71. Ibid.

72. Ex Parte Jianfeng Xu, Deborah Meyers, Sigun Zheng, Patrick C. Walsh, William B. Isaacs, Eugene Bleecker, and David Herrington, 2009 WL 819042 (Bd.Pat.App. & Interf.), 2009, 3.

73. Ibid.

74. Ibid.

75. Ibid.

76. Ex Parte Jennifer Jones McIntire, Rosemarie Dekruyff, Dale T. Umetsu, and Gordon Freeman, 2010 WL 250531 (Bd.Pat.App. & Interf.), 2010, 8.

77. Heinz-Joseph Lenz and Jan Stoehlmacher, Manganese superoxide dismutase gene polymorphism for predicting cancer susceptibility, U.S. Patent 6,716,581, filed April 2, 2001, and issued April 6, 2004.

78. Heinz-Joseph Lenz and Jan Stoehlmacher, Manganese Superoxide Dismutase Gene Polymorphism for Predicting Cancer Susceptibility, US Patent Application No. 20020039733, filed April 2, 2001, and issued April 4, 2004.

79. Heinz-Joseph Lenz and Jan Stoehlmacher, Manganese superoxide dismutase gene polymorphism for predicting cancer susceptibility, U.S. Patent 6,716,581.

80. Heinz-Joseph Lenz and Jan Stoehlmacher, Manganese superoxide, U.S. Patent 6,716,581; P.A.I.R. Docket # 13761–7001/App. Control # 09/824,629. Carla Myers. [Final Action] Office Action Responsive to Communication Filed on September 16, 2002. November 20, 2002, 3.

81. Ibid.

82. See, e.g., Genentech, Inc. v. Novo Nordisk, A/S, 108 F.3d 1361 (Fed. Cir. 1997).

83. Francis S. Collins, "What We Do and Don't Know about 'Race,' 'Ethnicity,' Genetics and Health at the Dawn of the Genome Era," *National Genetics Supplement* 36 (2004): S13–S15.

84. R. C. Lewontin and Daniel L. Hartl, "Population Genetics in Forensic DNA Typing," *Science* 254 (1991): 1745, 1749.

85. U.S. Patent 6,716,581, P.A.I.R. Docket # 13761–7001/App. Control # 09/824,629. David Maher. Amendment and Response Under 37 C.F.R. s. 1.111. September 16, 2002.

86. EPO communication, "Despatch of communication that the application is refused, reason: substantive examination," April 12, 2011. EP1509242 Treatment of hepatitis C in the Asian population with subcutaneous interferon β.

87. Ibid.

88. Ibid.

89. "Metes and bounds" is a legal description of a parcel of land that begins at a well-marked point and follows the boundaries, using directions and distances around the tract, back to the place of beginning. Schechter and Thomas, *Intellectual Property*, 404.

90. Harris, "Whiteness," 1720–1721.

91. Harris, "Whiteness," 1745–1757, citing Brown v. Board of Education, 347 U.S. 483 (1954).

92. Plessy v. Ferguson, 163 U.S. 537, 540 (1895).

93. Charles Lofgren, *The Plessy Case: A Legal-Historical Interpretation* (New York: Oxford University Press, 1987), 41.

94. Harris, "Whiteness," 1746–1750.

95. Lofgren, *Plessy Case*, 55.

96. Plessy v. Ferguson, 163 U.S. at 549.

97. Cheryl I. Harris, "Whiteness," 1750.

98. T. M. Baye and R. A. Wilke, "Mapping Genes That Predict Treatment Outcome in Admixed Populations," *Pharmacogenomics Journal* 10 (2010): 466.

99. Ibid., 473. Matthew Freedman of the Broad Institute and the Dana Farber Cancer Center in Boston presented an almost identical slide in which the chromosomes were explicitly labeled as "African" and "European" to a meeting of the Genetic Association Information Network and the NHGRI. Matthew Freeman, "8g24: Prostate Cancer," presentation at the Gain Analysis Workshop II, October 17–18, 2007, National Human Genome Research Institute, Bethesda, Maryland, http://www.genome.gov/27532174.

100. Baye and Wilke, "Mapping Genes," 466.

101. John O. Calmore, "Racialized Space and the Culture of Segregation: 'Hewing a Stone of Hope from a Mountain of Despair,'" *University of Pennsylvania Law Review* 143 (1995): 1235.

102. See generally Keith Aoki, "Space Invaders: Critical Geography, the 'Third World' in International Law and Critical Race Theory," *Villanova Law Review* 45 (2000): 913; Calmore, "Racialized Space"; Richard Thompson Ford, "The Boundaries of Race: Political Geography in Legal Analysis," 107 (1994): 1841, 1847–1857, 1870–1878.

103. Calmore, "Racialized Space," 1234.

104. Melissa Nobles, *Shades of Citizenship: Race and the Census in Modern Politics* (Palo Alto, Calif.: Stanford University Press, 2000), 135–136; see generally Michael Omi and Howard Winant, *Racial Formation in the United States: From the 1960s to the 1990s* (New York: Routledge, 1994).

105. Keith Aoki, "Race, Space, and Place: The Relation Between Architectural Modernism, Post-Modernism, Urban Planning, and Gentrification," *Fordham Urban Law Journal* 20 (1993): 699–830.

106. Ford, "The Boundaries of Race," 1877.

107. Aoki, "Space Invaders," 19.

6. NOT FADE AWAY

1. Friedrich Engels, *Anti-Durhing* (1878; Moscow: Progress Publishers, 1975), 333.

2. Buddy Holly and Norman Petty, "Not Fade Away," Brunswick Records. Originally released in 1957.

3. Troy Duster, "The Molecular Reinscription of Race: Unanticipated Issues in Biotechnology and Forensic Science," *Patterns of Prejudice* 40 (2006): 427–441. On the promissory

nature of genomics, see Mike Fortun, *Promising Genomics: Iceland and deCODE Genetics in a World of Speculation* (Berkeley: University of California Press, 2008); Adam Hedgecoe, *The Politics of Personalised Medicine* (New York: Cambridge University Press, 2004).

4. Catherine Elton, "Why Racial Profiling Persists in Medical Research," *Time*, August 22, 2009, http://www.time.com/time/health/article/0,8599,1916755,00.html.

5. Peter F. Zhu, "Renowned Af-Am Professor Gates Arrested for Disorderly Conduct," *Harvard Crimson*, July 20, 2009, http://www.thecrimson.com/article/2009/7/20/renowned -af-am-professor-gates-arrested-for/; Helene Cooper and Abby Goodnough, "Over Beers, No Apologies, but Plans to Have Lunch," *New York Times*, July 30, 2009, http:// www.nytimes.com/2009/07/31/us/politics/31obama.html?_r=1&scp=3&sq=%22beer %20summit%22&st=cse.

6. Kathy S. Albain, Joseph M. Unger, John J. Crowley, Charles A. Coltman Jr., and Dawn L. Hershman, "Racial Disparities in Cancer Survival among Randomized Clinical Trials Patients of the Southwest Oncology Group," *Journal of the National Cancer Institute* 101 (2009): 984–992.

7. Elton, "Why Racial Profiling."

8. Ibid.

9. Albain et al., "Racial Disparities," 985.

10. Katrina F. Trivers, Lynne C. Messer, and Jay S. Kaufman, "Re: Racial Disparities in Cancer Survival among Randomized Clinical Trials of the Southwest Oncology Group," *Journal of the National Cancer Institute* 102 (2010): 278–279.

11. Clarence C. Gravlee and Connie J. Mulligan, "Re: Racial Disparities in Cancer Survival among Randomized Clinical Trials of the Southwest Oncology Group," *Journal of the National Cancer Institute* 102 (2010): 280.

12. Elton, "Why Racial Profiling." Or, as the article itself concluded, "Our findings suggest that *unrecognized interactions* [italics added] of tumor biological, hormonal, and/or inherited host factors must be contributing to differential survival outcomes by race in sex-specific malignancies." Albain et al., "Racial Disparities."

13. This approach was echoed in some responses to the *JNCI* article. For example, Lisa A. Newman, director of the University of Michigan Breast Care Center, said, "There seems to be something associated with racial and ethnic identity that seems to confer a worse survival rate for African Americans. I think it's likely to be hereditary and genetic factors." Rob Stein, "Blacks with Equal Care Still More Likely to Die of Some Cancers," *Washington Post*, July 8, 2009, accessed October 5, 2010, http://www.washingtonpost .com/wp-dyn/content/article/2009/07/07/AR2009070702252.html. Yet, as David Williams, Harvard professor of public health, noted in commenting on the Albain et al. study, "The biology is a fall-back black box that many researchers use when they find racial differences. . . . It is knee-jerk reaction. It is not based on science, but on a deeply held, cultural belief about race that the medical field has a hard time giving up." Catherine Elton, "Why Racial Profiling."

14. Catherine Elton, "Why Racial Profiling."

15. Yin Paradies, Michael Montoya, and Stephanie Fullerton, "Racialized Genetics and the Study of Complex Diseases," *Perspectives in Biology and Medicine* 50 (2007): 216.

16. S-M. Huang and R. Temple, "Is This the Drug or Dose for You? Impact and Consideration of Ethnic Factors in Global Drug Development, Regulatory Review, and Clinical Practice," *Clinical Pharmacology and Therapeutics* 84 (2008): 291.

17. I am indebted to Karen-Sue Taussig for the idea of considering the "unknown" and "potential" as spaces for the production of meaning and assignment of value.

18. Cardiovascular and Renal Drugs Advisory Committee, Transcript, Food and Drug Administration, June 16, 2005, 355–356, accessed April 8, 2012, http://www.fda.gov/ohrms/dockets/ac/05/transcripts/2005-4145T1.pdf.

19. Ben Harder, "The Race to Prescribe: Drug for African Americans May Debut Amid Debate," *Science News*, April 16, 2005, http://findarticles.com/p/articles/mi_m1200/is_16_167/ai_n13724918/.

20. Ibid.

21. Robert Temple and Norman Stockbridge, "BiDil for Heart Failure in Black Patients: The U.S. Food and Drug Administration Perspective," *Annals of Internal Medicine* 146 (2007): 57–62.

22. Lea Harty, Keith Johnson, and Aidan Power, "Race and Ethnicity in the Era of Emerging Pharmacogenomics," *Journal of Clinical Pharmacology* 46 (2006): 405.

23. J. Yen-Revollo, J. T. Auman, and H. L. McLeod, "Race Does Not Explain Genetic Heterogeneity in Pharmacogenomic Pathways," *Pharmacogenomics* 9 (2008): 1639, 1644.

24. Ibid., 1643.

25. Ibid.

26. Myong-Jim Kim, Shiew-Mei Huang, Urs A. Meyer, Atiqur Rahman, and Lawrence J. Lesko, "A Regulatory Science Perspective on Warfarin Therapy: A Pharmacogenomic Opportunity," *Journal of Clinical Pharmacology* 49 (2009): 138–146.

27. B. F. Gage, C. Eby, J. A. Johnson, E. Deych, M. J. Rieder, P. M. Ridker, P. E. Milligan, et al., "Use of Pharmacogenetic and Clinical Factors to Predict the Therapeutic Dose of Warfarin," *Clinical Pharmacology and Therapeutics* 84 (2008): 328.

28. Matt Jones, "Francis Collins Addresses State of Personalized Medicine," *GenomeWeb Daily News*, January 30, 2009, http://www.genomeweb.com/dxpgx/francis-collins-addresses-state-personalized-medicine.

29. International Warfarin Pharmacogenetics Consortium, "Estimation of the Warfarin Dose with Clinical and Pharmacogenetic Data," *New England Journal of Medicine* 360 (2009): 753–764, esp. 754.

30. Next General Pharmaceuticals, "Pharmacogenetics and Warfarin Therapy," *Drug Discovery* 7 (2007), http://www.ngpharma.com/article/Issue-7/Drug-Discovery/Pharmacogenetics-and-warfarin-therapy/.

31. Kim et al., "A Regulatory Science Perspective," 139.

32. "Pharmacogenomics and Its Role in Drug Safety," *FDA Drug Safety Newsletter* 1 (2008), http://www.fda.gov/Drugs/DrugSafety/DrugSafetyNewsletter/ucm119991.htm; Ann K. Daly, "Pharmacogenomics of Anticoagulants: Steps Toward Personal Dosage," *Genome Medicine* 1 (2009): 10.1–10.4; FDA, "Critical Path Initiative—Warfarin Dosing," accessed April 8, 2012, http://www.fda.gov/ForConsumers/ConsumerUpdates/ucm077473

.htm?utm_campaign=Google2&utm_source=fdaSearch&utm_medium=website&utm _term=.

33. Ibid.; Turna Ray, "Warfarin-Dose Dx May Not Be Cost-Effective for 'Typical' Patient: May Be for At-Risk Cohort," *Pharmacogenomics Reporter*, January 21, 2009, http://www .genomeweb.com/dxpgx/warfarin-dose-dx-may-not-be-cost-effective-typical-patient -may-be-risk-cohort.

34. Bristol-Myers Squibb, Coumadin package inserts, http://packageinserts.bms.com/pi/pi _coumadin.pdf.

35. Julie A. Johnson, "Ethnic Differences in Cardiovascular Drug Response: Potential Contribution of Pharmacogenetics," *Circulation* 118 (2008): 1383. See also H. Takahashi and H. Echizen, "Pharmacogenetics of Warfarin Elimination and Its Clinical Implications," *Clinical Pharmacokinetics* 40 (2001): 587–603; S. El Rouby, C. Mestres, F. LaDuca, and M. Zucker, "Racial and Ethnic Differences in Warfarin Response," *Journal of Heart Valve Disease* 13 (2004): 15–21.

36. Bristol-Myers Squibb, Coumadin package inserts.

37. See, e.g., A. Nguyen, Z. Desta, and D. A. Flockhart, "Enhancing Race-Based Pre-scribing Precision with Pharmacogenomics," *Clinical Pharmacology and Therapeutics* 81 (2007): 324.

38. M. T. Dang, J. Hambleton, and S. R. Kayser, "The Influence of Ethnicity on Warfarin Dosage Requirement," *Annals Pharmacotherapy* 39 (2005): 1008–1012.

39. Anna Mathews, "In Milestone, FDA Pushes Genetic Tests Tied to Drug," *Wall Street Journal*, August 16, 2007, http://online.wsj.com/article/SB118722561330199147.html.

40. M. Teichert, R. H. N. van Schaik, A. Hofman, A. G. Uitterlinden, P. A. G. M. de Smet, B. H. C. Stricker, and L. E. Visser, "Genotypes Associated with Reduced Activity of *VKORC1* and *CYP2C9* and Their Modification of Acenocoumarol Anticoagulation Dur-ing the Initial Treatment Period," *Clinical Pharmacology and Therapeutics* 85 (2009): 379.

41. A. Wu, Ping Wang, Andrew Smith, Christine Haller, Katherine Drake, Mark Linder, and Roland Valdes, "Dosing Algorithm for Warfarin Using CYP2C9 and VKORC1 Genotyping from a Multi-Ethnic Population: Comparison with Other Equations," *Pharmacogenomics* 9 (2008): 169–170.

42. Kim et al., "Regulatory Science Perspective," 140.

43. Wu et al., "Dosing Algorithm," 169–170.

44. Ibid.

45. Fumihiko Takeuchi, Ralph McGinnis, Stephane Bourgeois, Chris Barnes, Niclas Er-iksson, Nicole Soranzo, Pamela Whittaker, et al., "A Genome-Wide Association Study Confirms *VKORC1*, *CYP2C9*, and *CYP4F2* as Principal Genetic Determinants of War-farin Dose," *PLoS Genetics* 5 (2009): e1000433; Hyun-Jung Cho, Kie-Ho Sohn, Hyang-Mi Park, Kyung-Hoon Lee, BoYoung Choi, Seonwoo Kim, June-Soo Kim, et al., "Fac-tors Affecting the Interindividual Variability of Warfarin Dose Requirement in Adult Korean Patients," *Pharmacogenomics* 8 (2007): 329–337; P. Ghadam, F. Sadeghian, R. Sharifian, S. Sadrai, B. Kazemi, and E. Nematipour, "*VKORC1* Gene Analysis in an Ira-nian Warfarin Resistant Patient," *Journal of Biological Sciences* 8 (2007); 691–692; K. Nakai,

Jyunichi Tsuboi, Hitoshi Okabayashi, Yoshiaki Fukuhiro, Takanori Oka, Wataru Habano, Noriko Fukushima, et al., "Ethnic Differences in the VKORC1 Gene Polymorphism and an Association with Warfarin Dosage Requirements in Cardiovascular Surgery Patients," *Pharmacogenomics* 8 (2007): 713–719.

46. American Medical Association, Critical Path Institute, and the Arizona Center for Education and Research on Therapeutics, "Personalized Health Care Report 2008: Warfarin and Genetic Testing," 2008, 1, accessed March 29, 2012, http://www.ama-assn .org/ama1/pub/upload/mm/464/warfarin-brochure.pdf.

47. Pharmacogenomics Knowledge Base, "Important Variant Information for VKORC1," accessed July 14, 2009, http://www.pharmgkb.org/search/annotatedGene/vkorc1/variant.jsp.

48. Turna Ray, "FDA Updates Warfarin Label to Explain Genetic Links to Response; Says Change Not Meant as 'Directive' for Doctors," *GenomeWeb Daily News*, August 16, 2007, http://www.genomeweb.com/fda-updates-warfarin-label-explain-genetic-links -response-says-change-not-meant-.

49. Matthew Arnold, "Warfarin Label Change Advises on Genetic Factors," *Medical Marketing & Media*, August 16, 2007, http://www.mmm-online.com/Warfarin-label -change-advises-on-genetic-factors/article/30045/.

50. Ray, "FDA Updates Warfarin."

51. See generally Philip Hilts, *Protecting America's Health: The FDA, Business, and One Hundred Years of Regulation* (New York: Knopf, 2003).

52. Mathews, "In Milestone."

53. Turna Ray, "Competition Heats Up in Warfarin Dx Market as New Tests Seek FDA OK," *Pharmacogenomics Reporter*, October 10, 2007, http://www.genomeweb.com/dxpgx /competition-heats-warfarin-dx-market-new-tests-seek-fda-ok.

54. Ibid.; Turna Ray, "23andMe Begins Reporting Three SNPs for Warfarin Sensitivity; Plans to Study Others," *Pharmacogenomics Reporter*, April 1, 2009, http://www.genomeweb.com /dxpgx/23andme-begins-reporting-three-snps-warfarin-sensitivity-plans-study-others. For a useful brief discussion of federal regulation of genetic testing, see Genetics and Public Policy Center, "Who Regulates Genetics Tests?" February 6, 2006, accessed August 2, 2009, http://www.dnapolicy.org/policy.issue.php?action=detail&issuebrief_id=10.

55. Centers for Medicare and Medicaid Services, "Proposed Decision Memo for Pharmacogenomic Testing for Warfarin Response (CAG-00400N)," May 4, 2009, http://www .cms.hhs.gov/mcd/viewdraftdecisionmemo.asp?from2=viewdraftdecisionmemo.asp& id=224&.

56. Ray, "Competition Heats Up."

57. Ibid.

58. AutoGenomics, "About Us," accessed July 13, 2009, http://www.autogenomics.com/1 /aboutUs.php.

59. AutoGenomics, "Warfarin XP: Enhanced Ethnic Characterization," accessed July 14, 2008, www.Autogenomics.com.

60. AutoGenomics, "Infiniti™ Warfarin XP: Because Ethnic Diversity Matters When Dosing with Warfarin," accessed July 14, 2008, http://www.Autogneomics.com, on file with author.

61. Ibid.

62. Ibid.

63. Ibid.

64. Anand Vairavan, personal communication to the author, May 20, 2009. On file with the author.

65. Ibid.

66. Ibid.

67. Buhlmann Laboratories, "AG, Pharmacogenetics Downloads," accessed April 8, 2012, http://www.dlmo.org/files/documents/molecular/autogenomics/flyer_2c9-vkorc1_v02 .pdf.

68. William Coty, CYP2C9*8 alleles correlate with decreased warfarin metabolism and increased warfarin sensitivity, U.S. Patent Application 20100130599, filed October 2, 2009, and issued May 27, 2010.

69. Ibid.

70. Pfizer Consumer Healthcare, Children's Advil suspension label, http://www.advil.com /childrens/pain/sus_label.asp.

71. International Warfarin Pharmacogenetics Consortium, "Estimation of the Warfarin Dose," 753–764.

72. Krista Conger, "Patients' Genetic Profiles Could Prevent Fatal Doses of Common Drug," *Stanford Report*, February 25, 2009, accessed March 29, 2010, http://news.stanford .edu/news/2009/february25/med-warfarin-022509.html.

73. International Warfarin Pharmacogenetics Consortium, "Estimation of the Warfarin Dose," 753.

74. Ibid., 754.

75. See, e.g., R. Hahn, "The State of Federal Health Statistics on Racial and Ethnic Groups," *Journal of the American Medical Association* 267 (1992): 268–271; R. Hahn, J. Mulinare, and S. Teutsch, "Inconsistencies in Coding of Race and Ethnicity between Birth and Death in U.S. Infants," *Journal of the American Medical Association* 267 (1992): 259–263; R. Hahn, B. I. Truman, and N. Barker, "Identifying Ancestry: The Reliability of Ancestral Identification in the United States by Self, Proxy, Interviewer, and Funeral Director," *Epidemiology* 7 (1996): 75–80.

76. International Warfarin Pharmacogenetics Consortium, "Estimation of the Warfarin Dose," 753–755.

77. Ibid., 753–756.

78. Ibid., 753.

79. Ibid., 758.

80. Ibid., 758.

81. Ibid., 759.

82. Ibid., Supplementary Appendix, S15. My thanks to Jay Kaufman for pointing this out and helping me interpret the statistical data.

83. Ibid., S6.

84. Rene Bowser, "Racial Profiling in Health Care: An Institutional Analysis of Medical Treatment Disparities," *Michigan Journal of Race and Law* 7 (2001): 111. For a broader

analysis of the operation of the "white norm" in American law, see Kimberle Williams Crenshaw, "Race, Reform, and Retrenchment: Transformation and Legitimation in Antidiscrimination Law," *Harvard Law Review* 101 (1988): 1331, 1377–1379.

85. Ursula Brown, *Multiracial Experience* (New York: Praeger, 2000), 18; For an excellent discussion of racial categories and "kinds," see Michael Root, "How We Divide the World," *Philosophy of Science* 67 (2000): 9628–9639.

86. Gage et al., "Use of Pharmacogenetic," 328.

87. Ibid.

88. Yen-Revollo et al., "Race Does Not Explain," 1643.

89. D. A. Flockhart, Dennis O'Kane, Marc S. Williams, Michael S. Watson, Brian Gage, Roy Gandolfi, Richard King, et al., "Pharmacogenetic Testing of CYP2C9 and VKORC1 Alleles for Warfarin," *Genetics in Medicine* 10 (2008): 139–150, 144.

90. C. Lee, J. Goldstein, and J. Pieper, "Cytochrome P450 2C9 Polymorphisms: A Comprehensive Review of the In-Vitro and Human Data," *Pharmacogenetics* 12 (2002): 251, 252, 263. See also "Important Variant Information for VKORC1," *Pharmacogenomics Knowledge Base*, accessed July 14, 2009, http://www.pharmgkb.org/search/annotatedGene/vkorc1/variant.jsp.

91. Flockhart et al., "Pharmacogenetic Testing."

92. G. Tai, F. Farin, M. J. Rieder, A. W. Dreisbach, D. L. Veenstra, C. L. Verlinde, and A. E. Rettie, "In-Vitro and In-Vivo Effects of the *CYP2C9*11* Polymorphism on Warfarin Metabolism and Dose," *Pharmacogenetics and Genomics* 15 (2005): 475–481.

93. Flockhart et al., "Pharmacogenetic Testing."

94. S. Y. Lee, M. H. Nam, J. S. Kim, and J. W. Kim, "A Case Report of a Patient Carrying *CYP2C9*3/4* Genotype with Extremely Low Warfarin Dose Requirement," *Journal of Korean Medical Science* 22 (2007): 557–559.

95. Ibid., 558.

96. S.-M. Huang, et al., "Application of Pharmacogenomics in Clinical Pharmacology," *Toxicology Mechanisms and Methods* 16 (2006): 93.

97. Ibid.

98. Ibid., 94.

99. "Pharmacodiagnostics and Personalized Medicine 2009 (Markets, Challenges, Forecasts and Key Players)," *Market Research.com*, http://www.marketresearch.com/product/display.asp?productid=2128157&xs=r&SID=95957877–452044944–524917733&curr=USD &kw=warfarin&view=abs.

100. Ray, "Competition Heats Up"; Turna Ray, "Personalized Rx Advocates Call on FDA, CMS to Align Standards after CMS' Restricted Coverage of PGx Warfarin Dosing," *Pharmacogenomics Reporter*, May 20, 2009, http://www.genomeweb.com/dxpgx/personalized-rx-advocates-call-evidence-guidelines-wake-cms-decision-restrict-co.

101. Mathews, "In Milestone."

102. International Warfarin Pharmacogenetics Consortium, "Estimation of the Warfarin Dose," 753–764.

103. Mathews, "In Milestone."

104. Secretary's Advisory Committee on Genetics, Health and Society, "Realizing the Potential of Pharmacogenomics: Opportunities and Challenges," 2008, 1, accessed March 29, 2012, http://oba.od.nih.gov/oba/SACGHS/reports/SACGHS_PGx_report.pdf.

105. Jones, "Francis Collins."

106. Ray, "FDA Updates Warfarin."

107. Centers for Medicare, "Proposed decision memo."

108. Ibid.

109. Turna Ray, "CMS Denies Medicare Payment for Warfarin PGx Testing; Proposes Limiting Coverage to Evidence Studies," *Pharmacogenomics Reporter*, May 6, 2009, accessed July 20, 2009, http://www.genomeweb.com/dxpgx/cms-denies-medicare-payment-warfarin-pgx-testing-proposes-limiting-coverage-evid, discussing M. H. Eckman, J. Rosand, S. M. Greenberg, and B. F. Gage, "Cost-Effectiveness of Using Pharmacogenetic Information in Warfarin Dosing for Patients with Nonvalvular Atrial Fibrillation," *Annals of Internal Medicine* 150 (2009): 73–83.

110. Turna Ray, "Warfarin-Dose Dx," critiquing Andrew McWilliam, Randall Lutter, and Clark Nardinelli, "Health Care Savings from Personalizing Medicine Using Genetic Testing: The Case of Warfarin," AEI–Brookings Joint Center for Regulatory Studies Working Paper 06–23, November 2006, accessed March 29, 2012, http://www.healthanddna.com/warfarinsavings.pdf?pid=1127. Another article, published in 2008, also criticized the AEI–Brookings study, asserting that "a close examination of this study reveals that the authors made several assumptions that may not be valid." Monica R. McClain, G. E. Palomaki, M. Piper, and J. F. Haddow, "A Rapid-ACCE Review of CYP2C9 and VKORC1 Alleles Testing to Inform Warfarin Dosing in Adults at Elevated Risk for Thrombotic Events to Avoid Serious Bleeding," *Genetics in Medicine* 10 (2008): 92.

111. "The Pharmacogenetics of Warfarin Dosing," *TheHeart.org*, 2008, accessed July 20, 2009, http://www.theheart.org/article/924397.do; FDA, "Critical Path Initiative—Warfarin Dosing," accessed April 8, 2012, http://www.fda.gov/ForConsumers/ConsumerUpdates/ucm077473.htm?utm_campaign=Google2&utm_source=fdaSearch&utm_medium=website&utm_term=.

112. Iverson Genetic Diagnostics, Inc., Warfarin dosing panel, accessed April 8, 2012, http://www.iversongenetics.com/Old/WarfarinPanel.html; Osmetech Molecular Diagnostics, "Osmetech Licenses VKOR Pharmacogenetic Marker for Warfarin Dosage," press release, 2007, accessed April 8, 2012, http://www.bionity.com/en/news/62694/osmetech-licenses-vkor-pharmacogenetic-marker-for-warfarin-dosage-management-from-university-of-washington.html.

113. Ray, "CMS Denies."

114. Ibid.

115. Ray, "Personalized Rx Advocates."

116. SourceWatch, "The Pacific Research Institute," http://www.sourcewatch.org/index.php?title=Pacific_Research_Institute.

117. Turna Ray, "NIH Launches Large Randomized Trial to Determine Utility of PGx-based Warfarin Dosing," *Pharmacogenomics Reporter*, February 18, 2009, http://www

.genomeweb.com/dxpgx/nih-launches-large-randomized-trial-determine-utility-pgx
-based-warfarin-dosing.

118. Turna Ray, "When Might Warfarin PGx Be Better Than Pradaxa? Stakeholders Weigh In," *Pharmacogenomics Reporter,* October 27, 2010, http://www.genomeweb.com/dxpgx /when-might-warfarin-pgx-be-better-pradaxa-stakeholders-weigh.

119. FDA, "Critical Path."

120. Yuan-Tsong Chen, Hsiang-Yu Yuan, and Jin-Jer Chen, Genetic variants predicting warfarin sensitivity, U.S. Patent Application 20060166239, filed December 21, 2005, and issued July 27, 2006.

121. Genomics Research Center, "Academia Sinica," http://www.genomics.sinica.edu.tw /index.php?t=13&article_id=33.

122. International Warfarin Pharmacogenetics Consortium, "Estimation of the Warfarin Dose," 753–764.

123. Yuan-Tsong Chen et al., Genetic variants.

124. Ibid.

125. Meg Chang, "Genetics May Hold the Key to Warfarin Dosing," *Taiwan Today,* March 13, 2009, accessed July 21, 2009, http://www.taiwantoday.tw/ct.asp?xItem=49357&Ct Node=429.

126. Ibid.

127. PTO, "Office Action," Serial No. 11/316,406, January 30, 2009, accessed through PTO Public Patent Application Information Retrieval (PAIR) web portal for U.S. Patent Application 20060166239, http://portal.uspto.gov/external/portal/pair.

128. Mark J. Rieder and Allan Rettie, Methods and compositions for predicting drug response, U.S. Patent Application 20080057500, filed March 16, 2007, and issued March 6, 2008.

129. Ibid.

130. Yuan-Tsong Chen, Inventor's Declaration under 37 C.F.R, s.1.132. Filed 3/10/09 with the PTO (emphasis original; citations omitted), accessed through PTO Public Patent Application Information Retrieval (PAIR) web portal for U.S. Patent Application 20060166239, http://portal.uspto.gov/external/portal/pair.

7. FROM DISPARITY TO DIFFERENCE

1. Brian D. Smedley, Adrienne Y. Stith, and Alan R. Nelson, eds., *Unequal Treatment: Confronting Racial and Ethnic Disparities in Health Care* (Washington, D.C.: National Academies Press, 2003).

2. Sarah K. Tate and David B. Goldstein, "Will Tomorrow's Medicines Work for Everyone?" *Nature Genetics* 36 (2004): S34.

3. Ibid.

4. Thomas H. Maugh II, "Drug for Only Blacks Stirs Hope, Concern," *Los Angeles Times,* November 9, 2004, http://articles.latimes.com/2004/nov/09/science/sci-blackdrug9.

NOTES

5. Anjana Ahuja, "We Can Treat Your Heart Disease . . . If You're Black," *Times* (London), October 29, 2004, 4.

6. "Toward the First Racial Medicine," *New York Times*, November 13, 2004, A14.

7. Tate and Goldstein, "Will Tomorrow's Medicines," S34.

8. Ibid.

9. Jonathan Kahn, "Misreading Race and Genomics after BiDil," *Nature Genetics* 37 (2005): 655.

10. Tate and Goldstein, "Will Tomorrow's Medicines," S37.

11. Ibid., S34.

12. University of Maryland Medical Center, "Experts Urge More Aggressive Treatment of Hypertension in African-Americans," March 10, 2003, accessed April 8, 2012, http://www.umm.edu/news/releases/hypertension_guidelines.htm#ixzz1rUbN8rFO.

13. Jon Entine, *Taboo: Why Black Athletes Dominate Sports and Why We Are Afraid to Talk About It* (New York: PublicAffairs, 2000).

14. Sally Satel, "I Am a Racially Profiling Doctor," *New York Times Magazine*, May 5, 2002, 56.

15. Jon Entine, "Welcome and Opening Presentation," presentation at the AEI Conference: Race, Medicine, and Public Policy, on November 12, 2004, Washington, D.C., accessed April 8, 2012, http://www.aei.org/files/2004/11/12/Race-Medicine-and-Public-Policy.html.

16. Sally Satel, presentation at the AEI Conference: Race, Medicine, and Public Policy, on November 12, 2004, Washington, D.C., accessed April 8, 2012, http://www.aei.org/files/2004/11/12/Race-Medicine-and-Public-Policy.html.

17. Sally Satel, "Race and Medicine Can Mix without Prejudice: How the Story of BiDil Illuminates the Future of Medicine," *Medical Progress Today*, December 10, 2004, http://www.medicalprogresstoday.com/spotlight/spotlight_indarchive.php?id=449.

18. Smedley et al., *Unequal Treatment*.

19. Richard A. Epstein, "Disparities and Discrimination in Health Care Coverage: A Critique of the Institute of Medicine Study," *Perspectives in Biology and Medicine* 48 (2005): S26.

20. Sally Satel and Jonathan Klick, "The Institute of Medicine Report: Too Quick to Diagnose Bias," *Perspectives in Biology and Medicine* 48 (2005): S22.

21. Ibid., S23.

22. Maxwell Gregg Bloche, "Health Care Disparities—Science, Politics, and Race," *New England Journal of Medicine* 350 (2004): 1568.

23. Ibid.

24. See Shankar Vedantam, "Racial Disparities Played Down," *Washington Post*, January 14, 2004, A17.

25. Bloche, "Health Care Disparities," 1568.

26. George Ellison and Ian Rees Jones, "Social Identities and the 'New Genetics': Scientific and Social Consequences," *Critical Public Health* 12 (2002): 267.

27. Dorothy Nelkin and M. Susan Lindee, *The DNA Mystique: The Gene as a Cultural Icon* (Ann Arbor: University of Michigan Press, 2004), 2.

28. Paul E. Farmer, Bruce Nizeye, Sara Stulac, and Salmaan Keshavjee, "Structural Violence and Clinical Medicine," *PLoS Medicine* 3 (2006): e449, doi:10.1371/journal.pmed.0030449.

29. Florida Agency for Health Care Administration, "Agency for Health Care Administration Announces the Addition of BiDil to Medicaid Preferred Drug List," press release, May 5, 2006, accessed April 8, 2012, http://ahca.myflorida.com/Executive/Communications/Press_Releases/archive/2006/05-01_BiDilFINAL.pdf.

30. Pamela Sankar, Mildred K. Cho, Celeste M. Condit, Linda M. Hunt, Barbara Koenig, Patricia Marshall, Sandra Soo-Jin Lee, and Paul Spicer, "Genetic Research and Health Disparities," *Journal of the American Medical Association* (2004): 2985–2989.

31. Ellison and Jones, "Social Identities," 277.

32. Frederick L. Hoffman, *Race Traits and Tendencies of the American Negro*, vol. 11 (New York: Publications of the American Economic Association, 1896).

33. Megan J. Wolff, "The Myth of the Actuary: Life Insurance and Frederick L. Hoffman's *Race Traits and Tendencies of the American Negro*," *Public Health Report* 121 (Jan–Feb 2006): 89.

34. Frederick L. Hoffman, *Race Traits*, 95.

35. Ibid., 1–329, *passim*.

36. Frederick L. Hoffman, "Vital Statistics of the Negro," *Arena* 29 (1892): 542.

37. See, e.g., L. Braun, "Race, Ethnicity, and Health: Can Genetics Explain Disparities?" *Perspectives in Biology and Medicine* 45 (2002): 160–163.

38. Excerpted from W. E. Burghardt DuBois, ed., *The Health and Physique of the Negro American. Report of a Social Study Made under the Direction of Atlanta University; Together with the Proceedings of the Eleventh Conference for the Study of the Negro Problems, Held at Atlanta University, on May the 29th, 1906*. Atlanta, Ga.: Atlanta University Press, 1906, as reprinted in "Voices from the Past: The Health and Physique of the Negro American by W. E. Burghardt DuBois," *American Journal of Public Health* 93 (2003): 272–276, http://ajph.aphapublications.org/cgi/content/full/93/2/272.

39. Wolff, "Myth of the Actuary," 84, 95.

40. Plessy v. Ferguson, 163 U.S. 537 (1896).

41. Plessy v. Ferguson, 551.

42. Ibid.

43. Ibid., 562.

44. Plessy v. Ferguson, 551.

45. J. Allen Douglas, "The 'Most Valuable Form of Property': Constructing White Identity in American Law, 1880–1940," *San Diego Law Review* 40 (2003): 889.

46. Brown v. Board of Education Topeka, Shawnee County, Kan., et al., 347 U.S. 483 (1954).

47. Ibid., 494.

48. Ibid., note 11; see also Herbert Hovenkamp, "Social Science and Segregation before Brown," *Duke Law Journal* 1985 (1985): 671–672, which argues that the real transition began with the 1948 case of *Shelly v. Kramer*, in which the petitioners relied extensively on the work of the anthropologists Franz Boas and Melville Herskovitz, as

well as Gunnar Myrdal, in arguing against racially restrictive covenants in housing transactions.

49. Mary L. Heen, "Ending Jim Crow Life Insurance Rates," *Northwestern Journal of Law and Social Policy* 4 (2009): 395.

50. Thomas Byrne Edsall and Mary D. Edsall, *Chain Reaction: The Impact of Race, Rights, and Taxes on American Politics* (New York: Norton, 1992), 7.

51. Alice Robbin, "The Politics of Representation in the U.S. National Statistical System: Origins of Minority Population Interest Group Participation," *Journal of Government Information* 27 (2000): 435; see also Alice Robbin, "Classifying Racial and Ethnic Group Data in the United States: The Politics of Negotiation and Accommodation," *Journal of Government Information* 27 (2000): 129.

52. King Center, http://www.thekingcenter.org/, accessed November 22, 2010.

53. Edsall and Edsall, *Chain Reaction*, 5, 143–144.

54. Kevin Phillips, *The Emerging Republican Majority* (New York: Arlington House, 1969).

55. Edsall and Edsall, *Chain Reaction*, 97.

56. Ibid., 188.

57. Griggs v. Duke Power Company, 401 U.S. 424 (1971).

58. Ibid., 431.

59. Edsall and Edsall, *Chain Reaction*, 252.

60. City of Richmond v. J. A. Croson Company, 488 U.S. 469 (1989).

61. Parents Involved in Community Schools v. Seattle School District No. 1, 551 U.S. 701 (2007).

62. Richmond v. J. A. Croson, 505–506 (italics added).

63. Plessy v. Ferguson, 551.

64. Parents v. Seattle, 723.

65. The *Plessy* court would later valorize laissez-faire economic theory in the 1906 case of Lochner v. New York, 198 U.S. 45 (1905).

66. Jonathan Kahn, "Controlling Identity: Plessy, Privacy and Racial Defamation," *DePaul Law Review* 54 (2005): 755–782.

67. 488 U.S. 469 (1989) at 505–506.

68. Grutter v. Bollinger, 539 U.S. 306, 343 (2003).

69. Ibid.

70. Adarand Constructors, Inc. v. Pena, 515 U.S. 200, 239 (1995).

71. Dorothy E. Roberts, "Is Race-Based Medicine Good for Us?: African American Approaches to Race, Biomedicine, and Equality," *Journal of Law, Medicine and Ethics* 36 (2008): 538.

72. Edsall and Edsall, *Chain Reaction*, 97.

73. Michael Omi and Howard Winant, *Racial Formation in the United States: From the 1960s to the 1990s*, 2nd ed. (New York: Routledge, 1994), 55–56.

74. Ibid.

75. Ibid., 82.

76. Smedley et al., *Unequal Treatment*, 3–4.

77. Ibid, 4.

78. Edsall and Edsall, *Chain Reaction*, 52–55.

79. William H. Frist, "Overcoming Disparities in U.S. Health Care," *Health Affairs* 24 (2005): 445–451.

80. Ibid.

81. Quoted in Jill Quadagno and J. Brandon McKelvey, "The Transformation of American Health Insurance," in *Health at Risk: America's Ailing Health System—and How to Heal It*, Jacob Hacker, ed. (New York: Columbia University Press, 2008), 19.

82. Philip Alcabes, "The Risky Genes: Epidemiology and the Evolution of Risk," *Patterns of Prejudice* 40 (2006): 424–425.

83. PhRMA, "Medicines in Development for Major Diseases Affecting African Americans 2007 Report: Nearly 700 Medicines in the Pipeline Offer Hope for Closing the Health Gap for African Americans," accessed April 8, 2012, http://www.phrma.org /sites/default/files/422/africanamericans2007.pdf.

84. Ibid.

85. Ibid.

86. PhRMA, "PhRMA Praises Congressional Leadership Alliance," press release, February 8, 2005, http://www.phrma.org/node/173.

87. National Minority Health Month Foundation, "Congressional Leadership Alliance to Eliminate Health Disparities," press release, accessed April 8, 2012, http://www.nmqf.org /press%5C2005%5C020805.pdf.

88. Joon-Ho Yu, Sara Goering, and Stephanie M. Fullerton, "Race-Based Medicine and Justice as Recognition: Exploring the Phenomenon of BiDil," *Cambridge Quarterly of Healthcare Ethics* 18 (2009): 58.

89. Ibid.

90. Ibid., 62–63.

91. Celeste Condit, "How Culture and Science Make Race 'Genetic': Motives and Strategies for Discrete Categorization of the Continuous and Heterogeneous," *Literature and Medicine* 26 (2007): 240–268, 244.

92. Ibid., 245.

93. Steven Epstein, *Inclusion: The Politics of Difference in Medical Research* (Chicago: University of Chicago Press, 2007), 4.

94. Ibid., 91.

95. Ibid., 6.

96. Ibid., 91.

97. Ibid., 92.

98. Anthony P. Cohen, *The Symbolic Construction of Community* (London: Ellis Harwood, 1985), 21.

99. Anne Fausto-Sterling, "Refashioning Race: DNA and the Politics of Health Care," *differences: A Journal of Feminist Cultural Studies* 15 (2004), 2.

100. PhRMA, "PhRMA Praises."

101. Linda Gottfredson, "The Health Disparities Myth: Diagnosing the Treatment Gap" presentation at a book event sponsored by the AEI, February 22, 2006, Washington, D.C., http://www.aei.org/EMStaticPage/1250?page=Summary.

102. Ibid.

103. Russell Jacoby and Naomi Glauberman, eds., *The Bell Curve Debate* (New York: Times Books, 1996), ix.

104. Jonathan Klick and Sally Satel, *The Health Disparities Myth* (Washington, D.C.: AEI Press, 2006).

105. Ibid., 42.

106. Ibid.

107. The literature on this phenomenon is extensive. A few recent and powerful analyses of these phenomena include: Ira Katznelson, *When Affirmative Action Was White: An Untold History of Racial Inequality in Twentieth-Century America* (New York: W.W. Norton, 2005); Douglas Massey and Nancy Denton, *American Apartheid: Segregation and the Making of the Underclass* (Cambridge: Harvard University Press, 1993); Douglas Massey, *Categorically Unequal: The American Stratification System* (New York: Russell Sage Foundation, 2007); Thomas Shapiro, *The Hidden Cost of Being African American: How Wealth Perpetuates Inequality* (New York: Oxford University Press, 2004).

108. Klick and Satel, *Health Disparities*, 4.

109. Smedley et al., *Unequal Treatment*, 19.

110. Ibid.

111. Satel and Klick, *Institute of Medicine Report*, S22.

112. Edsall and Edsall, *Chain Reaction*, 11–14.

113. Klick and Satel, *The Health Disparities Myth*, 7.

114. Jeffrey Temple, "Racism Is Not the Cause of Health Disparities," National Center for Public Policy Research, accessed October 29, 2010, http://www.nationalcenter.org/P21NVTempleHealth90609.html.

115. National Center for Public Policy Research, "About Us," accessed October 29, 2010, http://www.nationalcenter.org/NCPPRHist.html.

116. See, e.g., Edmund F. Haislmaier, "Medicare: It's About the Future, Stupid!" National Center for Public Policy Research, November 2003, accessed October 29, 2010, http://www.nationalcenter.org/NPA498.html; and Edmund F. Haislmaier, "Medicare's Fatal Weakness: Expensive New Technologies Are Rationed," March 2005, accessed October 29, 2010, http://www.nationalcenter.org/NPA525MedicareRationing.html.

117. P. Sankar et al., "Genetic Research and Health Disparities," 2985.

118. Ibid.

119. Ibid.

120. Ibid.

121. Ibid., 2986.

CONCLUSIONS AND RECOMMENDATIONS

1. Troy Duster, "Buried Alive: The Concept of Race in Science," *Chronicle of Higher Education*, September 14, 2001, B12.
2. Sheryl Gay Stolberg, "Skin Deep: Shouldn't a Pill Be Colorblind?" *New York Times*, May 13, 2001, 4. Venter, however, here goes to the extreme of denying the significance of race altogether. The logic of his argument compels us to overlook the significance of health disparities, such as varying rates of certain types of cancer or hypertension that do strongly correlate with certain *social* categories of race.
3. Stolberg, "Skin Deep," 4, quoting Joseph Graves.
4. Ibid.
5. See, e.g., Michael Sandel, "The Procedural Republic and the Unencumbered Self," *Political Theory* 12 (1984): 81.
6. Brian D. Smedley, Adrienne Y. Stith, and Alan R. Nelson, eds., *Unequal Treatment: Confronting Racial and Ethnic Disparities in Health Care* (Washington, D.C.: National Academies Press, 2003).
7. See, e.g., Chevron v. Echazabal, 537 U.S. 73, 80 (2002).
8. See generally Americans with Disabilities Act of 1990, 42 U.S.C. § 12112(b)(6) (2000). See also, e.g., Albertsons v. Kirkingburg, 527 U.S. 555 (1999); Automobile Workers v. Johnson Controls, Inc., 499 U.S. 187 (1990).
9. Chevron v. Echazabal, 537 U.S. 73.
10. The ADA defines a "direct threat" as "a significant risk to the health and safety of others that cannot be eliminated by reasonable accommodation." Americans with Disabilities Act of 1990.
11. Chevron v. Echazabal, 537 U.S. at 86.
12. This story is drawn largely from Troy Duster, "Buried Alive," 24–27; Daniel J. Kevles, *In the Name of Eugenics* (Cambridge, MA: Harvard University Press, 1995), at 277–279; Raymond R. Coletta, "Biotechnology and the Law: Biotechnology and the Creation of Ethics," *McGeorge Law Review* 32 (2000): 97; Americans with Disabilities Act of 1990.
13. Norman-Bloodsaw v. Lawrence Berkeley Lab, 135 F.3d 1260, 1261, 1264 (9th Cir. 1998).
14. Elizabeth Pendo, "Race, Sex and Genes at Work: Uncovering the Lessons of Norman-Bloodsaw," *Houston Journal of Health Law and Policy* 10 (2010): 234, citing Brief of Defendants-Appellees, Regents of the University of California, University of California, Lawrence Berkeley National Laboratory, Charles V. Shank, Henry H. Stauffer, M.D., Lisa Snow, M.D., T. F. Budinger, M.D., and William G. Donald, Jr., M.D., at 9–10, Norman-Bloodsaw v. Lawrence Berkeley Laboratory, No. 96–16526 (9th Cir. 1997).
15. National Collegiate Athletic Association, "NCAA Division I Sickle Cell Trait QA for Institutions," May 10, 2010, accessed June 6, 2010, http://www.ncaa.org/wps/portal/ncaahome?WCM_GLOBAL_CONTEXT=/ncaa/ncaa/academics+and+athletes/personal+welfare/health+and+safety/sicklecelltrait.

16. Julianne Hing, "NCAA's Mandatory Sickle Cell Testing Could Impact Black Athletes," *Colorlines,* April 13, 2010, accessed June 6, 2010, http://colorlines.com/archives/2010/04/ncaas_mandatory_sickle_cell_testing_could_impact_black_athletes.html.

17. Dennis Dodd, "NCAA to Recommend Schools Test for Sickle Cell Trait," *CBSSports.com,* June 29, 2009, accessed June 6, 2010, http://www.cbssports.com/collegefootball/story/11903550.

18. NCAA, "NCAA Division I Sickle."

19. Ibid.

20. Secretary's Advisory Committee on Heritable Disorders in Newborns and Children, *Screening of U.S. College Athletes for Their Sickle Cell Carrier Status,* June 14, 2010, 11. http://www.hrsa.gov/advisorycommittees/mchbadvisory/heritabledisorders/recommendations/correspondence/sicklecell061410.pdf.

21. Ibid., 10–11.

22. Mark Rothstein, "GINA's Beauty Is Only Skin Deep," *GeneWatch,* accessed June 6, 2010, http://www.councilforresponsiblegenetics.org/GeneWatch/GeneWatchPage.aspx?pageId=184&archive=yes.

23. Ibid.

24. Secretary's Advisory Committee, *Screening of U.S. College Athletes,* 12. http://www.hrsa.gov/advisorycommittees/mchbadvisory/heritabledisorders/recommendations/correspondence/sicklecell061410.pdf.

25. See, e.g., Nancy Kass, "The Implications of Genetic Testing for Health and Life Insurance," in *Genetic Secrets: Protecting Privacy and Confidentiality in the Genetic Era,* ed. Mark A. Rothstein (New Haven, Conn.: Yale University Press, 1999), 299–316; Mark A. Rothstein, "The Law of Medical and Genetic Privacy in the Workplace," in *Genetic Secrets,* 281–298.

26. Sandra Soo-Jin Lee, Joanna Mountain, and Barbara A. Koenig, "The Meanings of 'Race' in the New Genomics: Implications for Health Disparities Research," *Yale Journal of Health Policy, Law, & Ethics* 1 (2001): 55.

27. Martha Minow, *Making All the Difference: Inclusion and Exclusion in American Law* (Ithaca, N.Y.: Cornell University Press, 1990), 20.

28. For example, current 2002 fiscal year CDC appropriations for "minority health" totaled $747,472,000. CDC, "Minority Health Funding," accessed December 15, 2003, http://www.cdc.gov/washington/funding/minorhea.htm.

29. Duster, *Buried Alive.*

30. U.S. Patent and Trademark Office, "Manual of Patent Examining Procedure," § 1504.01(e), accessed May 20, 2003, http://www.uspto.gov/web/offices/pac/mpep/documents/1500_1504_01_e.htm#sect1504.01e.

31. Ibid., § 608.

32. "Census, Race and Science," editorial, *Nature Genetics* 24 (2000): 99.

33. C. Sullivan and E. Lilquist, "The Law and Genetics of Racial Profiling in Medicine," *Harvard Civil Rights–Civil Liberties Law Review* 39 (2004): 391–480; Sharona Hoffman, "'Racially-Tailored' Medicine Unraveled," *American University Law Review* 55 (2005):

395–452; J. Robertson, "Constitutional Issues in the Use of Pharmacogenomic Variations Associated with Race," in *Pharmacogenomics; Social, Ethical and Clinical Dimensions*, M. Rothstein, ed. (Hoboken, N.J.: Wiley, 2003), 391–418.

34. Grutter v. Bollinger, 539 U.S. 306 (2003).

35. Grutter v. Bollinger, 123 S.Ct. 2325, 2337–2338 (2003).

36. Osagie K. Obasogie, "Beyond Best Practices: Strict Scrutiny as a Regulatory Model for Race-Specific Medicines," *Journal of Law, Medicine, and Ethics* 36 (2008): 491–497.

37. David E. Winickoff and Osagie K. Obasogie, "Race-Specific Drugs: Regulatory Trends and Public Policy," *Trends in Pharmacological Sciences* 29 (2008): 278.

38. Ibid.

39. See, e.g., Timothy Caulfield, Stephanie M. Fullerton, Sarah E. Ali-Khan, Laura Arbour, Esteban G. Burchard, Richard S. Cooper, Billie-Jo Hardy, Simrat Harry, et al., "Race and Ancestry in Biomedical Research: Exploring the Challenges," *Genome Medicine* 1 (2009): 8, doi: 10.1186/gm8; Lundy Braun, Anne Fausto-Sterling, Duana Fullwiley, Evelynn M. Hammonds, Alondra Nelson, William Quivers, Susan M. Reverby, and Alexandra E. Shields, "Racial Categories in Medical Practice: How Useful Are They?" *PLoS Medicine* 4 (2007): e271, doi:10.1371/journal.pmed.0040271; Alexandra Shields, Michael Fortun, Evelynn M. Hammonds, Patricia A. King, Caryn Lerman, Rayna Rapp, and Patrick F. Sullivan, "The Use of Race Variables in Genetic Studies of Complex Traits and the Goal of Reducing Health Disparities: A Transdisciplinary Perspective," *American Psychology* 60 (2005): 77–103; Sandra Lee, Joanna Mountain, Barbara Koenig, Russ Altman, Melissa Brown, Albert Camarillo, Luca Cavalli-Sforza, et al., "The Ethics of Characterizing Difference: Guiding Principles on Using Racial Categories in Human Genetics," *Genome Biology* 9 (2008): 404 (doi:10.1186/gb-2008-9-7-404).

40. NIH, "NIH Policy and Guidelines on the Inclusion of Women and Minorities as Subjects in Clinical Research—Amended," October 2001, accessed March 23, 2005, http://grants.nih.gov/grants/funding/women_min/guidelines_amended_10_2001.htm.

41. Ibid.

42. Ibid.

43. International HapMap Consortium, "The International HapMap Project," *Nature* 426 (2003): 789–796.

44. Melissa Nobles, *Shades of Citizenship: Race and the Census in Modern Politics* (Palo Alto, Calif.: Stanford University Press, 2000).

45. See, e.g., Morris Foster and Richard Sharp, "Race, Ethnicity, and Genomics: Social Classifications as Proxies for Biological Heterogeneity," *Genome Research* 12 (2002): 844; Gary Marchant, "Genetics and Toxic Torts," *Seton Hall Law Review* 31 (2001): 949–982.

46. See, e.g., SA Hunt, DW Baker, MH Chin, MP Cinquegrani, AM Feldman, GS Francis, TG Ganiats, et al., "ACC/AHA Guidelines for the Evaluation and Management of

Chronic Heart Failure in the Adult: Executive Summary: A Report of the American College of Cardiology/American Heart Association Task Force on Practice Guidelines (Committee to Revise the 1995 Guidelines for the Evaluation and Management of Heart Failure)," *Circulation* 104 (2001): 2996–3007, accessed April 9, 2012, http://circ .ahajournals.org/content/104/24/2996.full.

INDEX

1.1:1 mortality rate, 77–78, 80
2:1 mortality rate, 20, 72–77

Academia Sinica, 188–190
ACE inhibitors. *See* Angiotensin-converting
   enzyme (ACE) inhibitors
Adarand v. Pena, 210
Affirmative action, 226
African-American Heart Failure Trial
   (A-HeFT): about, 51–52; as basis for
   BiDil approval, 48; completion of, 2; and
   NitroMed, 71, 92; racial framing in, 80;
   support by blacks, 67–68
African Americans: and *Brown v. Board of
   Education*, 149, 205; characterized as
   biological group, 226; and civil rights,
   206; health disparities for, 193–194;
   insurance statistics excluding, 202–203,
   205–206; Moynihan on, 213; and *Plessy v.
   Ferguson*, 149–150, 204; as race-specific
   targets, 108–109, 112–116, 121–122,
   141–142; and sickle cell discrimination,
   228–234
AIDS vaccine, 91

Albain, Kathy, 160–161
Alcabes, Philip, 214–215
Algorithms, dosing, 175–180
Alleles: in Caucasian data sets, 45–46;
   connecting race and genetics, 45–46,
   133–135, 153, 167, 181–183; in dosing
   algorithms, 176; in genetic testing,
   170–174; variations in groupings, 9
American Anthropological Association, 40
American College of Medical Genetics
   (ACMG), 181–183
American Pharmacists Association, 115
Americans with Disabilities Act (ADA),
   227–228, 298n10
Amgen v. Chugai Pharmeceuticals, 140
Angiotensin-converting enzyme (ACE)
   inhibitors: compared to H/I
   combination, 54; efficacy in black
   patients, 52–53; to manage heart failure,
   51; and racial framing, 20; statistics used
   for, 83–86
Annals of Internal Medicine, 185
Anticoagulation Forum, 169
Aquino, John, 142

Ashkenazi Jews, 74, 209

Asian population, 132–134, 135, 166, 189–191

Association of Black Cardiologists (ABC), 75–76, 101

Aumen, J.T., 164, 180, 181

AutoGenomics, 170–174, 184

Bate, Kenneth, 117–118

"Bayh-Dole" Act. *See* Patent and Trademark Laws Amendment Act (1980)

The Bell Curve, 220

Beta-blockers, 112–115

Bibbins-Domingo, Kirsten, 93

BiDil: and 2:1 mortality statistic, 74–77; 1997 FDA review, 95–96; 1999 patent application, 64–65; 2005 FDA review, 96–97; about, 3–5, 19–20, 51; and ACE therapy, 52–53; approved for African Americans, 6, 48; author's input on approval, 5; biological basis for, 225–226; case against, 53–57; case for, 50–53; cited as precedent, 111–113, 115–116; connected with other drugs, 194–196; controversy over, 6–7; determining race for, 209; as ethnic drug, 7, 21–22, 58–61; and failure of NitroMed, 116–123; genetic strategy for, 129–130, 155; legislation concerning, 61–69; limitations of racial designation for, 237; marketing of, 105–116, 120–121; Medco trademark application for, 55–57; media coverage on, 75, 276n120; named AHA top advance, 82–83; and novelty patent requirement, 137–138; off-label promotion of, 100–103; patent comparison with warfarin, 191; pharmacogenetics model for, 87–123; physicians' support for, 102–103; policy considerations for, 98–99; politics behind, 216–219; as possessive investment in blackness, 126; pricing of, 103–105; and racial interpretation of data, 63–65, 69–70; and self-reporting

of race, 43–44; similar drug referenced in media, 121; single-dose form, 62–63, 260n58; support for, 86; as surrogate marker, 105–109; sustained release form, 66; Yancy's connection to, 80–81

Biomedicine: arguments for including race, gender, 26–27; impact of federal mandates, 234–238; proposal for revising mandates, 239–246; race entering, 25–27; racial categories in, 2; racialized products in, 125, 132–134, 140, 153–156; racial structures in, 212

Board of Patent Appeals and Interferences (BPAI), 143–144

Borer, Jeffrey, 96

Bowker, Geoffrey, 33

Bowser, Rene, 134

Bragdon, Kathleen, 141–143, 146

Branding, 105–106, 111–112

Brawley, Otis, 27

Brown, Henry, 204, 208

Brown v. Board of Education, 149, 205, 294n48

Bystolic, 112–116

Calmore, John, 152

Carson, Peter, 58–62, 64, 71, 80, 225

Caucasian population, 135

cDNA, 128–129

Center for Medicine in the Public Interest (CMPI), 187

Centers for Disease Control and Prevention (CDC), 30

Centers for Medicaid and Medicare Services (CMS), 184, 186–187, 188

Chain Reaction, 221

"Changes in Mortality from Heart Failure—United States, 1980–1995," 79–80

Chevron, 228

Cho, M.K., 38, 266n41

Christensen, Donna, 101, 216

Christopher, Gail, 101

Civil rights movement, 67–68, 206–207

Clarification of Optimal Anticoagulation through Genetics (COAG), 187

Clinton, Bill, 1

Cohen, Anthony, 40

Cohn, Jay, 5, 49, 53, 54–62, 64–65, 69, 80, 91, 95, 103, 106–107, 191, 203, 225, 259n40, 259n50, 260n55

"Collection of Race and Ethnicity Data in Clinical Trials," 26, 84

Collins, Francis, 146, 165, 185

Commerce: and science, 16–17, 234; value of race, 159, 181–188, 234

Condit, Celeste, 217

Congestive heart failure, 50–51

Congressional Leadership Alliance to Eliminate Health Disparities, 216, 218–219

Cooper, R.S., 85–86

Coriell Institute for Medical Research, 45–46

Coumadin. See Warfarin

Cutting Edge Information, 110

Data, databases: care of, 15–16; EMBL, 30; genetic, 29–33; genetic information in, 131; HapMap, 152; neutrality of, 34; producing, organizing, 27–33; PubMed, 36; structuring racial characterization, 46

dbSNP database, 30–31, 251n29

deCode Genetics, 111–112

Deerfield Capital, 117, 123

Diabetes, 14

Diagnostic and Statistical Manual of Mental Disorders (DSM), 33

Diamond v. Chakrabarty, 128

Discriminatory practice, 73

DNA DataBank of Japan (DDBJ), 30

DNA Polymorphisms (dbSNP database), 29, 30–31

DNA samples, and race, 44–45

"Does Race Matter in Heart Failure?," 108

Dosing algorithms, 175–180

Dries, Daniel, 71–73, 78, 79–80, 81–82, 84

Drugs, failed, 90–92

DuBois, W.E.B., 203

Duster, Troy, 4, 9, 225, 234

Echazabal, Mario, 228

Eckman, Mark, 185

Edsall, Thomas and Mary, 206, 210–211, 221

Ellison, George, 198, 201

Ellison, G.T., 93

Enalapril, 54, 58–59, 84

Engels, Friedrich, 157

Entine, Jon, 195–196

Epstein, Richard, 197, 212

Epstein, Steven, 10, 26–27, 85, 217–218

Equal protection doctrine, 236, 238–239

Ethics, and genetic classification, 33–34

Ethnicity: categories of, 28; and niche marketing, 105, 109–116, 171–174; as term to avoid race, 35. See also Race

European Molecular Biology Laboratory (EMBL) database, 30

European Patent Office, 74, 148

Exner, Derek, 83–85

Farmer, Paul, 3

Fausto-Sterling, Anne, 35–36, 218–219

FDMA (1997). See Food and Drug Modernization Act (FDMA) (1997)

Federal Drug Administration (FDA): accepting race as reference, 162–163; approving BiDil, 20–21, 48–50, 98–99; approving genetic test kits, 170–171; on BiDil substitutions, 118–119; concerns on race issue, 94; connecting race and genetics, 183; defending BiDil approval, 93; failure to approve BiDil, 55–57, 95–96; guidances for race, ethnicity, 26; issues of inclusion and, 27; manipulating approval by, 92–99; on off-label drug use, 100; testing conflict with CMS, 184

Federal mandates: for biomedicine, 234–238; impact on biomedical practice, 234–235; key, 25; NIH and FDMA, 68; proposal for revising, 239–246; proposed revision of, 240–244; and racial categorization, 146–147, 155, 223. *See also* OMB (U.S. Office of Budget and Management) Directive

Feinstein Kean Healthcare, 76

Ferdinand, Keith, 51

Fernandez, Alicia, 93

Filipino population, 132–134

Flack, John, 270n30

Food and Drug Modernization Act (FDMA) (1997), 19, 25–26, 58, 68

Ford, Richard Thompson, 154

Forest Laboratories, 112–116

Formulary tier structure, 117–118

FoxKiser, 101, 118

Frank, D., 119

Fraser, Nancy, 216

Frazier, Elyse, 43–44

Frist, Bill, 213–214

Fullerton, S.M., 216–218

Fullwiley, Duana, 44–45, 180

Gage, Brian, 179–180

Gates, Henry Louis Jr., 159

GenBank, 30

Genetic essentialism, 199

Genetic Information Nondiscrimination Act (GINA)(2008), 224, 231–232, 278n3

Genetics: as basis for health disparity, 81; clinal variation in, 2–3; connected to race, 45–46, 133–135, 153, 167, 181–182; dangers of classifying, 33–34; databases for, 29–33; dosing algorithm, 41–42; and health disparities, 199; human variation in, 8–10; identifying specific variations, 167–170; linked to BiDil, 89; politics of, 18–19; testing for, 170–172, 184–185, 188–191

"Genetic Variants Predicting Warfarin Sensitivity," 188–191

GenMark Dx (Osmetech), 174, 186

Genomes. *See* Human genome

Ghosh, Shubha, 125

Gillum, Richard, 78–79, 81

Gingrich, Newt, 216

Goering, S., 216–218

Goldstein, David, 194–195

Gottfredson, Linda, 207, 219

Gratz v. Bollinger, 209–210

Graves, Joseph, 225

Griggs v. Duke Power, 207, 219–220

Hahn, Robert, 44

HapMap, 34–36, 130, 151–152. *See also* International Haplotype Map Project (IHMP)

Haraway, Donna, 35

Harlan, John Marshall, 204

Harris, Cheryl, 149

Hartl, Daniel, 146

Health disparities: for African Americans, 193–194; attributed to cognitive ability, 219–220; attributed to socioeconomic factors, 220–221; debate on, 197–199, 212–214, 298n2; and genetics, 222; King on, 206; personal responsibility for, 213–214; pharmaceutical response to, 215–216; politics of, 18–19, 211–223, 216–219; racial, 67–68, 200; responsibility for, 200–201; shift from access to outcomes, 206

The Health Disparities Myth: Diagnosing the Treatment Gap, 219–220

Healthy People initiatives, 234

Hernstein, Richard, 220

H/I combination, 54, 58–59, 62, 257n16. *See also* BiDil

Hoffman, Frederick, 202, 204

Holly, Buddy, 157

Hsiang-Yu Yuan, 188–189

Huang, Shiew-Mei, 162–163

Human Genetic Cell Repository, 30

Human Genetic Variation Collection, 30

Human genome: cataloguing, 31–32; defined, 8–9; as key object of knowledge, 35; role in disease, 107–108; segregated, 21–22, 152–156

Human Genome Project, 2, 6, 130

Hydralazine, 55, 119

Hypertension, 13–14, 73, 81

Hypodescent, 153

"I Am a Racially Profiling Doctor," 106, 196

Identity, 127–130

Inertial force, race as, 158–159

Institutional mandates, 15

Intellectual property, 125–126, 127–130, 148–155, 280n21

International Haplotype Map Project (IHMP), 29–312

International Nucleotide Sequence Database Collaboration, 30

International Society for Hypertension in Blacks (ISHIB), 113

International Warfarin Pharmacogenomics Consortium (IWPC), 41, 175–180

Isosorbide dinitrate, 55, 119

Iverson Genetic Diagnostics, 186

Jasanoff, Sheila, 129

Jin-Jer Chen, 188–189

Johnson, Gary, 58–59

Jones, B. J., 111

Jones, David, 36

Jones, Ian Rees, 198, 201

Journal of the American College of Cardiology, 187

Journal of Clinical Pharmacology, 164

Journal of the National Cancer Institute (JNCI), 160

Kalow, Werner, 36

Kaufman, Jay, 162

Kaufman, S., 85–86

King, Martin Luther Jr., 206

Kingston, Raynard, 187

Klick, Jonathan, 197–198, 219–221

Kong, B. Waine, 86, 101, 110

Konstam, Marvin, 96

Krieger, Nancy, 6

Lawrence Berkeley Laboratory (LBL), 229–230

Legislation: concerning BiDil, 61–69; concerning civil rights, 206–210; as impetus for *Race Traits*, 202; implications of race as biology, 226–233

Lesko, Lawrence, 163, 169, 183, 188

Levine, Alan, 200–201

Lewontin, Richard, 2, 40, 146

Lindee, M. Susan, 199

Lipicky, Ray, 96

Lipsitz, George, 126

Loberg, Michael, 103–104, 110, 216

"A Look at Personalized Medicine," 141

"Mapping Genes That Predict Treatment Outcome in Admixed Populations," 151–152

Marketing: of BiDil, 20, 63, 109–116, 120–121; of genetic test kits, 171–174; off-label promotion of BiDil, 100

Maxey, Randall W., 101

McLeod, H.L., 164, 180, 181

"Meantime" solution, race as, 157–192

Medco, 187

Medco Research Inc., 55–57, 90–91

Medical Marketing & Media, 115, 116, 169

"Medicines in Development for Major Diseases Affecting African Americans," 215

Metes and bounds, 283n89

"Methods and compositions for predicting drug response," 190

Minow, Martha, 233

Moore, Joseph Earle, 122
Mountain, J., 38, 266n41
Moussatos, Linda, 117
Moynihan, Daniel Patrick, 213
Moynihan Report: The Negro Family, 213
Murray, Charles, 220
Myriad Genetics, 74, 209

National Academy of Sciences (NAS), 229
National Center for Biotechnology Information (NCBI). See GenBank
National Center for Public Policy Research (NCPPR), 221–222
National Health and Nutrition Examination Survey (NHANES), 77
National Heart, Lung, and Blood Institute (NHLBI), 76–77
National Human Genome Research Institute (NHGRI), 30–31, 222–223
National Institute of General Medical Sciences (NIGMS), 29, 30
National Institutes of Health Revitalization Act (1993), 19. See also NIH Revitalization Act
National Minority Health Month Foundation (NMHMF), 101
Nature Biotechnology, 2
Nature/culture divide, 127–130
Nature Genetics, 2, 9–10, 194, 196, 235–236
NCAA, 230–232
Nebivolol, 112–113, 275n115
Nelkin, Dorothy, 199
Neurontin, 100
Nguyen, T.T., 85–86
NIH Revitalization Act (1993), 26–27, 68
Nissen, Steven, 89, 93–95, 97–98, 122, 163
Nitric oxide, 51
NitroMed: and 2:1 mortality statistic, 74–76; and 2.5 statistic, 83; 2009 patent application, 66; acquired by Deerfield Capital, 117; acquiring BiDil, 59–61;

author's contact with, 5; and BiDil FDA approval, 1–2, 48–49, 69, 226; and BiDil substitutions, 119; change of rhetoric, 82; commercial failure of, 116–123; compared with Academia Sinica, 191; concerns on race issue, 94; developing BiDil, 50–53, 91; early success of BiDil, 116–117; funds spent on BiDil approval, 92; genetic strategy for, 129–130; and A-HeFT trial, 71; marketing BiDil, 90, 105–116; off-label promotion of BiDil, 100–103; pricing of BiDil, 103–105; public offering for, 106; and racialization, 126; Yancy's connection to, 80–81
Nixon, Richard, 206
Non-obviousness requirement, in patents, 138–139
Norman-Bloodsaw v. Lawrence Berkeley Laboratory, 229
Novelty requirement, in patents, 137–138

Obasogie, Osagie, 236–237
O'Connor, Sandra Day, 207–208, 209–210
Office of Minority Health, 234
Off-label promotion, 100–103
OMB (U.S. Office of Budget and Management) Directive 15: about, 27–29; data contained in, 234; effects of, 46–47; recommendations concerning, 240, 244; used in patent law, 129, 130
OMB (U.S. Office of Budget and Management) Revised Standards, 240
Omi, Michael, 5, 211–212
Orphan disease, 98
Osmetech (GenMark Dx), 174, 186
Ota Wang, Vivian, 97

Pacific Research Institute, 187
Parents Involved in Community Schools v. Seattle School District No. 1, 207, 208
Patent and Trademark Laws Amendment Act (1980), 62

Patent and Trademark Office (PTO): on gene patents, 128–129, 188–191; prosecution process of, 64; race as surrogate for, 68; reasons for rejection by, 235; requiring racial categories, 21, 141–148; role of, 15

Patents: basics of law, 126–127; biotechnology, 132–134, 140, 148–156; genetic categorization affecting, 124–125; and nature/culture divide, 128–129; non-obviousness requirement in, 138–139; novelty requirement in, 137–138; process for, 64; race-specific, 125; rise in university, 260n54; rise of racial, 130–132; specification requirement in, 139–140; utility requirement in, 136–137

Patients: and ACE inhibitors, 52, 54; categorized by zip code, 160–161, 285n13; drugs given, 57; racializing, 124–156; and research, 26, 54, 58–59, 65–66, 80; self-reporting race, 42; taking BiDil, 69; trust of, 121

Perier, Frank, 114

Personalized medicine: announcing reality of, 169; enablement in, 141–142; framing BiDil marketing, 109–110; potential problems with, 169; testing for, 171

Pharmaceutical Research and Manufacturers of America (PhRMA), 215–216, 219

Pharmacogenetics, 248n16

Pharmacogenomics: affecting clinical trials, 88; genetic, racial preoccupation in, 36–41; narrowing market, 89–90; and personally tailored therapies, 109–110; politics of the meantime, 17–18, 22, 157–192; purpose of, 6; resurrecting failed drugs, 90–92

Pharmacogenomics Journal, 116, 151–152

Pharmacogenomics Knowledge Base (PharmGKB), 41, 168, 175, 254n73

PharmiGene Inc., 190

Philips, Kevin, 206

PHOSITA, 127

Plessy v. Ferguson, 149–150, 203–204, 209

Politics: debate on health disparities, 22–23; of disparity, 211–223; vs. economics, 198; and health disparities, 216–219; of the meantime, 17–18, 22; of race, genetics, disparities, 18–19; of racial medicine, 193–224

Population Pharmacokinetics (1999), 26

Prazosin, 54

Prescription benefit management corporations (PBMs), 117–118

PubMed, 36–37

Puckrein, Gary, 101, 216

Race: based on appearance, 44; as biology, 226–233; and biomedicine, 234; categories of, 28; commercial value of, 159; commodification, 148–149; complexities of, 7–8; defined, 151; and dosing algorithms, 175–180; and drug development, 5–7; effects on patents, 136–141; entering biomedicine, 19, 25–27; and equal protection doctrine, 236, 238–239; ethics of classifying, 33–34; exploiting, in drug development, 87–123; FDA concerns on politics of, 94; and FDA drug approval, 48–50; as genetic category, 67–68, 150–151, 284n99; in genetic databases, 29–33; implicating time, 43; indeterminacy of, 149–150; as inertial force, 15–16, 158–159; and marketing, 171–174, 192; as medical condition, 106; missing race, 177–180; mixed race, 177–180, in patent applications, 130–132; patenting, 124–156, 188–191; as pathology, 98; persistence of, in research, 17–18, 159–162; politics of, 194–225; profiling, 106–107; proposal for revised federal guidelines, 240–244; recursion, 34–36; as residual category, 158; responsibility for determining, 209;

Race (*continued*)
role in genetic research, 1; shifts in status
of, 35; as social construct, 40–41;
statements on, 254n68; as symbol, 40;
and technology, 41–46; used in
marketing, 111–116; use of data on, 28–29;
as weak genetic concept, 146. *See also*
Ethnicity; Racial framing; Self-
reporting, of race
"Race and Ethnicity in the Era of Emerging
Pharmacogenomics," 164
*Race Traits and Tendencies of the American
Negro*, 202, 204
Racial branding, 111–113
"Racial Differences in the Outcome of Left
Ventricular Dysfunction," 71–72
"Racial Differences in Response to Therapy
for Heart Failure: Analysis of the
Vasodilator-Heart Failure Trials," 58–59
Racial formation, 211
Racial framing: arguments against, 85; of
Ashkenazi Jewish women, 74; author
challenging, 95; for BiDil, 69–70, 74–75;
financial incentive for, 80–81;
implications of, 3; reasons for, 83; in
research articles, 77–79, 80; using
statistics for, 71–86
Racialization: intellectual property as site
for, 125–126; of medicine, 10–14, 23–24;
of patents, 130–132; of patients, 124–156
Racial profiling, 159–160, 226
Racial project, 211
"Racism Is Not the Cause of Health
Disparities," 222
Reagan, Ronald, 206–207
"Realizing the Potential of
Pharmacogenomics: Opportunities and
Challenges," 185
Recommendations, for federal directives for
biomedical research, 240–244
*Regents of the University of California v. Eli
Lilly*, 140–141

Regulation, tied to research, commerce,
184–188
Research: comparative, 51; concerns about,
97; Coriell Institute for Medical
Research, 45–46; databases for, 29–30;
diverse populations for, 26–27, 266n44;
federal funds for, 62; race persisting in,
158–162; race terms used in, 36–41;
racial, ethnic data in, 34; tied to
regulation, commerce, 184–188; white
norm in, 134
Residual category, race as, 158
Responder rate, for drugs, 89
Reverby, Susan, 122
Richmond v. Croson, 207–208, 209
Rieder, Mark, 190
Roberts, Dorothy, 210
Roberts, John, 207, 208
Roche Pharmaceuticals, 6
Rothstein, Mark, 231–232

Sam, Flora, 104–105
Sankar, Pamela, 38, 222–223, 266n41
Satel, Sally, 107, 195–198, 212, 219–222
Saunders, Elijah, 113–115
Scalia, Antonin, 210
Science, 6
Science, and commerce, 16–17
Segregated genomes, 152–156
Sehgal, Ashwini, 85
Self-identification, of race. *See* Self-
reporting, of race
Self-reporting, of race: for BiDil, 48–49;
and dosing algorithms, 176–180;
limitations of, 147–148; as surrogate
for genome, 163; variances in, 11–12,
42–43
Sickle cell trait, 12–13, 228–233
Socioeconomic status (SES), 52, 72–73
Souter, David, 228
Specification requirement, in patents,
139–140

"Standards for Maintaining, Collecting, and Presenting Federal Data on Race and Ethnicity," 27

Star, Leigh, 33

"Statement on Race," 40

Statistics: 1.1:1 mortality rate, 77–78, 80; 2:1 mortality rate, 72–77, 82; 2.5 mortality rate, 83; and ACE inhibitors, 83–86; author disclaimer on, 263n11; vs. clinical data, 96–98; inaccuracy in, 73

Stevenson-Wydler Technology Innovation Act (1980), 62

Stockbridge, Norman, 93, 94, 99, 164

Studies of Left Ventricular Dysfunction (SOLVD) trials, 51–52, 78, 79, 80, 84

Study of Pharmacogenetics in Ethnically Diverse Groups (SOPHIE), 45–46

Surrogate markers, 105–109

Tate, Sarah, 194–195

Temple, Jeffrey, 221–222

Temple, Robert, 93, 94, 96, 99, 119, 162–164, 188

Testing, genetic, 170–172, 184–185, 188–191

Thompson, Tommy, 198, 212

Tier structure, 117–118, 276n127

Time, and race definition, 43

Time magazine, 159

"Toward the First Racial Medicine," 194–195

Triano, Charles, 115

Tuskegee Syphilis Study, 58, 122, 259n42, 281n42

Uhl, Robert, 117

Underwood, Paul, 113–114

Unequal Treatment: Confronting Racial and Ethnic Disparities in Health Care, 197, 212

"Unexpectedness" in patent application, 64–66

U.S. Air Force Academy, 229

U.S. Census Bureau, 10, 28

Utility requirement, in patents, 136–137

Vairavan, Anand, 174

Vasodilator Heart Failure Trial (V-HeFT I and II), 54, 59, 61–62, 91, 259n40, 260n55

Vasodilators, 51

Vasotec. See Enalapril

VaxGen, 91

Venter, Craig, 1, 225, 298n2

Vocabularies, health, 35–41

Wall Street Journal, 76–77, 184–185

Ward, Leslie, 202

Warfarin: assumptions made for, 291n110; dosing for, 175–180, 187–188; as example in racial profiling, 192; and persistence of race, 158; pharmacogenomics of, 41–42, 165–169; regulatory clash over, 184; testing for, 188–191

Werner, Michael, 88

White norm, 134–136, 177–178, 281n43, 289n84

"Why Racial Profiling Persists in Medical Research," 159–162, 285n12

Williams, Patricia, 12

"Will Tomorrow's Medicines Work for Everyone?," 194–195

Winant, Howard, 5, 211–212

Winickoff, David, 237

Wittkowsky, Ann, 185

Woodcock, Jane, 169, 185

Worcel, Manuel, 110

Yancy, Clyde, 51–52, 80–81, 102, 108, 121–123, 256n10

Yen-Revollo, J., 164, 180, 181

Yu, J., 216–218

Yuan-Tsong Chen, 188–191

Zeische, Susan, 58–59